HIK

D1366245

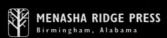

**MENASHA RIDGE PRESS**
Birmingham, Alabama

# 60 HIKES WITHIN 60 MILES

# PHILADELPHIA

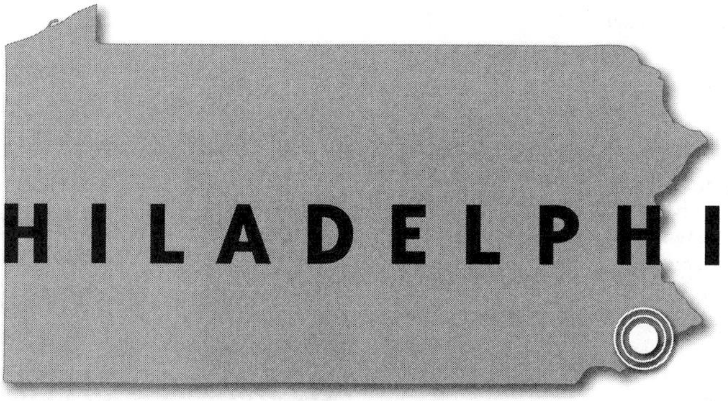

INCLUDING
SURROUNDING COUNTIES
PLUS HUNTERDON AND
MERCER, NEW JERSEY

SANDRA KEAR AND GARETH KEAR

60 Hikes Within 60 Miles: Philadelphia

Copyright © 2009 Sandra and Gareth Kear
All rights reserved
Printed in the United States of America
Published by Menasha Ridge Press
Distributed by Publishers Group West
First edition, third printing 2015

Library of Congress Cataloging-in-Publication Data

Kear, Sandra.
    60 hikes within 60 miles, Philadelphia: including surrounding counties plus Hunterdon and Mercer, New Jersey/Sandra Kear and Gareth Kear.
        p. cm.
    Includes index.
    ISBN-13: 978-0-89732-572-1
    ISBN-10: 0-89732-572-9
    1. Hiking—Pennsylvania—Philadelphia Region—Guidebooks. 2. Trails—Pennsylvania—Philadelphia Region—Guidebooks. 3. Philadelphia Region (Pa.)—Guidebooks. I. Kear, Gareth. II. Title. III. Title: Sixty hikes within sixty miles, Philadelphia.
    GV199.42.P4P554 2009
    917.4—dc22

                                    2009025254


Cover design by Steveco International and Scott McGrew
Text design by Steveco International
Cover and interior photos by Sandra Kear
Maps by Scott McGrew and Gareth Kear
Indexing by Jan Mucciarone

Menasha Ridge Press
P.O. Box 43673
Birmingham, AL 35243
www.menasharidge.com

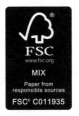
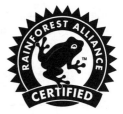

FSC
www.fsc.org
MIX
Paper from
responsible sources
FSC® C011935

DISCLAIMER
This book is meant only as a guide to select trails in the Philadelphia area and does not guarantee your safety in any way—you hike at your own risk. Neither Menasha Ridge Press nor Gareth and Sandra Kear are liable for property loss or damage, personal injury, or death that may result from accessing or hiking the trails described in the following pages. Please be aware that hikers have been injured in the Philadelphia area. Be especially cautious when walking on or near boulders, steep inclines, and drop-offs, and do not attempt to explore terrain that may be beyond your abilities. To help ensure an uneventful hike, please read carefully the introduction to this book, and perhaps get further safety information and guidance from other sources. Familiarize yourself thoroughly with the areas you intend to visit before venturing out. Ask questions and prepare for the unforeseen. Familiarize yourself with current weather reports, maps of the area you intend to visit, and any relevant area regulations.

WE DEDICATE THIS BOOK TO OUR LOVING AND CREATIVE CHILDREN, CLARISSA AND KAELYN.

—SANDRA AND GARETH KEAR

# TABLE OF
# CONTENTS

# ACKNOWLEDGMENTS

First and foremost, we would like to thank our parents, Diane, Jacqueline, and Bernard, for all their support and love throughout the years. We would also like to thank Molly Merkle and the editors at Menasha Ridge for their hard work, professionalism, and understanding. Last, but not least, we would like to extend an extra special thanks to our best hiking buddy, Andrew Kear, who contributed to the research and writing of this book.

# FOREWORD

Welcome to Menasha Ridge Press's *60 Hikes within 60 Miles,* a series designed to provide hikers with the information they need to find and hike the very best trails surrounding metropolitan areas typically underserved by outdoor guidebooks.

Our strategy was simple: First, find a hiker who knows the area and loves to hike. Second, ask that person to spend a year researching the most popular and very best trails around. And third, have that person describe each trail in terms of difficulty, scenery, condition, elevation change, and all other categories of information that are important to hikers. "Pretend you've just completed a hike and met up with other hikers at the trailhead," we told each author. "Imagine their questions; be clear in your answers."

Sandra and Gareth Kear have selected 60 of the best hikes in and around the Philadelphia metropolitan area. Including not only obscure and unknown trails but also in-depth information regarding the history, flora, and fauna of the most outstanding day escapes in the Greater Philadelphia area, the Kears provide hikers (and walkers) with a great variety of hikes—and all within roughly 60 miles of Philadelphia.

You'll get more out of this book if you take a moment to read the introduction explaining how to read the trail listings. The "Topographic Maps" section will help you understand how useful topos are on a hike and will also tell you where to get them. And though this is a "where-to," not a "how-to" guide, readers who have not hiked extensively will find the introduction of particular value.

As much for the opportunity to free the spirit as well as to free the body, let these hikes elevate you above the urban hurry.

**All the best,
The Editors at Menasha Ridge Press**

# ABOUT THE AUTHORS

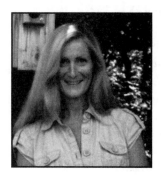

## SANDRA KEAR

A freelance writer and editor, Sandra specializes in academic and trade books on health care, technology, and the environment but has also worked in a variety of other genres. She is coauthor of the book *Coping with Grief* for teenagers, along with Dr. Robert W. Buckingham, one of the original founders of the hospice movement. She has written for such print and online publications as *CD-ROM World* and *Internet World* magazines; *Philadelphia House & Home;* Go2 Mobile; and PhiladelphiaRestaurants.com. Her most inspiring job has been as mother of her two beloved children, Clarissa and Kaelyn. She has primarily worked for book and magazine publishers, most recently as editorial director for a book packager with clients such as Reader's Digest Trade, the American Psychological Association, and Harcourt Press. You can find out more about Sandra at **www.keareditorial.com** or find more hiking updates and information at **www.trekalong.com**.

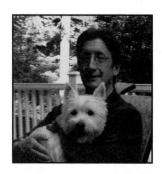

## GARETH KEAR

Outings director for the Bucks County chapter of the Sierra Club, Gareth is an avid hiker and outdoorsman as well as a talented musician. His recent CDs, *Bucks County Guitar* and *Bucks County Guitar II,* were largely inspired by the Greater Philadelphia countryside. A senior software analyst, he is involved in his local environmental-action committee and in organic community-supported agriculture. He also teaches folk, classical, and blues guitar in his spare time, when not immersed in his role as Number-one Dad. You can download Gareth's music from **CDBaby.com**.

# PREFACE

Shortly after my husband, Gareth, and I moved from Connecticut to the Philadelphia suburbs, he started leaving the house after work and disappearing for hours. He returned filled with a renewed zest for life. "Where have you been?" I'd ask. "I've been out hiking," he'd reply. *A likely story,* I thought. But before I knew it, Gareth had many of the major trails memorized much in the same way he would memorize a series of classical-guitar pieces.

Before we were married, Gareth and I often hiked together. In fact, in 1994, on one of our regular hikes through Weir Farm, in Wilton, Connecticut, Gareth proposed by an old apple tree that had fallen and re-rooted itself, growing back upward with a lush, widespread crown. Shortly after we were married, the National Park Service took cuttings from the historic apple trees at the Weir Farm, and now 12 new trees produce abundant fruit.

Unfortunately, natural areas like this disappear each day, and if pioneers of preservation had not persisted over the last hundred years, we might be facing environmental destruction more severe than we have seen in this 21st century, and the hikes that have influenced romantics and revived the great minds of our time might no longer exist.

The hikes in this book would not be possible without unsung heroes who realized that although this country has fallen environmentally, it is never too late to save what is precious. Through preservation, lands management, and education, we can once again cherish the outdoors as we did when we were children.

Remember riding bikes around the neighborhood, having crab-apple fights, and playing hide-and-seek past sundown? Most children today don't have these outdoor opportunities. The freedom we enjoyed has been stolen from our children by predators, fear, micromanaged schedules, hundreds of TV channels, urban sprawl, the Internet, and electronic games that offer a virtual world that has caused some people to forgo the outdoors—and reality in general.

But because of forward-thinking individuals in both the public and private sectors, there are secret havens of awesome beauty less than an hour from Philadelphia—places like Tohickon Valley Park, which spans from the lowlands of the Tohickon Creek to the high points of Ralph Stover State Park, shooting up 400 feet into the cliffs that overhang the glistening water below. Not only does the Greater Philadelphia area offer parks of immense beauty, but many of these parks also include preserved land with scenic views of stone houses, covered bridges, and old battlefields.

You can almost step into history in places like Valley Forge, Washington Crossing, the Daniel Boone Homestead, or the Howell Living History Farm. Other, less notable places feature unusual historical tidbits, such as the Evansburg Funkites, Warwick's Eight Arch Bridge, and Batsto Village in the New Jersey Pinelands.

Places like Peace Valley and Neshaminy Park offer not only water views but also an education in preservation, with kiosks and programs to help people to better understand the importance of saving our local lands and watersheds. Organizations such as the Natural Lands Trust and the Pennypack Ecological Restoration Trust go a step further, offering insight into land-preservation solutions.

Other points along this 60 Hikes repertoire include the best places to see a bald eagle, a blue heron, and a variety of butterflies. Did you know that Johns James Audubon was originally from Pennsylvania, and that he gained much of his inspiration for natural illustration on the grounds near Mill Grove?

Many of these hikes are near quaint historic and river towns and constitute an inexpensive weekend getaway or "staycation" that would surprise even the most astute world traveler. If you've never been to Longwood Gardens, for instance, or don't consider it a typical hiking experience, cover the perimeter in a day and visit its verdant meadows—and don't forget your camera, because you won't see plants and flowers like these anywhere else.

Each hike presented here is as unique as a beautiful song, as is the person who is reading this book. We hope this guide will help you connect with the Philadelphia countryside in ways you never thought possible. We know that if you make the effort, you too will find a renewed zest for life and for the land. We hope you will share this joie de vivre with those you love, and that, like the apple tree that fell at Weir Farm, the connection with the land that you once knew as a child can take root once again to sprout back up and form a luscious crown. Who knows? It may provide cuttings that will propagate for generations to come.

—Sandra Kear
Bucks County, Pennsylvania

# HIKING RECOMMENDATIONS

## HIKES 1 TO 3 MILES

## HIKES 3 TO 6 MILES

## HIKES 6 TO 8 MILES

## HIKES 8 TO 10 MILES

## STEEP HIKES

## COASTAL HIKE

## HIKES WITH VIEWS

## FAMILY HIKES

## HIKES FOR BIRDING

## HIGH-TRAFFIC HIKES

## LOW-TRAFFIC HIKES

## WILDLIFE HIKES

## HIKES WITH STRENUOUS CLIMBS

## HIKES WITH STRENUOUS CLIMBS (*continued*)

## HIKES FOR SPRING WILDFLOWERS

## HIKES FOR FALL COLORS

## HIKES FOR VERY YOUNG CHILDREN

## HIKES FOR DOGS

(Many sites allow dogs on leashes; call or check online for more information.)

## FLAT HIKES

## HIKES FOR SOLITUDE

## HIKES ALONG WATER

## HIKES ALONG WATER (*continued*)

## TRAILS FOR RUNNERS

## MULTIUSE TRAILS

## HIKES WITH HISTORIC INTEREST

# INTRODUCTION

Welcome to *60 Hikes within 60 Miles: Philadelphia*. If you're new to hiking, or even if you're a seasoned trailsmith, take a few minutes to read the following introduction as we explain how this book is organized and how to use it.

## HIKE DESCRIPTIONS

Each hike contains eight key items: a locator map, an In Brief description of the trail, a Key At-a-Glance Information box, directions to the trail, a trail map, an elevation profile, a trail description, and a listing of nearby activities. Combined, the maps and information provide a clear method to assess each trail from the comfort of your favorite reading chair.

### IN BRIEF

A "taste of the trail." Think of this section as a snapshot focused on the historical landmarks, beautiful vistas, and other sights you may encounter on the trail.

### KEY AT-A-GLANCE INFORMATION

The information presented here gives you a quick idea of the specifics of each hike. Fourteen basic elements are covered:

**LENGTH** The length of the trail from start to finish. There may be options to shorten or extend the hikes, but the mileage corresponds to the described hike. Consult the hike description to help decide how to customize the hike for your ability or time constraints.

**CONFIGURATION** A description of what the trail might look like from overhead. Trails can be loops, out-and-backs (trails on which one enters and leaves along the same path), figure eights, or balloons.

**DIFFICULTY** The degree of effort an average hiker should expect on a given hike. For simplicity, this category is classified as *easy, moderate, or hard*.

**SCENERY** A summary of the overall environs of the hike and what to expect in terms of plant life, wildlife, streams, and historic buildings.

**EXPOSURE** A quick check of how much sun you can expect on your shoulders during the hike. Descriptors used are self-explanatory and include terms such as *shady, exposed,* and *sunny.*

**TRAIL TRAFFIC** Indicates how busy the trail might be on an average day and if you might be able to find solitude out there. Trail traffic, of course, varies from day to day and season to season.

**TRAIL SURFACE** A description of the trail surface, be it paved, rocky, dirt, or a mixture of materials.

**HIKING TIME** The length of time it takes to hike the trail. Most of the estimates in this book reflect an average speed of 3 miles per hour. Difficult terrain and scrambling can add significantly to the amount of time required.

**DRIVING DISTANCE** Indicates expected distance from an easily identifiable point. In the case of this book, it's downtown Philadelphia (aka Center City).

**ACCESS** Operating hours and any fees or permits needed to access the trail.

**MAPS** Which maps are the best, or easiest, for this hike, and where to get them.

**WHEELCHAIR TRAVERSABLE** What to expect in terms of access to the trail and its facilities.

**FACILITIES** What to expect in terms of restrooms, water, and other amenities available at the trailhead or nearby.

**SPECIAL COMMENTS** Cover little extra details that don't fit into any of the above categories. Here you'll find trail-hiking options and facts, tips on how to get the most out of your hike, and helpful phone numbers/Web sites.

## DIRECTIONS TO THE TRAIL

The detailed directions given for each hike will lead you to its trailhead. If you use GPS technology, the UTM coordinates, latitude–longitude coordinates, and street addresses provided will allow you to navigate directly to the trailhead.

## DESCRIPTION

The trail description is the heart of each hike. Here we provide a summary of the trail's essence and highlights any special sights along the hike. Ultimately, the hike description will help you choose which hikes are best for you.

## NEARBY ACTIVITIES

Look here for information on nearby trails, other points of interest, or places to eat or shop.

# WEATHER

With the exception of rather short-lived extremes in weather, hiking can be done year-round in southeast Pennsylvania. Each season brings its own distinctive and pleasant features, all of which are worth exploring. Our favorite time of year for getting out is the fall, which tends to offer many clear and crisp days, and, for three or four weeks, colorful foliage. If you spend enough time trekking around, you'll notice that fall brings other events, such as harvest festivals, seasonal hawk migrations, the shortening of days, and a lot of activity around the forest as the animals prepare for winter. The fall is also accompanied by the constant crunching of leaves beneath your feet, making it difficult to be silent as you walk. Fall can also bring wet, cold rain—perfect conditions for hypothermia.

## AVERAGE TEMPERATURES (°F) BY MONTH: PHILADELPHIA

|      | JAN | FEB | MAR | APR | MAY | JUN |
|------|-----|-----|-----|-----|-----|-----|
| HIGH | 38° | 41° | 51° | 63° | 73° | 81° |
| LOW  | 23° | 25° | 33° | 42° | 51° | 61° |
|      | JUL | AUG | SEP | OCT | NOV | DEC |
| HIGH | 86° | 84° | 76° | 64° | 53° | 42° |
| LOW  | 66° | 64° | 57° | 45° | 36° | 28° |

Winter brings short days, rather stark lighting as the leaves have fallen from the trees, and occasional snowfalls. A snowpack of a foot or so is not uncommon in the high country, but it tends to be rather short-lived. With the absence of foliage, this is an especially good time of year for seeing foxes and watching birds. Some of our nicest days out have been during the winter, though you do want to be prepared for sudden changes in weather and dips in temperature. At this time of year, take special care around stream crossings and near ledges, which are often icy, as a slip could have unpleasant or even fatal consequences.

Spring in southeast Pennsylvania can be a little muddy and wet, but this part of the state is home to many species of surprising and beautiful wildflowers. Birds and other animals become more active as they begin raising young, and the seasonal migrations can be extraordinary. Be prepared for sudden changes in weather, particularly in March and April, when cold rains are not atypical. This is also the time of year when streams run high, making some hikes impassable or more hazardous.

Finally, summers are characteristically warm and can be rather humid, especially getting into August. This is a great time of year to hike along the high ridges the Tohickon Valley, but take care to hike early to avoid afternoon thunderstorms and midday heat. Carry plenty of water with you as the humidity can deplete your strength quickly, and don't forget your sunscreen.

# ALLOCATING TIME

On flat or lightly undulating terrain, we average 3 miles per hour when hiking. That speed drops in direct proportion to the steepness of a path. Navigation of obstacles such as brush and boulders, off-trail exploration of flora and fauna, photography, and rest stops also extend a hike. Give yourself plenty of time. Few people enjoy rushing through a hike, and fewer still take pleasure in scrambling down a rocky chute after dark. Remember, too, that your pace naturally slackens over the back half of a long trek.

# MAPS

## TOPO MAPS

The maps in this book have been produced with great care and, when used with the hiking directions, will direct you to the trail and help you stay on course. However, you will find superior detail and valuable information in the 7.5-minute series topographic maps produced by the United States Geological Survey (USGS). Topo maps are available online in many locations, including **terraserver -usa.com** and **maps.google.com** (click "terrain"). You can view and print topos of the entire United States at these sites and view aerial photographs of the same areas. The downside to topos is that many of them are outdated, having been created 20 to 30 years ago. But they still provide excellent topographic detail.

Digital topographic map programs such as DeLorme's TopoUSA enable you to review topo maps of the entire United States on your PC. You can also plot your own hikes by gathering GPS data out on the trail and then downloading it into the software.

If you're new to hiking, you might be wondering, "What's a topographic map?" In short, a topo indicates linear distance, as well as elevation, using contour lines. Contour lines spread across the map like dozens of intricate spiderwebs. Each line represents a particular elevation, and at the base of each topo, a contour's interval designation is given. If the contour interval is 200 feet, then the height difference between each contour line is 200 feet. Follow five contour lines up on the same map, and the elevation has increased by 1,000 feet.

Let's assume that the 7.5-minute series topo reads "Contour Interval 40 feet," that the short trail we'll be hiking is 2 inches in length on the map, and that it crosses five contour lines from beginning to end. What do we know? Well, because the linear scale of this series is 2,000 feet to the inch (roughly 2.75 inches representing 1 mile), we know our trail is approximately 0.8 miles long (2 inches translate to 4,000 feet). We also know we'll be climbing or descending 200 vertical feet (five contour lines are 40 feet each) over that distance. The elevation designations written on occasional contour lines will tell us if we're heading up or down.

In addition to outdoor shops and bike shops, major universities and some public libraries have topos; you might try photocopying the ones you need to avoid buying them. If you want your own and can't find them locally, visit the USGS Web site at **topomaps.usgs.gov.**

## GLOBAL POSITIONING SYSTEM (GPS) TRAILHEAD COORDINATES

To collect accurate map data, the authors hiked each trail with a handheld GPS unit (Garmin eTrex series). Data collected was then downloaded and plotted onto a digital USGS topo map. In addition to rendering a highly specific trail outline, this book also includes the GPS coordinates for each trailhead in two formats: latitude–longitude and Universal Transverse Mercator (UTM). Latitude–longitude coordinates tell you where you are by locating a point north or south of the 0-degree (latitude) line that belts the earth (aka the equator) and a point west of the 0-degree meridian (longitude) line that passes through Greenwich, England.

Topographic maps show latitude–longitude as well as UTM grid lines. Known as UTM coordinates, the numbers index a specific point using a grid method. The survey datum used to arrive at the coordinates in this book is WGS84 (versus NAD27 or WGS83). For readers who own a GPS unit, whether handheld or onboard a vehicle, the latitude–longitude or UTM coordinates provided on the first page of each hike may be entered into the GPS unit. Just make sure your GPS unit is set to navigate using WGS84 datum. Now you can navigate directly to the trailhead.

Most trailheads, which begin in parking areas, can be reached by car, but some hikes still require a short walk to reach the trailhead from a parking area. In these cases, a handheld unit is necessary to continue the GPS navigation process. That said, however, you can easily access all trailheads in this book by using the directions given, the overview map, the regional maps, and the trail maps, which show at least one major road leading into the area. But for those who enjoy using the latest GPS technology to navigate, the necessary data has been provided. A brief explanation of the UTM coordinates for Hike 27: Binky Lee Preserve (page 138), follows:

UTM Zone   18T
Easting   o448664
Northing   4438685

The UTM zone number, 18, refers to one of the 60 vertical zones of the UTM projection. Each zone is 6 degrees wide. The UTM zone letter, **T**, refers to one of the 20 horizontal zones that span from 80 degrees south to 84 degrees north. The easting number, **0448664**, indicates in meters how far east or west a point is from the central meridian of the zone. Increasing easting coordinates on a topo map or on your GPS screen indicate that you are moving east; decreasing easting coordinates indicate you are moving west. The northing number, **4438685**, references in meters how far you are from the equator. Above and below the equator, increasing northing coordinates indicate that you are traveling north; decreasing northing coordinates indicate you are traveling south.

## LATITUDE AND LONGITUDE

A more commonly used coordinate system specifies each point on the globe with a pair of angular measurements—latitude and longitude. Similar to x–y coordinates that specify points on a two-dimensional plane, the latitude and longitude coordinates specify a point on our spherical planet. These coordinates are also given in the trailhead coordinates box.

*Latitude* is specified in degrees and measures the north–south angular distance between a point on the map and the earth's equatorial plane, which divides the earth into a northern hemisphere and a southern hemisphere. A point on the equator has a latitude of 0 degrees, while the North Pole has a latitude of 90 degrees. Points of equal latitude trace out concentric circles called *parallels*. (The 38th Parallel, for example, became a well-known latitude during the Korean War.) Because the United States lies in the northern hemisphere, latitudes for points within the United States will be some number between 0 and 90.

*Longitude* is also specified in degrees and measures the east–west angular distance between a point on the map and an arbitrary reference point—the Royal Observatory at Greenwich in England—designated as having 0 longitude. Points of equal longitude form *meridians* and run vertically from the North Pole to the South Pole. The 0-degree longitudinal line is also known as the Prime Meridian. Longitude values increase as you move away horizontally from the Prime Meridian. Everything to the east of the Prime Meridian is in the eastern hemisphere, and everything to its west is in the western hemisphere. For arbitrary reasons, points in the western hemisphere are given a negative longitude. So 111 degrees west is the same thing as –111 degrees longitude. The longitudinal line at 180 degrees—points farthest from the Prime Meridian—also serves (roughly) as the International Date Line.

Because longitude and latitude are angular coordinates, they are sometimes noted in degrees (°), minutes ('), and even seconds (") for better readability. A typical GPS unit comes from the factory set to display latitude–longitude coordinates in degrees and minutes. Therefore, all latitude–longitude coordinates in this book are specified in degrees and minutes. Make sure your GPS unit is set to use the WGS84 datum when using latitude–longitude coordinates. Again, WGS84 is a typical default setting on many GPS units.

For the same example given from page 138, the trailhead for Binky Lee Preserve has the following latitude–longitude coordinates:

Latitude   N 40° 5' 48.69"
Longitude   W 75° 36' 8.17"

These coordinates specify a point in the northern hemisphere, 40 degrees, 5 minutes, and 48.69 seconds north of the equator, and in the western hemisphere, 75 degrees, 36 minutes, and 8.17 seconds west of the Prime Meridian.

To learn more about how to enhance your outdoor experiences with GPS technology, refer to *GPS Outdoors: A Practical Guide for Outdoor Enthusiasts* (Menasha Ridge Press).

# WATER

How much is enough? Well, one simple physiological fact should convince you to err on the side of excess when deciding how much water to pack: a hiker working hard in 90-degree heat needs approximately 10 quarts of fluid per day. That's 2.5 gallons—12 large water bottles or 16 small ones. In other words, pack along one or two bottles even for short hikes.

Some hikers and backpackers hit the trail prepared to purify water found along the route. This method, while less dangerous than drinking untreated water, comes with risks. Purifiers with ceramic filters are the safest. Many hikers pack along the slightly distasteful tetraglycine–hydroperiodide tablets (sold under the names Potable Aqua, Coughlan's, and others) to debug water.

Probably the most common waterborne "bug" that hikers face is *Giardia,* which may not hit until one to four weeks after ingestion. It will have you living in the bathroom, passing noxious rotten-egg gas, vomiting, and shivering with chills. Other parasites to worry about include *E. coli* and *cryptosporidium,* both of which are harder to kill than *Giardia.*

For most people, the pleasures of hiking make carrying water a relatively minor price to pay to remain healthy. If you're tempted to drink "found water," do so only if you understand the risks involved. Better yet, hydrate prior to your hike, carry (and drink) 6 ounces of water for every mile you plan to hike, and hydrate after the hike.

# CLOTHING

Use common sense when dressing for a hike, and be prepared for sudden changes in weather. Check the forecast before you go out, and then count on it being worse than predicted. Getting caught without the appropriate clothes can be not only uncomfortable but dangerous.

In the summertime, hike in shorts and T-shirt. In your pack, carry raingear (both a jacket and pants), and a wool sweater or some type of synthetic pullover (polypropylene, Capilene, Thermax, or the like). Wear a broad-brimmed hat during the summer as the sun can be strong. In the winter, dress in layers, and carry a Gore-Tex jacket and wind pants. Wear gloves, a wool hat, and wool socks. If you often hike alone, ask yourself, "What if?" Pack enough clothes to spend a night if doing so should become necessary. In the winter, carry an extra set of dry pile pants, as Pennsylvania winters can be notoriously damp and stream crossings can be troublesome.

Footwear is something that needs to be taken rather seriously when hiking around southeast Pennsylvania. For most of the rail-trails, you can get away with a good pair of sneakers or a lightweight pair of hiking books. When you get into the backcountry, you would be foolhardy not to wear a sturdy pair of boots. Many of the trails are extremely rocky and rugged. By wearing lightweight boots, not only do you risk a sprained ankle, but you can develop some very painful foot injuries (like heel spurs) that take a long time to heal. If you wear a traditional pair of one-piece leather hiking boots, you shouldn't have any problems.

## THE TEN ESSENTIALS

One of the first rules of hiking is to be prepared for anything. The simplest way to be prepared is to carry the "Ten Essentials." In addition to carrying the items listed below, you need to know how to use them, especially navigation items. Always consider worst-case scenarios like getting lost, hiking back in the dark, broken gear (for example, a broken hip strap on your pack or a water filter getting plugged), twisting an ankle, or a brutal thunderstorm. The following items don't cost a lot of money, don't take up much room in a pack, and don't weigh much, but they might just save your life:

> **WATER:** durable bottles and water treatment such as iodine or a filter
>
> **MAP:** preferably a topo map and a trail map with a route description
>
> **COMPASS:** a high-quality model
>
> **FIRST-AID KIT:** a good-quality kit including first-aid instructions
>
> **KNIFE:** a multitool device with pliers is best
>
> **LIGHT:** flashlight or headlamp with extra bulbs and batteries
>
> **FIRE:** windproof matches or lighter and fire starter
>
> **EXTRA FOOD:** bring enough that you still have some in your pack when you've finished hiking
>
> **EXTRA CLOTHES:** rain protection, warm layers, gloves, a warm hat
>
> **SUN PROTECTION:** sunglasses, lip balm, sunblock, sun hat

## FIRST-AID KIT

A typical first-aid kit may contain more items than you might think necessary. The following are just the basics. Prepackaged kits in waterproof bags (Atwater Carey and Adventure Medical make a variety of kits) are available. Even though there are quite a few items listed here, they pack down into a small space:

Ace bandages or Spenco joint wraps

Antibiotic ointment (Neosporin or the generic equivalent)

Aspirin or acetaminophen

Band-Aids

Benadryl or the generic equivalent, diphenhydramine (in case of allergic reactions)

Butterfly-closure bandages

Epinephrine in a prefilled syringe (for people known to have severe allergic reactions to bee stings and the like)

Gauze (one roll)

Gauze compress pads (a half dozen 4- by 4-inch pads)

Hydrogen peroxide or iodine

Insect repellent

Matches or pocket lighter

Moleskin/Spenco "Second Skin"

Sunscreen

Whistle (it's more effective in signaling rescuers than your voice)

## HIKING WITH CHILDREN

No one is too young for a hike in the outdoors, just be mindful, though. Flat, short, and shaded trails are best with an infant. Toddlers who haven't quite mastered walking can still tag along, riding on an adult's back in a child carrier. Use common sense to judge a child's capacity to hike a particular trail, and always count on the child tiring quickly and needing to be carried.

When packing for the hike, remember the child's needs as well as your own. Make sure children are adequately clothed for the weather, have proper shoes, and are protected from the sun with sunscreen. Kids dehydrate quickly, so make sure you bring along plenty of fluid for everyone. To assist an adult with determining which trails are suitable for children, a list of hike recommendations for young children is provided on page xvi, and hikes for families on page xiv.

## GENERAL SAFETY

In addition to the wonderful places you come across in the backcountry, much of the excitement of going for a hike stems from having to make decisions and having to be somewhat self-reliant. There is no reason why exploring the woods should not be as safe as or safer than traveling around an urban area. Yet being safe requires a certain presence of mind. Try to assume an "expedition mentality"— always behave and make decisions as if rescue or assistance were days away. Getting hurt or lost isn't an option from this mind-set, and rather than doing something foolhardy, you'll find it in your best interest to just turn back. Here are some things that you can do to help make your excursions safe and enjoyable:

- **ALWAYS LET SOMEONE KNOW YOUR ITINERARY. Leave word about where you are going, when you will return, and what should be done if you are overdue. No matter how careful you are, things do happen. Someone knowing your plans can be critical if an emergency arises. That said, always let the person know when you have returned.**

- **ALWAYS CARRY FOOD AND WATER, whether you are planning an overnight trip or not. Food will give you energy, help keep you warm, and sustain you in an emergency situation until help arrives. You never know if you will have a stream nearby when you become thirsty. Bring potable water or treat water before drinking it from a stream.**

- **STAY ON DESIGNATED TRAILS. Most hikers get lost when they leave the path. Even on the most clearly marked trails, there is usually a point where you have to stop and consider in which direction to head. If you become disoriented, don't panic. As soon as you think you may be off-track, stop, assess your current direction, and then retrace your steps back to the point where you went awry. Using a map, a compass, this book, and keeping in mind what you have passed thus far, reorient yourself and trust your judgment on which way to continue. If you become absolutely unsure of how to continue, return to your vehicle the way you came in. Should you become completely lost and have no idea how to return to the trailhead, staying where you** are and waiting for help is most often the best option for adults and always the best option for children.

- **BE ESPECIALLY CAREFUL WHEN CROSSING STREAMS.** Whether you are fording the stream or crossing on a log, make every step count. If you have any doubt about maintaining your balance on a foot log, go ahead and ford the stream instead. When fording a stream, use a trekking pole or stout stick for balance and face upstream as you cross. If a stream seems too deep to ford, turn back. Whatever is on the other side is not worth risking your life for.

- **BE CAREFUL AT OVERLOOKS.** While these areas may provide spectacular views, they are potentially hazardous. Stay back from the edge of outcrops and be absolutely sure of your footing; a misstep can mean a nasty and possibly fatal fall.

- **WATCH OUT FOR STANDING DEAD TREES** and storm-damaged living trees—both pose a real hazard to hikers and tent campers. These trees may have loose or broken limbs that could fall at any time. When choosing a spot to rest or a backcountry campsite, look up.

- **KNOW THE SYMPTOMS OF HYPOTHERMIA.** Shivering and forgetfulness are the two most common indicators of this insidious killer. Hypothermia can occur at any elevation, even in the summer, especially when the hiker is wearing lightweight cotton clothing. If symptoms arise, get the victim shelter, hot liquids, and dry clothes or a dry sleeping bag.

- **TAKE ALONG YOUR BRAIN.** A cool, calculating mind is the single most important piece of equipment you'll ever need on the trail. Think before you act. Plan ahead. Avoid accidents before they happen.

- **ASK QUESTIONS.** Forest and park employees are there to help. It's a lot easier to gain advice beforehand and avoid a mishap away from civilization when it's too late to amend an error. Use your head out there, and treat the place as if it were your own backyard.

## BLACK BEAR

It should be fairly obvious that you shouldn't stop to photograph or feed a black bear, but many people don't realize that running away or even quietly skulking behind a tree might pique that bear's interest even more. When hiking, if you suspect that a bear is nearby, make lots of loud noises and wave your arms. These actions will likely scare the bear.

## SNAKES

Southeast Pennsylvania is home to one type of poisonous snake: the copperhead. This snake is rare; nonetheless, copperheads are out there and you should bear this in mind, particularly when traveling the rocky, mountainous areas. Be careful if you move rocks and when climbing around outcrops, as these places are where snakes like to sun themselves. If you see any snake with a diamond-shaped head

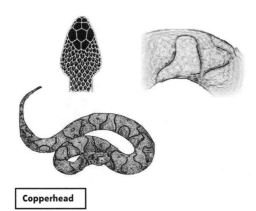

**Copperhead**

(characteristic to many poisonous snakes) or have any doubts, give it a wide berth.

## POISON IVY, OAK, AND SUMAC

Recognizing these plants and avoiding contact with them is the most effective way to prevent the painful, itchy rashes associated with them. In southeast Pennsylvania, poison ivy ranges from a thick, tree-hugging vine to a shaded groundcover, three leaflets to a leaf; poison oak occurs as either a vine or a shrub, with three leaflets as well; and poison sumac flourishes in swampland, each leaf containing 7 to 13 leaflets. Urushiol, the oil in the sap of these plants, is responsible for the rash. Usually within 12 to 14 hours of exposure (but sometimes much later), raised lines and/or blisters will appear, accompanied by a terrible itch. Refrain from scratching, as hard as that may be, because bacteria under your fingernails can cause infection and you will spread the rash to other parts of your body. Wash and dry the rash thoroughly, applying calamine lotion or other product to help dry the rash. If itching or blistering is severe, seek medical attention.

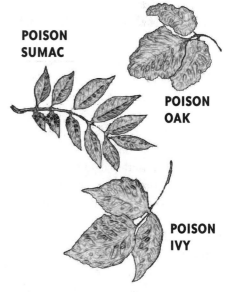

**Common poisonous plants**

POISON SUMAC

POISON OAK

POISON IVY

Remember that oil-contaminated clothes, pets, or hiking gear can easily cause an irritating rash on you or someone else, so wash not only any exposed parts of your body, but also clothes, gear, and pets.

## MOSQUITOES

Although it's an uncommon occurrence, individuals can become infected with the West Nile virus after being bitten by an infected mosquito. Culex mosquitoes, the primary varieties that can transmit West Nile virus to humans, thrive in urban rather than natural areas. They lay their eggs in stagnant water and can breed in any standing water that remains for more than five days. Most people infected with West Nile virus have no symptoms of illness, but some may become ill, usually 3 to 15 days after being bitten.

In southeast Pennsylvania, late spring and summer are the times thought to be the highest risk periods for West Nile virus. At this time of year—and anytime you expect mosquitoes to be buzzing around—you may want to wear protective clothing, such as long sleeves, long pants, and socks. Loose-fitting, light-colored clothing is best. Spray clothing with insect repellent. Remember to follow the instructions on the repellent and to take extra care with children.

## CLIFFS AND MOUNTAINOUS AREAS

Some of the hikes in this book include high elevations and cliffs with dangerous drops. Avoid walking to a cliff's edge, and stay on the trail, especially in windy weather. Although the view may be outstanding, it takes only a momentary loss of footing to spawn a fatal accident. Although this sounds obvious, accidental falls occur yearly in our state and national parks.

## TICKS AND LYME DISEASE

Until you are struck with this malady, you cannot imagine that something the size of a pinhead could make you feel so awful. Left undiagnosed, Lyme disease can cause neurological damage, joint pain, and heart problems. Not everyone will present with the trademark bulletlike rash. Most of the hikes in this book are in high-risk areas; therefore, take precautions to avoid the ticks that cause this virus.

Tiny deer ticks (black-legged ticks) carry Lyme disease; if you find a tick attached to your skin, gently remove it with tweezers, taking care to pull it off gently so the mouth part does not break off and remain attached. Always shower after a hike to wash off any ticks you might not have caught earlier, and check your hair thoroughly with your fingers.

If possible, wear long pants and long-sleeved shirts. (It's also a good idea to wear a hat to prevent ticks from falling from above and burrowing into your scalp.) Use a non-DEET tick wipe or spray prior to hiking. Stay on dirt and paved trails, and avoid grassy trails whenever possible. Ask a partner or family member to do a visual inspection. Become familiar with the symptoms of Lyme disease, and if you feel that you have been exposed to or are exhibiting any of the symptoms, see your doctor immediately and be assertive in your own treatment.

## TIPS FOR ENJOYING YOUR HIKE

Consider a few tips that will make your hike enjoyable and more rewarding:

- **Take your time along the trails. Pace yourself for the longer hikes. The forests, fields, and wetlands of the greater Philadelphia area are filled with wonders both big and small. Keep watch on the ground for box turtles, blue-lined skinks, and butterflies. Stop and enjoy the delicate blooms of trout lilies. Imagine what the day was like when that enormous mass of stone fell into the valley. Enjoy listening to the banter of birds** or the wind at an overlook. Shorter hikes allow you to stop and linger more than long hikes. Take close notice of the elevation maps that accompany each hike. If you see many ups and downs or large altitude changes, you'll obviously need more time. Inevitably you'll finish some of the "hike times" long before or after what is suggested. Nevertheless, leave yourself plenty of time for those moments when you simply feel like stopping and taking it all in and letting it all out.

- We can't always schedule our free time when we want, but try to hike during the week and avoid the traditional holidays if possible. Trails that are packed in the summer are often clear during the colder months. If you are hiking on a busy day, go early in the morning; it'll enhance your chances of seeing wildlife. The trails really clear out during rainy times; however, don't hike during a thunderstorm. Hiking in winter is also a good time to have the trail all to yourself. The best time to hike is after a snow and during a snowfall of fluffy snow, which muffles the noises of daily life and lets you enjoy a few moments of serenity. (Just remember to turn off the cell phone.)

- Participate in some online wildlife-observation counts. The Cornell University Lab of Ornithology operates www.ebird.org, where you can log in at no cost and submit bird lists from your hikes or find out what's being seen at some of the area's birding hot spots. A similar count is being done for butterflies at the North American Butterfly Association's Web site, www.naba.org. If you have a favorite hiking location, speak with the property manager or naturalist to see if he or she needs assistance conducting counts.

## TRAIL ETIQUETTE

Following are some suggestions to improve not only your hiking experience, but also the environment for those who follow you. Whether you're on a city, county, state, or national park trail, always remember that great care and resources (from nature as well as from your tax dollars) have gone into creating these trails. Treat the trail, wildlife, and fellow hikers with respect:

- **Hike on designated trails only.** Respect trail and road closures (ask if not sure), avoid trespassing on private land, and obtain all required permits and authorizations. Also, leave gates as you find them or as marked. Note that some of the trails in this book include sections off the main trails. Clear directions are provided.

- **Leave only footprints.** Be sensitive to the ground beneath you. Pack out what you pack in. No one likes to see the trash someone else has left behind.

- **Never spook animals.** An unannounced approach, a sudden movement, or a loud noise startles most animals. A surprised snake or skunk can be dangerous to you, others, and themselves. Give animals extra room and time to adjust to your presence.

- **Plan ahead.** Know your equipment, your ability, and the area in which you are hiking—and prepare accordingly. Be self-sufficient at all times; carry necessary supplies for changes in weather or other conditions. A well-executed trip is a satisfaction to you and to others.

- **Be courteous to other hikers, bikers, or equestrians you meet on the trails.** It is customary to yield to equestrians, hikers going uphill, and faster hikers.

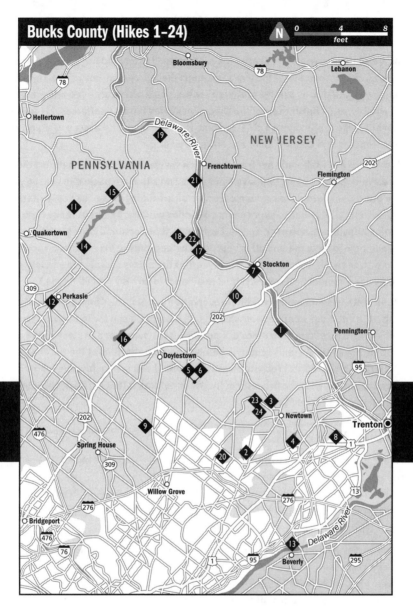

Bloomsbury

Lebanon

78

78

Hellertown

Delaware River

NEW JERSEY

19

PENNSYLVANIA

Frenchtown

Flemington

202

21

15

11

18  22

Quakertown

17

14

Stockton

7

309

12  Perkasie

10

Pennington

202

16

95

Doylestown

5   6

23   3

Newtown

Trenton

202

24

9

476

4

8

Spring House

2

1

309

20

Willow Grove

276

13

Bridgeport

276

476

13

Delaware River

76

1   95   295

Beverly

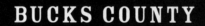

**BUCKS COUNTY**

# 01 BOWMAN'S HILL TOWER AND WILDFLOWER PRESERVE

## KEY AT-A-GLANCE INFORMATION

**LENGTH:** 3 miles

**CONFIGURATION:** Balloon

**DIFFICULTY:** Hard

**SCENERY:** Tower view, wildflowers, pond, creek, woods

**EXPOSURE:** Full sun–full shade

**TRAIL TRAFFIC:** Light

**TRAIL SURFACE:** Dirt, gravel, pavement (parts of trail not well blazed)

**HIKING TIME:** 1.5 hours

**DRIVING DISTANCE FROM CENTER CITY:** 35 miles

**ACCESS:** The Preserve is open daily year-round, except Thanksgiving, Christmas, and New Year's Day. The grounds are open 8:30 a.m.–sunset, and the visitor center and Twinleaf Shop are open 9 a.m.–5 p.m. Admission (nonmembers): $5 adults, $3 seniors age 62+, $2 children ages 4–14, free for children under age 4.

**MAPS:** USGS Lambertville; maps at visitor center

**WHEELCHAIR TRAVERSABLE:** No, although other trails within the preserve, such as Woods Edge Walk, are paved and accessible. See staff at the preserve's visitor center for more information.

**FACILITIES:** Restrooms in nature center at wildlife preserve

**SPECIAL COMMENTS:** More information: (215) 862-2924; www.bhwp.org.

---

## GPS Trailhead Coordinates

UTM Zone (WGS84) 18T

Easting 0505245

Northing 4464427

Latitude N 40° 19' 49.30"

Longitude W 74° 56' 17.78"

## IN BRIEF

This is like two hikes in one: first an outstanding view of the Delaware River Valley atop Bowman's Hill Tower, and then a one-of-a-kind wildflower preserve with the lush horticulture of the Bucks County area at its best. Don't forget to bring $5 per person for the tower-access fee.

*Note:* Stop at the visitor center, just inside the gates from the parking lot, to pick up trail maps, which will give you detailed information about the flowers in the preserve.

## DESCRIPTION

During the American Revolutionary War, George Washington needed to find a high vantage point in Pennsylvania before his famous crossing of the Delaware and subsequent attack upon loyalist and Hessian troops on the other side. The hill where Bowman's Hill Tower stands may well have been that high point; and even if it was not, the view from the top of the tower, at 380 feet above sea level, with the river and green valley below, certainly gives one pause to appreciate the history and richness in this part of the country.

---

## Directions ⟶

Take Interstate 95 north from Philadelphia to Exit 51, New Hope (old Exit 31). Turn left (north) onto Taylorsville Road. Go north on Taylorsville Road for 7 miles, crossing PA 532 at 5 miles. Turn left (north) onto PA 32–River Road and go 2.5 miles, past the road to Bowman's Hill Tower on the left and then the Thompson-Neely House on the right. The entrance to the preserve is on your left—look for the large brown sign that reads BOWMAN'S HILL WILDFLOWER PRESERVE. *1635 River Road, New Hope, PA 18938.*

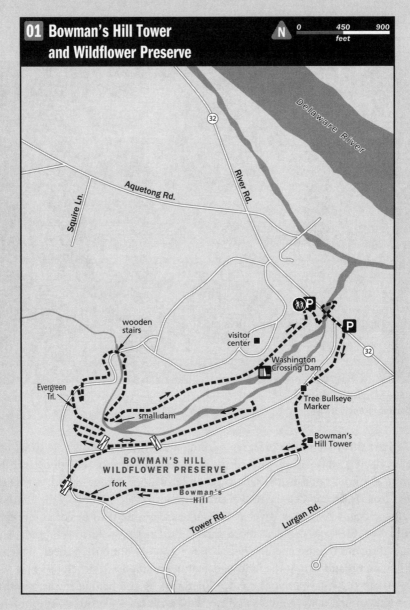

N

0      450      900
feet

Delaware River

32

Aquetong Rd.

Squire Ln.

River Rd.

wooden stairs

visitor center

Washington Crossing Dam

P

P

32

Evergreen Trl.

small dam

Tree Bullseye Marker

Bowman's Hill Tower

BOWMAN'S HILL
WILDFLOWER PRESERVE

fork

Bowman's Hill

Tower Rd.

Lurgan Rd.

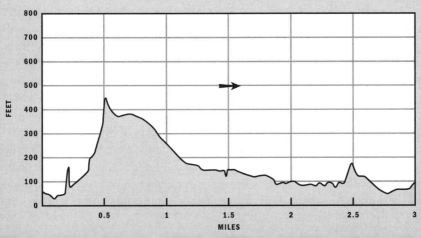

FEET

800
700
600
500
400
300
200
100
0

0.5      1      1.5      2      2.5      3

MILES

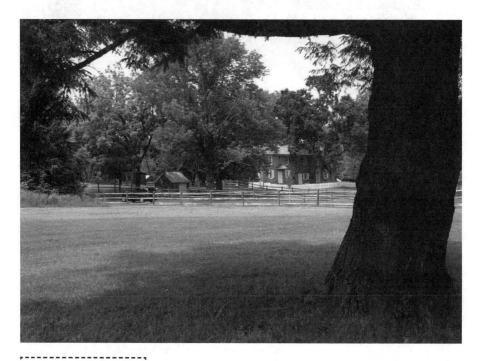

Thompson-Neely House

Start this hike at the preserve parking area, directly off River Road. From the trailhead, walk south toward a white stucco farmhouse. Follow the trail behind the house and to the left to go under a stone bridge, which goes under River Road. Once under the bridge, walk up onto the road and to the south end of the bridge. Cross over River Road and pick up the trail beside the preserve fence. The preserve protects more than 1,000 native wildflowers and plants, some of them rare and endangered. The fence keeps out hungry deer, which are left to chomp and stomp the landscapes of nearby housing developments.

About 0.2 miles along the fence-lined trail is an opening in the woods, to your left, strewn with boulders and carpeted with ferns. At this point, look for a faded bull's-eye marker, painted on a large oak tree—it's blue in the middle and white on the outside, with an arrow. If you do not want to visit Bowman's Hill Tower and are in the mood for a less strenuous hike, continue to hug the fence all the way to the entrance of the wildflower preserve. If you do want to see the tower, follow the arrow to the left, where there is no place to go but up, up, up—slowly and carefully, side-footing your way to the top of the hill—where the tower awaits. You will value this ultimate lookout point even more after you have ascended the hill by foot like the muddied soldiers of Washington's army.

At the top of the hill, you may need to sit and break out your water bottle; at this point you've completed the most strenuous climb of this hike. Give yourself a pat on the back, and then enter the visitor center to pay the $5 admission fee to the top of Bowman's Hill Tower. The structure was completed in June

View from atop Bowman's Tower

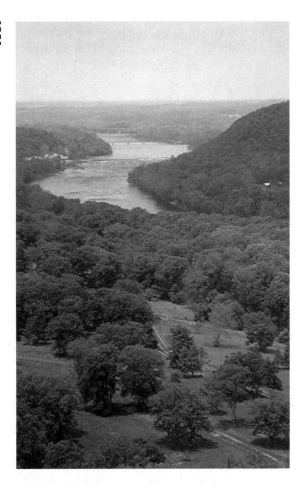

of 1931 to commemorate George Washington and his army. Several improvements at the tower and the surrounding grounds were completed in the 1930s as part of President Franklin Roosevelt's New Deal, which gave work to the unemployed and recovery to the weak economy. Relief workers did tree and grounds work, cleared trees to provide better views from the tower, and placed large rocks and boulders in the banks near the tower to prevent soil erosion. New Deal workers also repaired and waterproofed the tower itself. The current tower staff will encourage you to take the elevator to the top level, so that the stairway stays intact.

At the tower's top level, take a small stone stairway to the lookout, where you will see green in spring and summer, and an array of reds, oranges, and yellows in the fall. The valley below is peppered with enormous homes that look like little cabins, and your car in the lot may resemble a bug. If you look carefully you will see a large American flag, which marks the graves of Revolutionary War soldiers. You will also notice two bridges that span the Delaware River: the New Hope–Lambertville Bridge and the toll bridge that brings you to Route 202. You can also view the Thompson-Neely House, barn, and gristmill on the opposite side of River Road.

The colonial history of this parcel of land where the tower and reserve are now located starts with a fur trader named John Pidcock, who lived here in the late 17th century, until a Quaker named John Simpson acquired the land. Simpson built a modest stone house and gristmill near what is now known as Pidcock Creek. After Simpson died, his hired miller, a Scottish Presbyterian named Robert Thompson, married Simpson's widow, Hannah, and expanded the business. The couple enlarged the house for their daughter, Elizabeth, and her husband,

William Neely. In 1776, patriot soldiers retreating through New Jersey set up camp nearby, and the Thompson-Neely House served as a hospital for wounded and disease-stricken soldiers. In fact, James Monroe and George Washington's cousin, William Washington, both convalesced here after the Battle of Trenton.

After you've fully absorbed this unique view, descend the stairs to the elevator to continue your hike. From the entrance, walk straight toward the parking lot, which ascends into a roadway; this is the route that less adventurous people take to the tower area. Take the one and only gravel trail that splits from the road, and watch for the deer that safely graze on this side of the fence. Pass over the paved road at the bend, and regain the trail until you pick up the tall chain-link fence once again.

There are three entrances to the wildflower preserve—if you descend to the third one, you can follow a lightly blazed, unmarked trail to Pidcock Creek, where clear, flowing waters make a meditative spot for a bag of trail mix and a cool refreshment. (If you want to save the wildflower preserve for another day, simply continue downhill on the trail.)

Once you've finished your snack, retrace your route uphill to the second entrance, which provides access to 2.5 miles of wildflower trails that wind in and out of a horticulturist's dream date. Follow along until you reach the Everglades Trail, where you turn right. The general rule at the preserve, however, is to stay near the creek so you don't get lost, especially if you don't have a map. If you secured your map at the start of this hike, you may want to explore the more than two dozen paths that the park has to offer, such as the Violet Trail, the Penn's Woods Tree Trail, and the Woods Edge Walk (which is handicapped accessible). Depending on the time of the year, you will see bursting purple irises, pink rhododendrons, bluebells, various types of azaleas, and a plethora of butterflies.

Continue on the trail you were on until you come to a stone bridge over Pidcock Creek. At the end of the bridge, turn right and climb the wooden stairs to a paved trail that hugs the creek all the way back to the parking lot. A small Walden-like cabin nearby serves as a shelter for park staff. Take another right after the cabin toward the end of the trail. A stone bridge and a gushing waterfall provide one last scenic wonder to enjoy before you end this hike.

## NEARBY ACTIVITIES

WASHINGTON CROSSING HISTORIC PARK
*(See Hike 51, page 266)*
1112 River Road, Washington Crossing
(215) 493-4076
**www.ushistory.org/washingtoncrossing**

HISTORIC NEW HOPE BOROUGH
*(Boutiques, restaurants, art community, and much more. To get here, follow River Road south about 6 miles.)*
**www.newhopepa.com**

# CHURCHVILLE NATURE CENTER  02

## IN BRIEF

This easy walk through 2 miles of diverse nature trails next to the Churchville Reservoir affords the opportunity to learn about local nature, history, and ecology in a tranquil setting.

## DESCRIPTION

Churchville Nature Center provides short, easy-to-follow trails suitable for the whole family. The center's programs foster an appreciation for the natural beauty that can so easily be mowed down and made into football fields, developments, and shopping malls.

Open spaces like this one make people want to move into the Philadelphia suburbs and outlying rural areas, but urban sprawl and the profit motive all too often destroy such spaces, which are so crucial to natural ecology and future well-being. It is the locals who pay in the end: with increased development comes an overtaxed infrastructure, and soon the area no longer resembles that cozy town-and-country spot homeowners dreamed of when purchasing their house or lot.

### Directions ⟶

**Take Interstate 95 north from Philadelphia to Exit 37 for PA 132–Street Road. Turn left onto Street Road and follow it west 6 miles to Bustleton Pike. Turn right on Bustleton Pike and get into the left lane. At the second traffic light, get into the left-turn lane (look for the Buck Hotel in front of you) and go left to continue on Bustleton Pike. Follow Bustleton Pike another 2 miles to the next traffic light at Bristol Road. Continue straight, now on Churchville Lane. Follow Churchville Lane 1 mile, just past a reservoir, to the nature-center parking lot, on your left.**
***501 Churchville Lane, Churchville, PA 18966.***

### KEY AT-A-GLANCE INFORMATION

**LENGTH:** 1.3 miles
**CONFIGURATION:** 2 loops
**DIFFICULTY:** Easy
**SCENERY:** Small woods, lake, protected habitats
**EXPOSURE:** Mostly shaded
**TRAIL TRAFFIC:** Light
**TRAIL SURFACE:** Dirt, wooden planks
**HIKING TIME:** 45 minutes
**DRIVING DISTANCE FROM CENTER CITY:** 23 miles
**ACCESS:** Trails open daily, dawn–dusk, year-round; visitor center open Tuesday–Sunday, 10 a.m.–5 p.m.; free admission
**MAPS:** USGS Langhorne; trail map at Web site (see below)
**WHEELCHAIR TRAVERSABLE:** Yes (with some maneuvering)
**FACILITIES:** Restrooms in visitor center
**SPECIAL COMMENTS:** Exhibits in the visitor center feature local ecology. More information: (215) 357-4005; www.churchvillenaturecenter.org.

### GPS Trailhead Coordinates

UTM Zone (WGS84) 18T
Easting 0500636
Northing 4448286
Latitude N 40° 11' 12.64"
Longitude W 74° 59' 33.36"

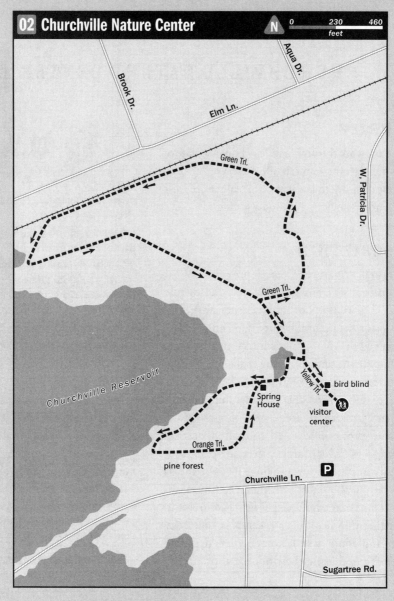

**02 Churchville Nature Center**

N

0   230   460
feet

Brook Dr.

Aqua Dr.

Elm Ln.

W. Patricia Dr.

Green Trl.

Green Trl.

Churchville Reservoir

Yellow Trl.

bird blind

Spring House

visitor center

Orange Trl.

pine forest

Churchville Ln.

P

Sugartree Rd.

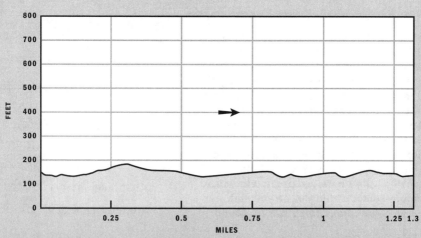

800

700

600

500

400

300

200

100

0

FEET

0.25   0.5   0.75   1   1.25  1.3

MILES

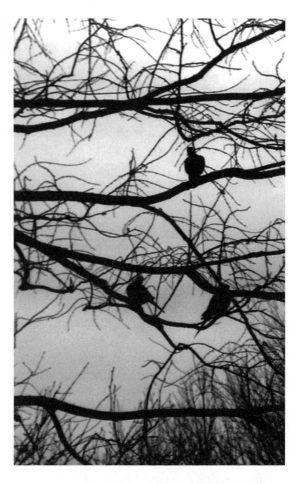

Native birds perching along the
Green Trail

When you arrive at the center's parking lot, pause to take a long look at the exquisite painted totem pole that welcomes visitors to the park. Native American totem poles once told stories or conveyed meanings, and the layers of this pole seem to express a holistic representation of the layers of nature—from the fish in the sea all the way up to the spirit world—all intertwined and eternally connected.

Continue your connection to nature with a quick stop at the visitor center for a map and a collection of brochures. You can double back to the visitor center toward the end of this hike to browse the educational dioramas and stop at the Laura Yeager Dragonfly Niche Gift Shop.

The Yellow Trail forks just behind the center, to its right. Stay to your left. Near this fork, visit the bird blind that overlooks a protected field habitat northwest of the nature center. From the blind, many birds native to the area have been spotted, including northern cardinals, ruby-throated hummingbirds, and occasionally a European goldfinch, most probably an escaped captive.

After you leave the blind, continue on the trail until you reach the wooden-plank walkways. On your right, you will pass an entrance to the Brown Trail and a Lenape Village, a re-creation of a Native American village from before European settlers arrived. You can see this village in detail after the hike, but for now, continue straight on the Green Trail, passing the Yellow Trail on your left. At a fork where the Green Trail splits to begin a broad loop, stay right. Continue on the Green Trail about 0.5 miles. Near a junction with the Red Trail stands a grove of rather old beech trees. A bit farther along the Green Trail stand sour gum trees, also called tupelos. These are easy to spot in fall, because their foliage turns fire-engine red.

Soon you approach an overlook with a view of Churchville Reservoir. This reservoir supplies much of the local water, so no fishing or swimming is allowed. At the overlook, break out the binoculars and enjoy the hawks swooping and ascending in front of tall pines. Continue east on the Green Trail, through the woods and eventually closing the loop. Now retrace your route to the junction with the Yellow Trail, where you turn right.

Springhouses, one just around the corner, are an interesting feature of the Greater Philadelphia area. In the 18th and 19th centuries, some of the local settlers were lucky to discover natural springs bubbling up from the ground. The water from these deep springs is always cold, even in mid-August. A springhouse traps some of the cold spring water in a pool, in effect creating a natural refrigerator. Because the temperature of the water and the surrounding walls was always in the mid-to-low 50s, settlers could cool their ale and store perishables for a long period of time. (You can visit another springhouse, at Tyler State Park, by following the hike described on page 119.)

Join the Orange Trail, a loop, by going straight at the next junction. On the first part of the loop, the reservoir is on you right. The trail then curves almost 180 degrees left and traverses a small planting of red pines and white pines. Soon rejoin the Yellow Trail, turn right, and retrace your route to the nature center by turning right again at the next junction.

Once you're back at the center, you may want to stroll through the field habitat to its northwest. Here you'll find some small artificial ponds inhabited by turtles and frogs. In the spring and summer, various butterfly species make this small field their temporary home.

On your way out of the Churchville Nature Center, don't forget to read about its green building expansion. This ambitious new facility will utilize new renewable-energy sources (such as geothermal and solar) to help minimize the impact of new construction on the environment. Smart, eco-friendly development can help offset the impact of urban sprawl and create a respect for the environment once embraced by the Native Americans of this area, who conveyed their respect of nature creatively through the tales of the totem.

## NEARBY ACTIVITIES

THE CHURCHVILLE INN
*(Restaurant)*
Bustleton Pike at Bristol Road,
Southampton
(215) 357-3967

RITA'S ITALIAN ICE
*(Snack spot; great frozen custard, too)*
722 Second Street Pike, Richboro
(215) 355-9676

# CLARK NATURE CENTER:
## Wilderness Trail

**03**

## IN BRIEF

Rich in nature and easily accessible from Inter-state 95, this brief hike makes a quiet stopping spot for a trip eastward from Philadelphia and points west.

## DESCRIPTION

This 50.6-acre park was once named Mount Pleasant, and for good reason. You almost expect to see the Cottingley fairies buzzing around its fields of bracken, green meadows, and towering trees. The park is cool in summer and effervescent in spring; it holds a special stillness in the winter and an intense embrace of color during fall. A well-kept secret in this part of Bucks County, the land of the Clark Nature Center was sold to Newtown Town-ship in 1997 and was preserved in perpetuity as open space. An unassuming blue sign marks the park's driveway off Durham Road, but if you blink, you'll surely miss it. You won't find any maps of this park or elaborate discussions regarding its hidden nooks and brooks on the Internet.

A private residence and an old farmhouse border the driveway, but a small parking lot awaits around the bend for visitors, which are few and far between despite the overwhelming

### KEY AT-A-GLANCE INFORMATION

**LENGTH:** 0.9 miles

**CONFIGURATION:** Balloon

**DIFFICULTY:** Beginner

**SCENERY:** Grassy fields, wooded brush, seasonal streams, wildflowers, historic buildings

**EXPOSURE:** Full sun–full shade

**TRAIL TRAFFIC:** Light

**TRAIL SURFACE:** Grass and dirt

**HIKING TIME:** 1 hour or less

**DRIVING DISTANCE FROM CENTER CITY:** 40 miles

**ACCESS:** Daily, dawn–dusk, year-round; free admission

**MAPS:** USGS Langhorne

**WHEELCHAIR TRAVERSABLE:** No

**FACILITIES:** No restrooms

**SPECIAL COMMENTS:** A short hike in a small park, but one that is rich with nature. More information: (215) 968-2800, x239.

## Directions ⟶

From Interstate 95 northbound from Philadel-phia, take Exit 49 and follow PA 332 toward Newtown/Yardley. Bear left off the exit ramp onto PA 413–Newtown Bypass. After about 4 miles, keep right to stay on PA 413 (near the entrance to Tyler Park). Go a few blocks, then keep left at a stop light to stay on PA 413–Durham Road. Go another 1 mile to the Clark Nature Center entrance driveway, on the left. *Durham Road (PA 413), Newtown, PA 18940.*

### GPS Trailhead Coordinates

UTM Zone (WGS84)  18T
Easting  0504008
Northing  4455097
Latitude  N 40° 14' 46.72"
Longitude  W 74° 57' 10.33"

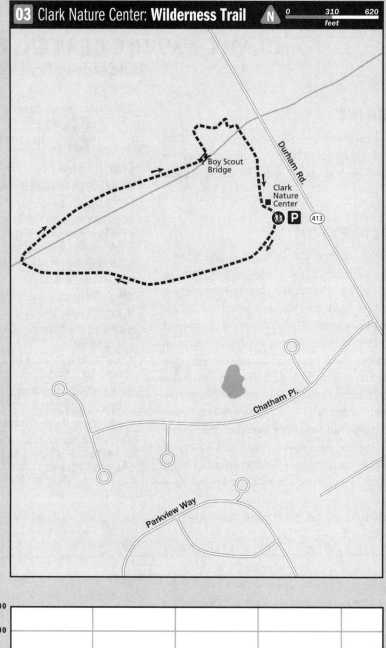

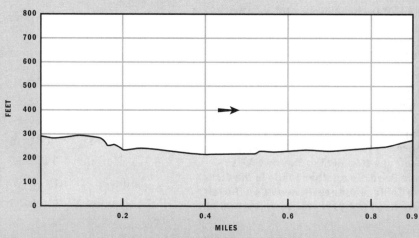

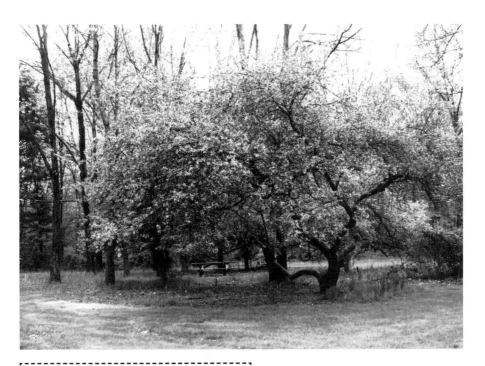

Flowering tree in spring at the Clark Nature Center

development that this area has seen over the past few decades. To the side of the house, the original 19th-century stone garage-barn stands like a giant white ghost telling stories of another time. Toward the back of the farmhouse, picnic benches provide the perfect place to break for a bagged lunch after a long morning of hard work in the office. A rich kelly-green field with a carpetlike quality welcomes you to the Wilderness Trail, which can be accessed from two different trailheads. Stay to the left toward the outermost part of the trail. The trail is clean and well maintained, and the park's close proximity to I-95 makes it an ideal stop for a breather when traveling to New Jersey and points east.

The best time to come is in July, when the sweet wild raspberries, in full ripeness, stand waiting for you to pluck them off the vines. As you stroll the dirt trail, watch the chipmunks dart in and out of the hollows of fallen trees. An occasional rabbit may also stop in stillness before scampering off under the brush. On the left side of the trail, a small seasonal stream weaves in and out of a green gully, where red-winged blackbirds stop to bathe.

As you circle the main trail, several side paths ascend toward the middle of the park. At any point you can follow one of these paths to a unique spot in the middle of the woods, where log benches lie in churchlike formation for visitors to stop and pray or just meditate in complete peace, where no traffic horns or screaming children threaten to cloud their rejuvenation. The breeze softens your demeanor as the canopy of tall elms and oaks sway ever so slightly in this outdoor cathedral.

Also in the middle of the park, a bird blind with openings at various heights allows hikers to stop and admire the many goldfinches, blue jays, and northern cardinals that spatter this wilderness with color. Many visitors have seen leaping white-tailed deer in these woods, and some have been lucky enough to spot wild turkeys.

After heavy rains, the flowing stream beside the far leg of the Wilderness Trail rids your head of the noise pollution of television, ringing phones, and rattling business meetings. As you round a bend, a wooden bridge that crosses the stream brings you into a less manicured area of the park. Be wary of poison ivy as you curve right and cross over the rocks on the thin side of the stream to pick up the trail on the other side.

This leg of the trail showcases blooming flowers in springtime and ample opportunities for photographs. In fact, this small park provides a wealth of material for both amateur and professional photographers. Wild rhododendrons provide pink pastels, while white lilacs fill the air with perfume. Near the end, you can loop around the trail and cross the Boy Scout bridge if it's not too overgrown. Near trail's end, an old structure on the right, probably the chimney from some summer kitchen, still stands erect, stacked with well-cut stones. And the ghostly old farmhouse peeks forth to wave you back to the start of the trail.

## NEARBY ACTIVITIES

JULES THIN CRUST PIZZA
300 Sycamore Street, Newtown
(215) 579-0111
www.julesthincrust.com

ROSEBANK WINERY
258 Durham Road, Newtown
(215) 860-5899
www.rosebankwinery.com

THE SUMMER KITCHEN
Route 232 at Penns Park Road,
Wrightstown
(215) 598-9210
www.thesummerkitchen.net

TYLER STATE PARK
101 Swamp Road, Newtown
(215) 968-2021
dcnr.state.pa.us/stateparks/
parks/tyler.aspx

WRIGHTSTOWN FARMERS' MARKET
(Fresh and organic meat and produce;
natural soaps and sprays; music and
much more)
2203 Second Street Pike, adjacent to
the Wrightstown municipal offices, at
Chippewa Farm; held every Saturday
from May 23 to November 21, 9 a.m.
to 1 p.m.
(215) 860-7081
www.buckscountyfoodshedalliance.org

# CORE CREEK PARK 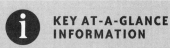 04

## IN BRIEF

Though this hike stays mostly on paved trails, Core Creek Park offers wooded retreats and paths that can be easily explored using Lake Luxembourg as a landmark. This park is great for family gatherings, as it offers exceptional facilities and recreation for all.

## DESCRIPTION

Core Creek Park is a perfect leisure spot for the entire family. The hiker who wants to explore trails can do so, whereas less adventurous family members can relax in comfort under the shelter of one of the park's many pavilions, with restrooms nearby. Benches are scattered throughout the park, offering walkers respite as needed.

Activities and facilities within the park—hiking, bicycling, tennis, picnicking, playgrounds, and ball fields—also make it well suited for company picnics and play-group gatherings. In May, Lake Luxembourg buzzes with boats carrying anglers reaping the benefits of the glistening waters. The lake is stocked with trout annually, and those wielding hook or fly can also expect to catch bass,

### KEY AT-A-GLANCE INFORMATION

**LENGTH:** 2.8 miles

**CONFIGURATION:** Figure-8

**DIFFICULTY:** Beginner

**SCENERY:** Glistening lake and forest with big glimpse of civilization

**EXPOSURE:** Full sun–full shade

**TRAIL TRAFFIC:** Moderate

**TRAIL SURFACE:** Mostly paved

**HIKING TIME:** 1 hour or less

**DRIVING DISTANCE FROM CENTER CITY:** 40 minutes

**ACCESS:** Daily, dawn–dusk, year-round; free admission

**MAPS:** USGS Langhorne

**WHEELCHAIR TRAVERSABLE:** Most of the trails are paved or smooth enough for wheelchairs.

**FACILITIES:** Several restrooms throughout park

**SPECIAL COMMENTS:** Paved trails and wooded paths with plenty of facilities; great picnic spot for large parties and families. More information: (215) 757-0571; www.buckscounty.org/government/ departments/ParksandRec/Parks/ CoreCreek.aspx.

## Directions

From Interstate 95 northbound/southbound from central Philadelphia, take Exit 44 for PA 413 toward Levittown/Penndel. Keep right at fork, follow signs for Levittown, and merge onto PA 413; after 1 mile, turn left at Woodbourne Road. Go 2.9 miles and turn left at Ellis Road. Go 0.4 miles and turn left at Fulling Mill Road, and then take a left at Fulling Mill Rd; go 0.2 miles and turn left at Tollgate Road. Park in the last lot on the left, directly in front of the lake near the boat-rental shack.
*901 Bridgetown Pike, Langhorne, PA 19047.*

## GPS Trailhead Coordinates

UTM Zone (WGS84) 18T

Easting 0507065

Northing 4449940

Latitude N 40° 12' 6.1"

Longitude W 74° 55' 1.3"

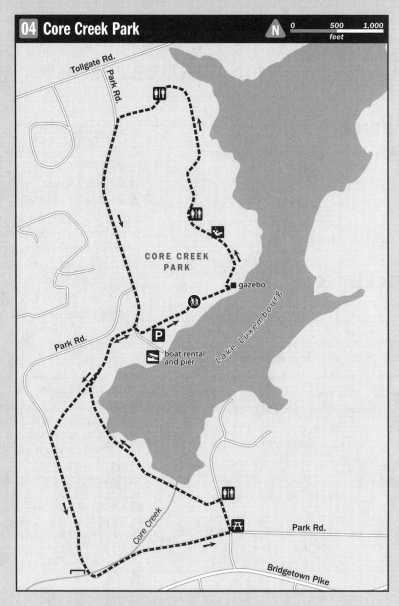

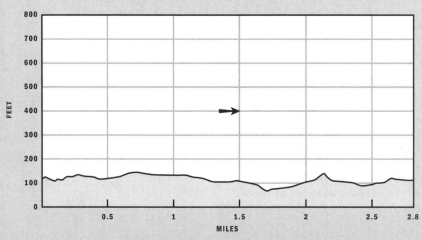

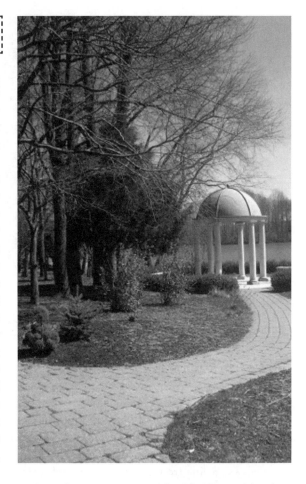

A classical-style gazebo looks out on Lake Luxembourg.

walleye, catfish, bluegill, carp, and other native species. Powerboats are limited to those with electric motors, which keeps the park relatively serene.

Take a canoe or an aqua-cycle to a marshy inlet and spot blue herons as they seek privacy amongst the cattails. Host a family cookout, but don't forget to bring your own charcoal. Teach the kids how to ride their bikes on one of the park's many paved trails. Bring a pair of binoculars and enjoy a variety of resident and migratory birds. But even if you're just looking for a new hike, Core Creek offers a variety of trails, both paved and not.

Start from the commemorative arbor entranceway, beside the parking lot. The arbor is dedicated to Bucks County crime victims and their families. In 1998, the Network of Victim Assistance (NOVA) came together with victims, Bucks County commissioners, Bucks County Park & Recreation officials, and police chiefs to designate a five-acre space in Core Creek Park for the memorial. Since 1998, 30 trees and three benches have been placed in memory or in honor of loved ones lost to or affected by violence. In partnership with Mothers Against Drunk Driving of Bucks County, an entranceway was added to this arbor in the fall of 2004.

As you continue along the arbor path, you will see a classical-style gazebo with six roman columns and a dome rooftop. Enjoy the view from its stone bench and look out toward the meditative waters. Stay as long as you like, then continue along the path and around the bend, where there is a view of the children's playground, to the left. Pause to refresh at a nearby water fountain. Soon afterward, the path splits. If you want a shorter hike, take the trail to the left; for a longer walk, stay right.

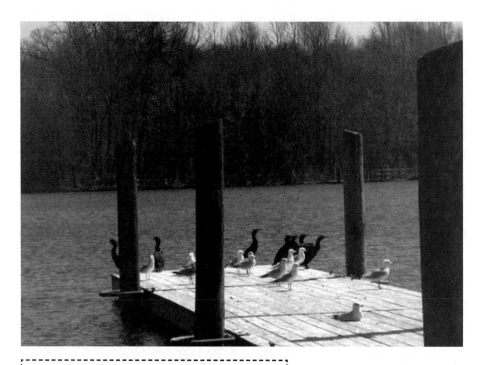

The pier by the boat rental attracts all kinds of spectators.

Watch for squirrels as they scamper from tree to tree, or spot an occasional northern cardinal as it brightens up the brush. Sparrows, starlings, and robins are also common year-round residents. For a closer look at the birds, amble along one of the many dirt paths that lead toward the lake. In clearings, you may see birds swooping from oak to maple, and from pine to birch.

Once you have had your birding moment and have circled the next bend, a parking lot ahead provides access to the road from which you entered the park. Wheelchair travelers can easily maneuver this roadway because the traffic is reasonably light, especially on the weekdays, and the speed limit is low. Once you arrive at the road, you will be near the rear of St. Mary's Medical Center on your right. Hospital workers and visitors may emerge, looking for a break from long shifts of caring for others, remembering that the best caretakers are those who take care of themselves.

An area to your left, surrounded by a fence and marked with Pennsylvania Department of Environmental Protection (DEP) signs, is called a pocket wetland. Funding for the wetland, which is intended to reduce pollution from nitrogen, phosphorous, and other nutrients, was awarded to the Bucks County Conservation District through the DEP and the U.S. Environmental Protection Agency. Princeton Hydro, a water and wetland resources-management firm, provides consulting services for the project. According to Dr. Fred Lubnow of Princeton Hydro, this is one of many such projects implemented in the park during the last ten years.

"Once the wetland is established," Lubnow said, "the plants aid in slowing storm water flow and allowing solids to drop out as well as assimilate nutrients that otherwise enter the lake and stimulate algal growth. Once complete, it will aid in improving the water quality of Lake Luxembourg."

Directly ahead is the lake's boat-rental shack and pier, indicating that you are close to your parking lot. You may stop your hike here or set off on another loop that will add an extra mile. (If you are disabled, please note that the last quarter mile of this hike is not paved.) The field adjacent to the parking lot catches the wind coming off the lake, thus making it a popular spot for kite flyers. Turn right at a junction, onto a path that angles toward the bath facilities and a pavilion, bringing you a view of the western part of the lake.

This trail leads to another park road that hugs the back of a nearby housing development and eventually leads to the opposite side of the lake. Before you turn the bend on the left, stop and listen to the trickling waters of the creek that flow beneath the road and off into the neighboring woodlands.

Continue along the road until you reach the Duchess Lane picnic area. This well-equipped park-within-a-park offers a view across the lake to the boat-rental shack where you began this walk. This mesmerizing lake view may distract you from noticing the majestic white birch tree that reaches out from the left. Adventurous hikers can explore dirt paths to the right that cut through the woods and provide other fine views. After you've explored this area, continue through the picnic area and pick up a path on your left that hugs the lake's southern end.

Unfortunately, your path stops at a grassy area, making a full figure-eight inaccessible to wheelchairs. This area does, however, provide a different vantage point for lake viewing. From here, a northern trek leads you back to the paved trail on the side of the lake and, ultimately, to the parking lot where you started. Here you can get a last look at the pier and the gulls that gather and bask, hoping for stray French fries to highlight their day.

## NEARBY ACTIVITIES

HISTORIC NEWTOWN
*(Restaurants, boutiques,
quaint Victorian architecture)*
**www.newtownhistoric.org**

THE BRICK HOTEL *(Restaurant)*
1 East Washington Avenue, Newtown
(215) 860-8313
**www.brickhotel.com**

ROUGET *(French cuisine)*
2 Swamp Road, Newtown
(215) 860-4480

TEMPERANCE HOUSE INN &
RESTAURANT AND TAVERN
5 South State Street, Newtown
(215) 860-9975
**www.temperancehouse.com**

SESAME PLACE
*(Children's theme park;
can be especially busy on weekends)*
100 Sesame Road, Langhorne
(215) 752-7070
**www.sesameplace.com**

## 05 DARK HOLLOW:
### Neshaminy Creek Palisades to Fields and Forests

**KEY AT-A-GLANCE INFORMATION**

**LENGTH: 3.9 miles**

**CONFIGURATION: Balloon**

**DIFFICULTY: Medium–hard**

**SCENERY: Tree-lined hills, cliffs, vistas of rolling hills and farmland**

**EXPOSURE: Full sun in fields, shade near cliffs**

**TRAIL TRAFFIC: Light**

**TRAIL SURFACE: Dirt, grass**

**HIKING TIME: 1.5 hours**

**DRIVING DISTANCE FROM CENTER CITY: 30 miles**

**ACCESS: Daily, dawn–dusk, year-round; free admission**

**MAPS: USGS Buckingham**

**WHEELCHAIR TRAVERSABLE: No**

**FACILITIES: No restrooms**

**SPECIAL COMMENTS: Be prepared for a steep scramble up a cliff. More information: (215) 757-0571.**

## IN BRIEF

Although close to a commercial area, this hidden area presents opportunities for a hike with views of cliffs, agricultural fields, and perhaps even soaring hawks.

## DESCRIPTION

The dark secret of Dark Hollow remains its location. Most people would never know that this sanctuary, with its diverse terrain, even exists behind the guise of a suburban township and its commercial surroundings. It's a location that is so close to perfect seclusion and yet so far. Some people drive for miles to find a piece of uninterrupted nature, whereas others enjoy the best of both worlds, grabbing groceries one minute, then enjoying the calming white noise of a rushing creek and chirping birds the next. Dark Hollow provides one of those dual escapes.

As you forge forward toward the trailhead, it can puddle in some areas, especially

------------------------------------------------

### *Directions*

**Merge onto Interstate 95 north via the ramp on the left toward Trenton–Northeast Philadelphia. Take Exit 37 for PA 132–Street Road. Turn left at Street Road; follow it 12 miles. Then turn right at PA 263–York Road. Continue on York Road 3.7 miles into Warwick Central. You will see banks and gas stations, but look for the Golden Arches on the right: McDonald's is the secret doorway into this hidden sanctuary. Take a right before the McDonald's and follow the entryway to the left, behind the restaurant. Continue along Mill Road, for about 1 mile past the town houses, until you see the iron Mill Road Bridge. Just before the bridge, take a left into a parking lot and walk across the street to the trailhead.** *Bridge Valley Road, Warwick, PA 18929.*

---

GPS Trailhead
Coordinates
UTM Zone (WGS84) 18T
Easting    0493600
Northing   4457400
Latitude   N 40° 16' 9.3"
Longitude  W 75° 4' 30.6"

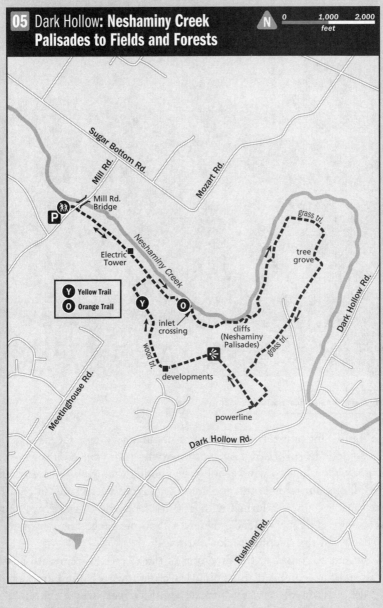

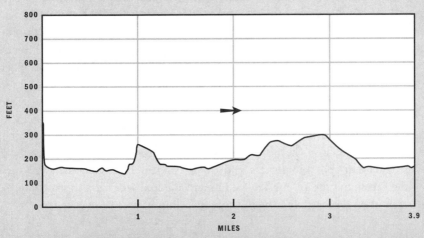

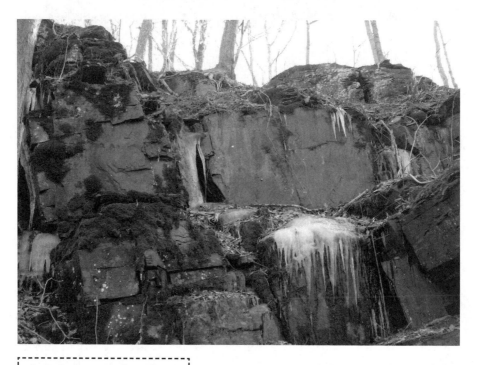

The Neshaminy Palisades in winter

after a significant rainstorm, making it a popular feeding spot for small garter snakes, so don't be surprised if one of those twigs near your boot starts to hiss at you slightly. Continue to wind around the puddles (being extra careful that you do not fall on your fanny) until you come to one of the last signs of civilization: a rusted electric tower adorned with graffiti. Don't be alarmed by the nearby gunshots—it isn't gang violence, merely a shooting range far east of the park. (They don't call this "Pennsyltucky" for nothin'.)

Continue to follow in the direction of the electric towers until just before the trail starts to climb. At this point, leave the towers behind and take a left-hand turn, walking directly toward Neshaminy Creek, where the shade of the trees and air off the water provide a waft of freshness. This is the start of the Orange Trail. In the creek, catfish, carp, sunfish, bass, trout, and crayfish swim freely until some clever angler makes them a meal. An occasional mallard floats by, and fortunate hikers will spot a heron or two. Follow the dirt trail that hugs the creek, then weaves left and right toward a glistening inlet.

After heavy rains, the water in this inlet can prove inconvenient and even a little threatening. If the inlet waters look entirely too high to cross along the rocks, double back to the electric towers and look for the Yellow Trail, which leads to the fields above the nearby palisades. This route offers a woodsy path where hikers can spot kingfishers and other resident bird species in the surrounding brush, but the Yellow Trail skims a residential area for a short distance, which can often detract from the illusion of seclusion.

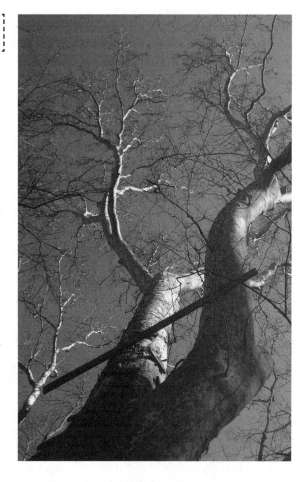

A majestic sycamore towers over a Neshaminy Creek inlet.

Crossing the water inlet along the Orange Trail will provide a premium view, offering tall pines, mature maples, and majestic sycamore trees, not to mention the towering Neshaminy Palisades. Scaling the palisades is not for the faint of heart, however, and the climb should be taken slowly— loose slate and branches may masquerade as safety handles but, once grasped, can easily come loose, taking you with them. If hiking with others, make sure to spread out so as not to injure anyone with a dislodged rock. There is no route to follow but up. Stop halfway up to explore the ferns, moss, and, seasonally, wood asters that adorn the rocky ledges. Your patient climbing pays generously at the top: a wide-open field, often planted with corn or soy, provides an expansive vista, often with hawks and osprey hovering overhead.

The Orange Trail circles the field, and the wind blows cold during the winter months. The field makes a popular feeding stop for a variety of birds and wildlife. The animal activity makes the open exposure to either sun or wind more tolerable. Look on your right for a grass trail, which you will turn onto and stay on through the whole field walk. Farther along the grass trail, when turning right again, you pass an enormous stump with a painted arrow—which points in the direction from which you just came. Ignore this instruction and continue through the field toward a grove of extremely tall pine trees.

At the pines, swing left and then look for the trail's continuation on the right, which leads you through more agricultural fields, across a driveway, and then more fields. Continue on the grass trail until it ends at a **T**-junction, then turn left and ascend a sloping field—with the knowledge that you are more than halfway through this diverse hike.

With open fields on your left, veer right toward a line of electric towers. When you reach the towers, turn right back toward the trailhead. In fact, at any point should you get lost along this hike, simply look to the towers to guide you.

Continue through the fields with the towers in front of you until you reach the top of a hill with yet another vista. At this point, head for an opening in the woods to your left. When you reach the woods, turn left on a dirt trail that is sometimes shared by equestrians and an occasional red fox.

Follow the trail to a corner, where for a brief moment you will edge close to a nearby development. But fear not, because a right-hand turn brings you back into the woods onto the Yellow Trail. This path gives you another opportunity to spot white-tailed deer prancing through the woods and to walk through a cathedral of color in the fall. Continue on the Yellow Trail, crossing a small stream via stones or fallen trees. Stay straight about 100 feet to where you can see the electric towers again. Walk toward the towers, which will bring you to the initial path that leads back to the parking lot and a last glimpse of the Mill Road Bridge, surrounded by trees and wildflowers, before heading back toward the fast-paced commercial world just down the road.

## NEARBY ACTIVITIES

BARLEY SHEAF FARM ESTATE & SPA
*(Inn and spa)*
5281 Old York Road, Holicong
(215) 794-5104
**www.barleysheaf.com**

JUSTEAT BY BROWNGOLD (RESTAURANT)
OR JUSTFOOD (TAKEOUT)
Buckingham Green Shopping Center,
Buckingham
4950 York Road (JustEat)
4920 York Road (JustFood)
(215) 794-1818 (JustEat)
(215) 794-3663 (JustFood)
**www.justeatbybrowngold.com**
**www.justfoodcatering.com**

NONE SUCH FARM MARKET
4493 York Road, Buckingham
Market: (215) 794-5201
Pick Your Own: (215) 794-5200
**www.nonesuchfarms.com**

RITA'S ITALIAN ICE
*(Snack spot; great frozen custard, too)*
790 Edison Furlong Road, Furlong
(215) 794-8388

RUSHLAND RIDGE VINEYARD & WINERY
2665 Rushland Road, Rushland
(215) 598-0251
**www.rushlandridge.com**

# DARK HOLLOW: Eight Arch Bridge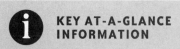

## IN BRIEF

This out-and-back hike to Eight Arch Bridge—at 218 feet the longest stone-arch bridge in Bucks County—was once a secret known only to Warwick-area residents. Not only is this bridge one of the last of its kind in Pennsylvania, but important Revolutionary War history was made nearby.

## DESCRIPTION

If you've hiked in Washington Crossing State Park or visited Princeton Battlefield, this short hike to Eight Arch Bridge in Warwick Township visits yet another Revolutionary War site. A bridge that predates the current Eight Arch Bridge, and which stood on the same spot, provided Generals Washington and Lafayette access to their nearby encampment in Hartsville and later to Brandywine and Germantown. Approximately 11,000 Revolutionary War soldiers passed over this very spot, some camping on the banks of Neshaminy Creek.

The Eight Arch Bridge stood under Old York Road until the early 1970s, when the road was rerouted. The road dates from 1710, when it was the primary thoroughfare between Philadelphia and New York. It's seen everything from market wagons and stagecoaches to Hummers and Smart Cars.

### KEY AT-A-GLANCE INFORMATION

**LENGTH:** 1 mile

**CONFIGURATION:** Out-and-back

**DIFFICULTY:** Moderate

**SCENERY:** Neshaminy Creek, vine-rich woodland, bridge

**EXPOSURE:** Mostly shade

**TRAIL TRAFFIC:** Light

**TRAIL SURFACE:** Dirt; some areas are a little overgrown.

**HIKING TIME:** About 1 hour

**DRIVING DISTANCE FROM CENTER CITY:** 30 miles

**ACCESS:** Daily, dawn–dusk, year-round; free admission

**MAPS:** USGS Buckingham

**WHEELCHAIR TRAVERSABLE:** No

**FACILITIES:** No restrooms

**SPECIAL COMMENTS:** There are deep gullies and steep cliffs along the trail, so watch your footing. More information: (215) 757-0571.

*Directions*

See Hike 5 (page 34)—you will drive to the same parking area, but the hike goes in a different direction. *Bridge Valley Road, Warwick, PA 18929.*

GPS Trailhead
Coordinates
UTM Zone (WGS84) 18T
Easting 0493620
Northing 4457610
Latitude N 40° 16' 8.8"
Longitude W 75° 4' 29.9"

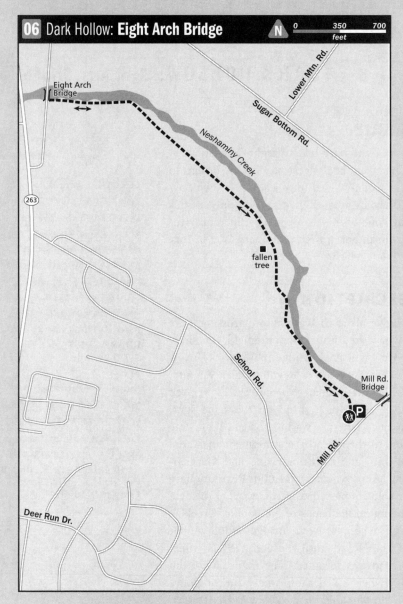

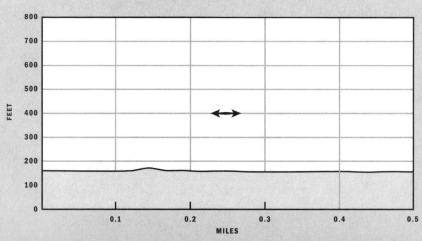

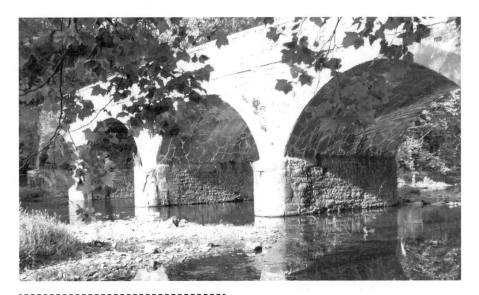

Eight Arch Bridge over the Neshaminy Creek

Visitors to Philadelphia often enjoy touring the nearby scenic covered bridges, but few realize that the stone-arch bridges in this area predate the covered ones. The Warwick Eight Arch Bridge was built in 1804 (the one used by Washington was built in 1710). The 1804 bridge resembles ancient European construction in its use of the Roman arch. Building it involved a monumental engineering and construction effort from many Warwick-area citizens.

The bridge took 290 days to build and cost $15,561.40. This budget included room and board and 70 gallons of whiskey for the workers. The structure has withstood several severe floods, including the Great Flood of 1865, which ruined all the bridges to its south. Eight Arch Bridge is included in the Bucks County Conservancy's Register of Historic Places.

Bridge and photography buffs alike will find this scenic hike worthwhile. The bridge makes an interesting picture, as its arches leap from Neshaminy Creek and combine with the water's reflection to create perfect ovals. And because the iron Mill Road Bridge is to the south, the hike is sandwiched between two scenic bridges.

The trailhead is on the northern corner of the Mill Road Bridge parking lot. Walk northward on the trail, away from the Mill Road Bridge. The trail, which may not be well maintained during summer and early fall, goes through a stretch of marsh grass. Visit during late spring and summer to see Neshaminy bluebells dotting the grasslands, along with sprigs of goldenrod and shoots of butterfly flowers, which add a symphony of color. Snapdragons and Queen Anne's lace also sway in the summer breeze, and if you look closely you may find vines with plump blackberries ready for picking.

Approximately 50 yards beyond an electrical tower on your left, the trail starts to become more distinct and enters a shady, vine-strewn woodland, with rare ferns sprouting under mature oaks, tulips, beeches, and hickories. Maples, ashes, walnuts, and box elders also line Neshaminy Creek, and the trail you walk on is sometimes used by muskrats, skunks, and opossums: look for their tracks. Watch out for deep drainage gullies that you will need to leap over, and don't stray too close to the creek—its steep bank could cause a fall and severe injury. Maneuver around or cross any downed trees carefully.

Evergreens here include white pines, red cedars, and old hemlock. Mallards swim in the creek below, looking for their share of crayfish and mussels. A disturbed heron may shoot over the creek to safety, while hawks and ospreys may hover overhead looking for lunch. Beavers sometimes swim in full view in the morning, and bucks often leap through the nearby woodlands, occasionally stopping for refreshment. The creek is stocked with trout in the spring, but anglers can also expect to catch catfish, carp, sunfish, and bass.

Continue northward until you start to see the Eight Arch Bridge's stone-and-mortar arches in the distance, where you will end the out part of this out-and-back. You can see six of the bridge's eight arches in clear view, with the other two disappearing into the hillside across the creek. Since this part of the hike is not steep, when the creek is low, you can tiptoe out to its pebbly bank to catch a better view.

After you've taken your photographs, you can head back the way you came, or you can walk across the top of the bridge and imagine Revolutionary War soldiers filling their canteens in the creek below after a long summer march from points in New York and New Jersey. Down the road from this bridge, at the Moland House, George Washington held a Council of War in which he mapped the crucial movements of the Continental army toward the fight for freedom. The 13-starred "Betsy Ross flag" was first unfurled at the Cross Roads, which is less than a few miles from this spot.

(A special thanks to Dave Mullen, president of the Warwick Township Historical Society, for providing documents on the bridge's historical significance; these were prepared by Christian Horn in January 1983.)

## NEARBY ACTIVITIES

CRAVEN HALL HISTORICAL SOCIETY
(Museum and 1840s restored manor house; former home of John Fitz, who built the first model of the steamboat)
House tours on the second Sunday of each month, noon to 3 p.m.
599 Newtown Road, Warminster
(215) 675-4698

LUIGI'S RISTORANTE ITALIANO
York Road (just south of Almshouse Road and north of Meyer Way),
Jamison
(215) 491-2001

MOLAND HOUSE
1641 Old York Road, Hartsville
Open second Sunday of every month
(215) 345-6439
**www.moland.org**

# DELAWARE CANAL: Pennsylvania Side 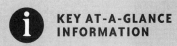 07

## IN BRIEF

This is a long but unique hike along the historic Delaware Canal on the Pennsylvania side of the Delaware River. What was once a path for mules pulling barges now offers beautiful vistas of the Delaware River and interesting buildings in New Hope, Pennsylvania.

## DESCRIPTION

This historical hike offers a glimpse into the region's economic past and a unique perspective about life on the canal more than a century ago. Just before the Centre Bridge, stairs lead down to the trail, which heads south (downstream) into historic New Hope. The trail is the towpath once used by mules pulling barges up and down the canal. Today most of this section of the channel is dry, but at one time it was a vital transportation link for consumer goods.

Inspired by the success of the Erie Canal in New York, builders completed the Delaware Canal in 1832. The hand-dug channel eventually ran between Bristol and Easton, and its primary cargo was coal.

---

### Directions ──────────→

**Take Interstate 95 north from Philadelphia 29.7 miles and enter New Jersey. Take Exit 1 and merge onto NJ 29. Continue 13.5 miles north on 29 (except when one-way streets force a three-block detour onto NJ 165 in Lambertville), then turn left in Stockton, New Jersey, onto Bridge Street and cross the bridge into Pennsylvania. You can park at Dilly's Corner ice-cream shop, on the right, just on the Pennsylvania side of the bridge. (Dilly's won't mind as long as you buy some ice cream.) After parking, walk toward the bridge and take the stairs down to the canal.**

### KEY AT-A-GLANCE INFORMATION

**LENGTH:** 7.16 miles

**CONFIGURATION:** Out-and-back

**DIFFICULTY:** Moderate

**SCENERY:** Canal, river views, downtown New Hope

**EXPOSURE:** Partial sun

**TRAIL TRAFFIC:** Medium

**TRAIL SURFACE:** Dirt

**HIKING TIME:** 2.5 hours

**DRIVING DISTANCE FROM CENTER CITY:** 45 miles

**ACCESS:** Year-round, daily, dawn–dusk; free admission

**MAPS:** USGS Stockton; maps along canal entrances

**WHEELCHAIR TRAVERSABLE:** No

**FACILITIES:** Restrooms at Dilly's

**SPECIAL COMMENTS:** The canal goes right through historic New Hope. For more information, visit dcnr.state.pa.us/stateparks/parks/delaware canal.aspx.

---

### GPS Trailhead Coordinates

UTM Zone (WGS84)  18T

Easting  0501660

Northing  4472140

Latitude  N 40° 24' 6.6"

Longitude  W 74° 58' 49.2"

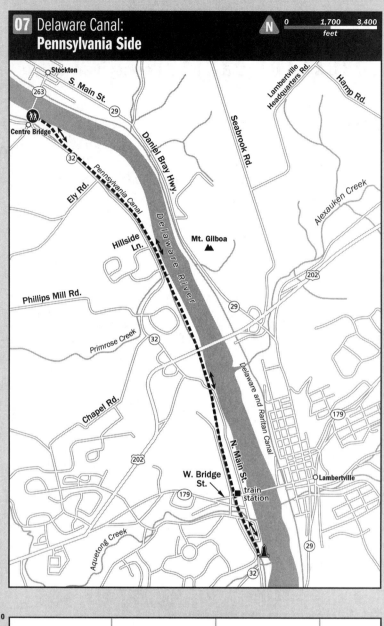

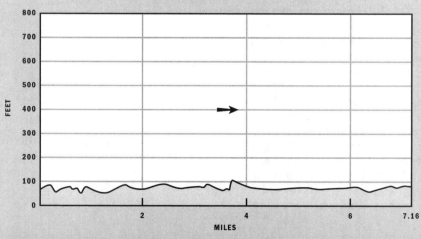

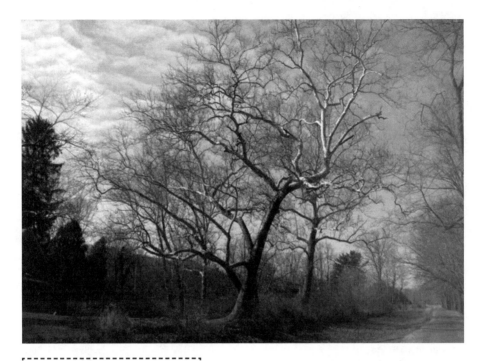

A variety of trees align the towpath.

On the left side of the towpath is the Delaware River. In the past two decades, the river has been dramatically cleaned up. In fact, the annual Shad Festival, across the river in Lambertville, New Jersey, celebrates the recovery of the shad's spring spawning run. The river is also known for periodic flooding. Still, many of the beautiful cottages along the river remain popular as year-round residences and seasonal homes.

At about the 2-mile mark, the US 202 overpass spans the river. Past the overpass, several small bridges cross the canal. Be careful; the bridges have barely more than six feet of clearance. Just before the 3-mile mark, you may see some old railcars and steam locomotives on the right. They belong to the New Hope & Ivyland Railroad, which offers rides on vintage equipment along the Buckingham Valley out of New Hope. The small train station is on the right at the 3-mile mark. You may see beautifully restored steam engines waiting to accept passengers, or hear the train whistle echoing in the distance.

Since its founding in 1962, this tourist railroad has also transported freight, for which it uses vintage diesel locomotives and freight cars. In the 1850s, the railroads began taking over freight transportation along the Delaware River, eventually making the canal obsolete.

Past the train station, the trail continues under the West Bridge Street bridge and into central New Hope. The town's shops and art galleries are so popular that it is hard to find a parking spot on Main Street on weekends. The restaurants overlooking the Delaware River are especially busy.

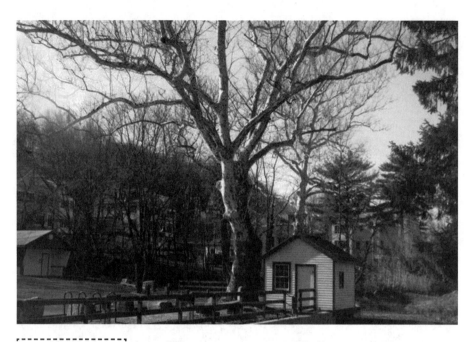

Locktender's House

The towpath continues into a shaded area of New Hope, where cottages and other buildings seem to hug the path. At around the 3.5-mile mark is the Locktender's House. Tending the locks was a full-time job, and entire families sometimes lived in tenders' houses. The tender also supplied mules to the canal's barge operators. Today, the Locktender's House is a museum that gives a good historical account of the area and of how the lock system worked. It also displays a detailed model of a canal barge. Past the Locktender's House, the trail leads down stairs to reach River Road. When you see the green dinosaur sculpture on the right, it is time to turn around and retrace your steps north to Centre Bridge.

## NEARBY ACTIVITIES

BOWMAN'S TOWER AND
WILDFLOWER PRESERVE
1635 River Road, New Hope
(215) 862-2924
**www.ushistory.org/washingtoncrossing/**
**visit/bowman.htm**

PEDDLER'S VILLAGE
*(Rustic-themed shopping and dining)*
81 Peddler's Village Road, Buckingham
(215) 794-1629
**www.peddlersvillage.com**

WASHINGTON CROSSING HISTORIC PARK
Box 103, Washington Crossing
(215) 493-4076
(215) 493-4820 (fax)
**www.ushistory.org/washingtoncrossing**

# FIVE MILE WOODS NATURE PRESERVE  08

## IN BRIEF

Although this hike is short, it offers a variety of plants and wildlife. It can be combined with a visit to the nearby Garden of Reflection 9-11 Memorial, which honors victims and heroes from Bucks County, from Pennsylvania, and from around the world who perished prematurely that day—may we never forget!

## DESCRIPTION

These 285 acres of preserved woods lie along the geological fall line between the Coastal Plain and Piedmont Plateau regions. Although Five Mile Woods Nature Preserve is small, the two different ecosystems supply a variety of naturally decorative plants, such as bloodroot, pink lady's slipper orchids, and honeysuckle, along with a variety of tree species. The fall line in the Philadelphia area has been highly developed, so the preserve constitutes a rare remaining landform with both sandy soil and rich forest.

A grassroots group of nature enthusiasts saved the woods by inspiring the residents of Lower Makefield to vote to preserve them forever. The township and the Friends of Five Mile Woods maintain and line the trails, prune, and repair; they also host guided

### KEY AT-A-GLANCE INFORMATION

**LENGTH:** 1.85 miles

**CONFIGURATION:** Loop

**DIFFICULTY:** Easy

**SCENERY:** Woods

**EXPOSURE:** Shade

**TRAIL TRAFFIC:** Light

**TRAIL SURFACE:** Gravel, dirt, boardwalks

**HIKING TIME:** 35 minutes

**DRIVING DISTANCE FROM CENTER CITY:** 27.4 miles

**ACCESS:** Daily, dawn–dusk, year-round; free admission

**MAPS:** USGS Trenton West; maps at kiosk or headquarters. See also www.lmt.org/parkrecfmwmap.htm.

**WHEELCHAIR TRAVERSABLE:** No

**FACILITIES:** Restrooms in nature center, when open; call before you visit.

**SPECIAL COMMENTS:** No pets, biking, hunting, or fishing. More information: (215) 493-6652; www.lmt.org/parkrecfmw.htm.

## Directions

Take Interstate 95 north from Philadelphia. After 23.7 miles, take Exit 46A to merge onto US 1 heading north toward Morrisville. After 0.7 miles, take the Oxford Valley exit. Turn left at the end of the ramp onto Oxford Valley Road. After 0.4 miles, take the first right onto Big Oak Road. The park entrance is on the right in 0.9 miles. The trail begins behind the kiosk, near the headquarters.
*1305 Big Oak Road, Yardley, PA 19067.*

### GPS Trailhead Coordinates

UTM Zone (WGS84)  18T

Easting  0512761

Northing  4450428

Latitude   N 40° 12' 14.93"

Longitude   W 74° 51' 0.18"

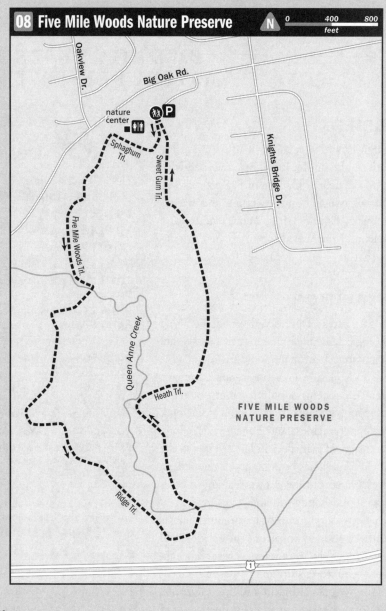

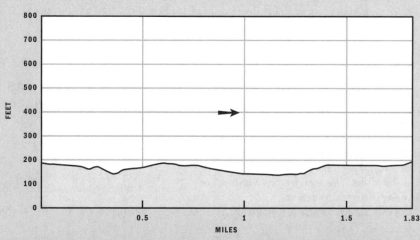

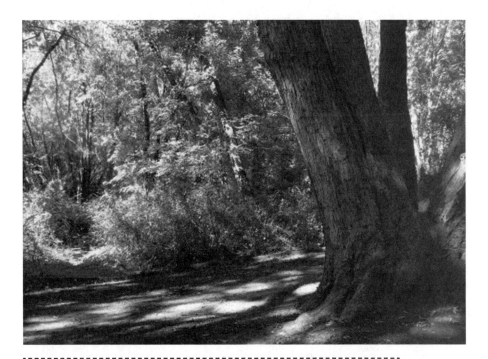

An unusually large sweet gum tree stands beside the preserve's outdoor classroom.

tours and special events. The Roving Nature Center, a mobile environmental-education program, conducts Nature Day Camps for preschool and grade-school children during the summer.

The trails are well marked and well maintained. A gravel walkway off the small parking lot brings you to the main trails. Take the Sphagnum Trail west over planks and boardwalks, and in about 0.1 mile you cross over a bog lined with sphagnum (peat moss), thus the trail name. This is a great place to listen for the loud peeping of the New Jersey chorus frog, which is critically imperiled in Pennsylvania, or to see the spotted salamander, most prominent in late winter or early spring. The preserve is also alive with gray squirrels and white-tailed deer. There is life under every rock.

Continue from boardwalk to boardwalk, following the yellow trail markers as the trail bends southward. The Sphagnum Trail intersects with the Five Mile Woods Trail, which, contrary to the name, does not extend 5 miles. Continue along the Five Mile Woods Trail, heading south, still following the yellow markers, and cross the Queen Anne Creek, which can be dry in summer. Follow the Five Mile Woods Trail to its end, past the intersections with the Evergreen and Ridge trails as it bends left and heads east. At the end of the Five Mile Trail, turn left onto the Creek Trail and head north, following the green trail markers. When the Creek Trail intersects the Heath Trail, turn right onto the Heath Trail, following the red trail markers northeast.

Turn right onto the Sweet Gum Trail and follow the blue markers. On this trail you can see the Five Mile Woods Nature Center's outdoor classroom. Not many classrooms are surrounded by a lush forest, and this small space boasts an unusually large sweet gum tree that spreads its branches over the benches like a wise old teacher delivering its lessons.

Sweet gums burst forth in red, orange, and yellow colors in the fall, and these trees will be part of the National 9/11 Memorial Plaza in New York City, not only for their fall colors but also because they are generally healthy and durable, symbolizing life and longevity.

Eighteen residents of Bucks County lost their lives during the 9/11 attacks; Victor Saracini, the pilot of United Airlines Flight 175, came from Yardley. There were nine victims from Lower Makefield Township. The nearby Garden of Reflection honors all the victims who lost their lives that day, the philosophy being that landscapes heal. So as you leave that sweet gum tree and follow the trail back toward the parking lot, may you cherish each day and each landscape, and may you never forget the heroes and victims of 9/11.

## NEARBY ACTIVITIES

9-11 MEMORIAL GARDEN OF REFLECTION
950 Woodside Road
Yardley
**www.9-11memorialgarden.org**

PENNSBURY MANOR
*(Re-created country home of William Penn)*
400 Pennsbury Memorial Road
Morrisville
(215) 946-0400
**www.pennsburymanor.org**

SHADY BROOK FARM
*(Pick-your-own, special events, farmers' market, deli)*
931 Stony Hill Road
Yardley
(215) 968-1670
**www.shadybrookfarm.com**

# GRAEME PARK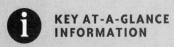

## IN BRIEF

This short nature trail features an interesting dichotomy between its historic, pastoral surroundings and the nearby mecca of stores, with an occasional loud boom of planes leaving Willow Grove Air Force Base. Include this walk as part of your trip to the area; it will prove especially interesting for history buffs.

## DESCRIPTION

A far cry from a strenuous trek, Graeme Park offers a peaceful and historic nature trail that can be completed in less than 20 minutes. But its brevity is not without beauty, because a great blue heron could be standing around the next corner to cast its massive shadow upon flowing creek waters. And those with a nose for history will enjoy the old homes in the park grounds, especially the Keith House, which is the only remaining residence of a colonial Pennsylvania governor, Sir William Keith.

The Keith residence and barn, which can be viewed as you drive deep into the park's entrance, mark the start of this short walk. William Keith was born in 1669 in Aberdeenshire, Scotland, into a family with strong Jacobite sympathies. The Jacobites supported Kings James II and VII (James Stuart), favoring monarchical succession. James VII favored

### KEY AT-A-GLANCE INFORMATION

**LENGTH:** 0.53 miles
**CONFIGURATION:** Loop
**DIFFICULTY:** Easy
**SCENERY:** Historic stone buildings, cornfields, natural wetlands, adjacent fields, and woods
**EXPOSURE:** Full sun–full shade
**TRAIL TRAFFIC:** Light on weekdays–moderate on weekends; heavy during special events
**TRAIL SURFACE:** Dirt
**HIKING TIME:** 15–20 minutes
**DRIVING DISTANCE FROM CENTER CITY:** 18.7 miles
**ACCESS:** Visitor center open Friday and Saturday, 10 a.m.–4 p.m.; Sunday, noon–4 p.m. Last tour starts at 3 p.m. Free to visit the grounds, fee charged for tour of Keith House
**MAPS:** USGS Ambler
**WHEELCHAIR TRAVERSABLE:** No
**FACILITIES:** Restrooms inside visitor center
**SPECIAL COMMENTS:** Very short walk that can be combined with other nearby activities (see Nearby Activities). More information: (215) 343-0965; www.ushistory.org/graeme.

*Directions*

From central Philadelphia, take PA 611 north. After 18.7 miles, take a left at County Line Road. The park is 0.5 miles on the left.
*859 County Line Road, Horsham, PA 19044.*

GPS Trailhead Coordinates

UTM Zone (WGS84) 18T
Easting 0486944
Northing 4451780
Latitude N 40° 12' 58.80"
Longitude W 75° 9' 12.49"

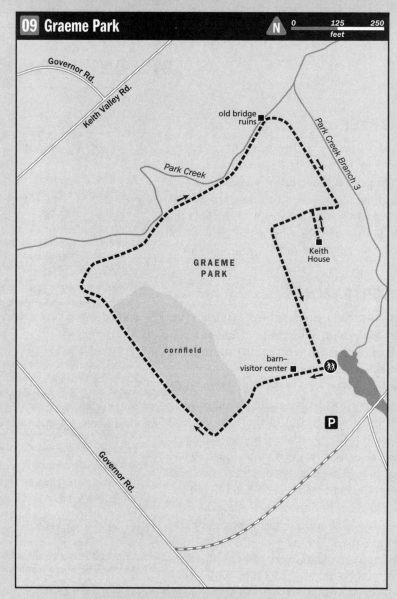

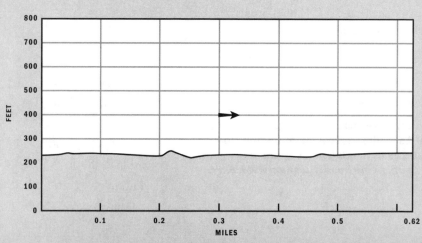

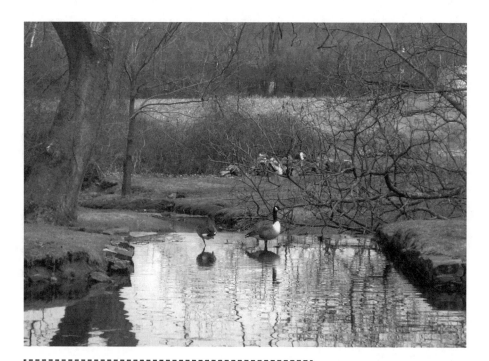

Canadian geese wade in the pond just outside the Keith House.

religious tolerance but was later replaced through a bloodless revolution by William of Orange and Mary II, James's eldest daughter. Despite Queen Anne's eventual succession to the throne, Keith lobbied for a government position and, in 1713, was appointed Surveyor-General for the Southern District of the Americas, which included Pennsylvania, Maryland, Virginia, the Carolinas, Jamaica, and the Bahamas.

Queen Anne died in 1714, and Charles I did not trust the Jacobites, who wanted to restore James's son to the throne. So the new king led a purge of all Tory officials, including William Keith. Keith then returned to England where he wined and dined his way into the then-open position of lieutenant governor of colonial Pennsylvania and Delaware. Keith and his family settled in Philadelphia, where he continued to accumulate debt through an expensive lifestyle and failed business ventures.

An acquaintance and victim of one of these business failures, Benjamin Franklin, remarked on Keith in his autobiography: "He wish'd to please everybody; and, having little to give, he gave Expectations. He was otherwise an ingenious sensible Man, a pretty good writer, and a good Governor for the People. . . . Several of our best laws were of his Planning, and pass'd during his Administration."

As lieutenant governor, Keith established a militia, despite the high Quaker (pacifist) population in the area. He also arranged peace conferences with the

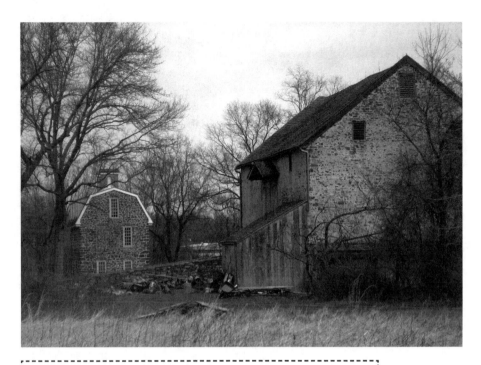

The side of the Keith House (left) and the adjacent stone barn and visitor center

local Native Americans, settled other local disagreements, and maintained an economically stable colony. The grounds, today known as Graeme Park, were offered to Keith as a partial salary for his government position. He dubbed the property "Fountain Low" because of its many natural springs and built his summer mansion and a malt house there.

After the death of William Penn in 1718, however, Keith became involved in disputes with Penn's widow, Hannah, regarding the conduct of the colony. Mrs. Penn later joined forces with her late husband's supporters and other heirs to nominate a new lieutenant governor. Keith attempted to form an opposition party but failed to gain power within its ranks. At this point, overwhelmed by debt, Keith fled his creditors and sailed back to England, leaving his family behind in Philadelphia. In 1719, a good friend of the Keith family, Dr. Thomas Graeme, married Keith's stepdaughter, Ann Diggs. In 1739, Graeme purchased Fountain Low as his own summer residence and renamed it Graeme Park. Meanwhile, back in England, Keith continued to assist in governmental affairs but died penniless in 1749, never returning to the Colonies or to his family.

Upon Graeme's death, Graeme Park was passed down to Graeme's daughter, Elizabeth Graeme Fergussen. During the Revolutionary War, the property was seized from the Fergussen family because of the family's loyalist ties. Elizabeth eventually reclaimed the property, selling it to her niece's husband. Since that time, the property had seen only a few owners before being donated to the

Pennsylvania Historical and Museum Commission in 1958. Other than minor renovations and restorations, the house retains its historic merit, and the grounds and surrounding buildings offer a glimpse into the birth of our country.

This trek walks to the back of the stone-and-wood barn, which currently serves as the visitor center. Field maps are available at the start of the hike during off-hours, and in the barn during operating hours. Bear left and then go straight to the opening of the Nature Trail. Admire the white birches, pines, and oaks, some of which are more than 100 years old. At this point, the stress of the booming modern civilization that surrounds this historic park will start to melt as the robins, cardinals, and blue jays flit around you and hawks hover high above.

Turn right at the line of trees that parallels the cornfield, and continue all the way to the end, where a clearing in the woods leads to Park Creek. You may need to navigate the brush a little to hug the creek line, but this short stretch provides the park's best bird-watching, and blue herons are often spotted in this corner of the park. Their nocturnal neighbor, the great horned owl, can often be heard in the early morning as it hoots in preparation for rest.

Continue to follow the creek's path, and you may see the abutment to an old bridge still standing amongst the flowing waters. The path soon veers to the right, leaving the creek behind for wooded brush, where you can count bird's nests in the trees. At the end of this walkway, you can view the back of the Keith mansion, with its many windows and light-blue sills. Now turn and retrace your route to the path where, in a widening field, sycamores line the way back to the Keith House and you can catch a fine view of two venerable trees, a pin oak and an ash.

Your short walk has ended, but your exploration of the historic grounds can certainly continue. Tours are available Fridays, Saturdays, and Sundays.

## NEARBY ACTIVITIES

COLD STONE CREAMERY
110 Easton Road, Warrington
(215) 491-7385

HAPPY TIMES FAMILY FUN CENTER
(Indoor play for children;
good on rainy days)
2071 County Line Road, Warrington
(267) 927-0570

WEGMANS
(Gourmet grocery store)
1405 Main Street, Warrington
(215) 918-3100

WINGS OF FREEDOM AVIATION MUSEUM
1155 Easton Road, Willow Grove
(215) 672-2277
**www.dvhaa.org/museum.html**

# 10 HONEY HOLLOW

## KEY AT-A-GLANCE INFORMATION

**LENGTH:** 1.9 miles

**CONFIGURATION:** Loop

**DIFFICULTY:** Easy

**SCENERY:** Tree-lined hills, ponds, birds

**EXPOSURE:** Full sun on hills, shade in short woods walk

**TRAIL TRAFFIC:** Light

**TRAIL SURFACE:** Grass, dirt paths

**HIKING TIME:** 1 hour or less

**DRIVING DISTANCE FROM CENTER CITY:** 46 miles

**ACCESS:** Visitor center open Monday–Saturday, 9 a.m.–5 p.m.; trails open daily, 9 a.m.–5 p.m., year-round (but see below); free admission

**MAPS:** USGS Buckingham

**WHEELCHAIR TRAVERSABLE:** No

**FACILITIES:** Restrooms in Audubon building

**SPECIAL COMMENTS:** This park is home to the Bucks County Audubon Society, a chapter of the National Audubon Society; bring binoculars for bird-watching. *Note:* Part of the described route is closed on weekends because it crosses a private Christmas-tree farm that is open to hikers only during the week. More information: (215) 297-5880; www.bcas.org.

GPS Trailhead
Coordinates

UTM Zone (WGS84)  18T

Easting  0499097

Northing  4468898

Latitude  N 40° 22' 21.15"

Longitude  W 75° 0' 38.30"

## IN BRIEF

A hidden treasure in the hills of Solebury, this park offers bird-watching, an open, rolling vista, and a meditative pond. Home to the Bucks County Audubon Society, the visitor center provides educational programs and community outreach year-round.

## DESCRIPTION

Honey Hollow is a classic example of successful conservation. This tract of land was the first small upland agricultural watershed area to demonstrate that water, soil, and wildlife can be safeguarded through local action.

## *Directions*

Take Interstate 76 west from Philadelphia toward Valley Forge. After approximately 13 miles, take Exit 331B onto I-476 for Plymouth Meeting and go 4.4 miles; then exit onto the Pennsylvania Turnpike–I-276, heading east. After 9.1 miles, take Exit 343 for Willow Grove, and proceed north on PA 611 toward Doylestown. After 2 miles, turn right at Meetinghouse Road; after 1.3 miles, turn right onto West County Line Road. Go 0.9 miles and turn left onto PA 263–York Road. Stay on PA 263 for 13.3 miles; along the way, PA 263 and PA 202 overlap, then split at a Y-intersection in Lahaska—look for Buckingham Friends School on the left just before the split. Keep left on PA 263 for 1.1 more miles: Pass through Peddler's Village; cross Street Road, then Aquetong Road. Go past the first sign you see for Honey Hollow, as this is the entrance to the administrative office. Pass Creamery Road on the left (you'll see a sign for Solebury Orchards), then go 100 yards and turn right onto Creamery Road (you'll see a sign for Audubon Visitor Center). Proceed on Creamery Road 0.33 miles to the Honey Hollow entrance, on the right. *2877 Creamery Road, Solebury, PA; 18938.*

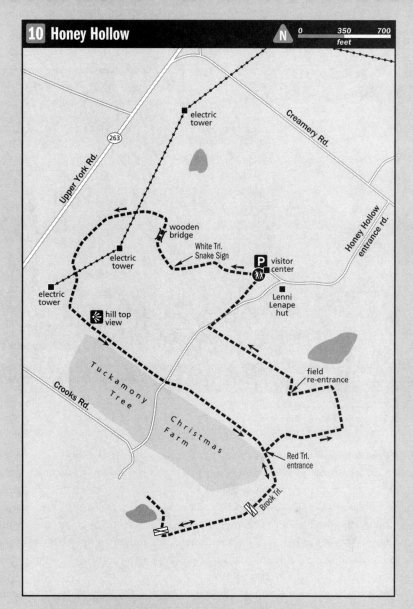

N

| 0 | 350 | 700 |

*feet*

Creamery Rd.

electric tower

Upper York Rd.

263

Honey Hollow entrance rd.

wooden bridge

White Trl. Snake Sign

electric tower

P visitor center

electric tower

Lenni Lenape hut

hill top view

field re-entrance

Crooks Rd.

T u c k a m o n y   T r e e

C h r i s t m a s   F a r m

Red Trl. entrance

Brook Trl.

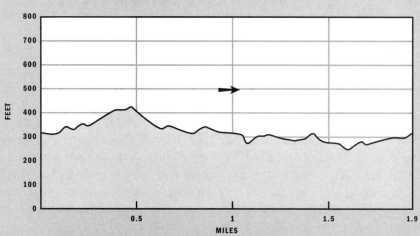

| 800 | | | |
| 700 | | | |
| 600 | | | |
| 500 | | | |
| 400 | | | |
| 300 | | | |
| 200 | | | |
| 100 | | | |
| 0 | | | |

FEET

| 0.5 | 1 | 1.5 | 1.9 |

MILES

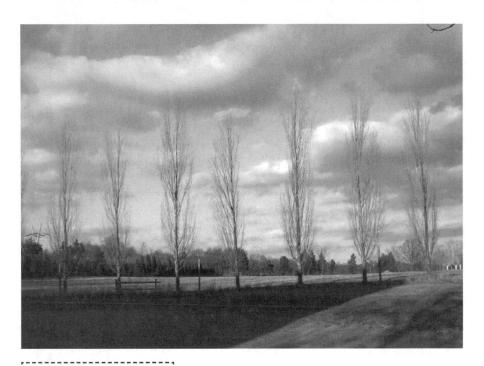

Swath of trees at Honey Hollow

During the late 1930s, farmers in Solebury applied to the U.S. Soil Conservation Service for assistance after experiencing soil erosion in their fields; these upland acres held the key to saving their farms. Through their efforts, the farmers saved almost 700 acres for posterity and preservation. This event attracted national attention and served as an example for other farmers throughout the country. Had these farmers not banded together when they did, developers most certainly would have gobbled up this tract of Bucks County, now a historic landmark, during the sprawl of the 1970s and 1980s.

Only when you visit this park, now the home of the Bucks County Audubon Society (BCAS), can you truly appreciate the determination put forth during that Depression-era effort. Honey Hollow, with its diverse terrain and wildlife, feels almost sacred.

The hike begins at the attractive stone home base of the BCAS nature center. Information regarding tours, programs, and events is available inside the building; announcements are posted outside the building as well for after-hours visitors. The trailhead is to the north side of the building, next to a kiosk.

Near the start of the trail is a bird blind. Bird blinds are shelters that allow up-close observation of birds and other animals. This one contains a guide to the more than 100 species recorded at Honey Hollow, including pileated woodpecker, winter wren, blue jay, northern cardinal, red-winged blackbird, and American robin. Here you can watch the birds eat from suet feeders. This type of feeder usually contains a piece of beef fat or other protein; the rich nutrition

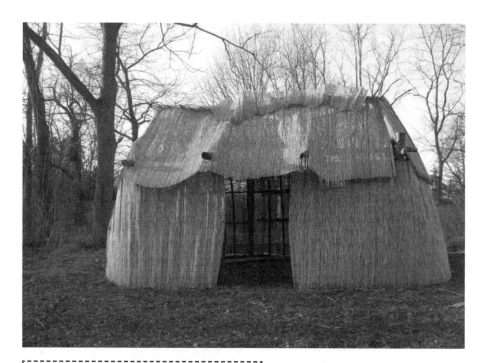

Re-creation of a Lenni Lenape Native American hut

helps the birds stay warm during cold temperatures. When you've finished your observation, continue on the trail and cross a babbling brook via a wooden bridge.

Near the brook is a sign that illustrates the 14 species of snakes found in the Philadelphia suburbs. Of the 14, only one, the northern copperhead, is poisonous. A tan-and-brown snake with eyes that have vertical, elliptical pupils, the northern copperhead is a denizen of wooded hillsides and plays an important role in the complex ecosystem of the area. The copperhead, like most poisonous snakes, will use its venom only when hunting or defending itself. Should you come across one of these rarely seen slithery creatures, give it a wide berth and continue on your way; unprovoked snakes are not likely to harm you.

When you come to the White Trail, turn right. This trail winds along the woods for a few hundred yards. After a series of small footbridges, stay straight until you reach the electric towers. Walk under them, off the White Trail, and turn left around a stand of small pines. Soon you reach a clearing with a majestic view of Solebury Mountain. The hazier hills in the distance are actually in New Jersey. This is a good place to stop and watch raptors soar and swoop over the meadow. If you're visiting after the harvest, round hay bales will be stacked in nearby fields.

Stay on the right side of the first field and walk straight. Cross a paved road beside the Tuckamony Christmas Tree Farm, which grows Douglas-firs and blue spruces. After crossing the road, continue straight beside a second field until you reach the lower right corner. Here is the entrance to the Red Trail, which starts as a wooded path. On the Red Trail, cross a footbridge and pass through two gates, about 200 yards apart. Just beyond the second gate is a little pond that buzzes with dragonflies and is alive with jumping frogs in the summer. Water trickles from a nearby brook, lending a soothing sound to this meditative spot year-round.

After pausing at the pond to rest, retrace your route to the start of the Red Trail. Here you'll take an alternate route onto the Brook Trail, which loops around more woods until you reenter a section of the field different from the one where you initially entered the Red Trail. To your right is another pond, which in the dead of winter freezes over and is used by skaters, who glide at their own risk.

Across the pond, in the distance, stands a re-creation of a Lenni Lenape Native American thatched hut. Bear right until you come to the paved road. Now turn right to return to the BCAS nature center, just 100 yards ahead.

On your way out of the driveway, keep a look out for the previously mentioned Lenni Lenape hut. This 10- by 20-foot structure is a realistic approximation of what an indigenous dwelling looked like before European settlement. It stands in dramatic contrast to nearby subdivisions, where 4,000-square-foot-plus homes accommodate modern American families that are similar in size to their native counterparts.

## NEARBY ACTIVITIES

DILLY'S CORNER
(Burgers, ice cream, and more)
Corner of PA 263 and PA 32,
New Hope
(215) 862-5333

HISTORIC NEW HOPE VISITOR CENTER
1 West Mechanic Street, New Hope
(215) 862-5880
**www.newhopevisitorscenter.org**

PEDDLER'S VILLAGE
(Rustic-themed shopping and dining)
81 Peddler's Village Road, Buckingham
(215) 794-1629
**www.peddlersvillage.com**

# LAKE TOWHEE PARK 11

## IN BRIEF

This short out-and-back provides different perspectives on a 50-acre lake named after the orange-sided sparrow known as the eastern towhee. The park also offers camping, fishing, skating, and picnic areas.

## DESCRIPTION

This 549-acre park in Haycock Township, purchased by Bucks County in the early 1960s, has become a forgotten spot for many Bucks County travelers. With so many other places to see and visit in the Greater Philadelphia area, the park gets little attention. In fact, the Yellow Trail that traces the perimeter of the lake disappears on the northeastern side because of flooding, making the hike an out-and-back rather than the loop it once was.

The eastern towhee, a large sparrow indigenous to the Haycock area, resembles the American robin, although it is smaller. Its red eyes and its chirp, which sounds something

### KEY AT-A-GLANCE INFORMATION

**LENGTH:** 2.27 miles

**CONFIGURATION:** Out-and-back

**DIFFICULTY:** Moderate

**SCENERY:** Lake, woodlands, barn

**EXPOSURE:** Mostly shade

**TRAIL TRAFFIC:** Light

**TRAIL SURFACE:** Dirt, gravel, downed trees

**HIKING TIME:** 1 hour

**DRIVING DISTANCE FROM CENTER CITY:** 52.8 miles

**ACCESS:** Daily, dawn–dusk, year-round; free admission

**MAPS:** USGS Quakertown; no maps at park

**WHEELCHAIR TRAVERSABLE:** No

**FACILITIES:** Restrooms on south side of park near dam

**SPECIAL COMMENTS:** Trail can be muddy in spots. More information: (215) 757-0571; www.buckscounty .org/government/departments/ parksandrec/Parks/Towhee.aspx.

---

## Directions ⟶

Take Interstate 76 west from Philadelphia. After 12.7 miles, take Exit 331B and merge onto Interstate 476. After 28.4 miles, take Exit 44. At the end of the ramp, turn left onto PA 663. After 3.4 miles, the road changes to PA 313 at Quakertown; continue on 313 for 2.5 miles, then turn left onto West Thatcher Road. After 0.3 miles, make a slight left to stay on West Thatcher. After 1.8 more miles, West Thatcher turns into Creamery Road; continue straight for 0.4 more miles, then turn right onto Cider Press Lane. After 0.9 miles, turn left onto Old Bethlehem Road. The park entrance is on the right in about 1 mile. The trailhead is behind a picnic pavilion north of the parking lot. *Old Bethlehem Road, Applebachsville, PA. 18951.*

---

GPS Trailhead
Coordinates
UTM Zone (WGS84)  18T
Easting  0477252
Northing  4480702
Latitude  N 40° 28' 43.27"
Longitude  W 75° 16' 4.78"

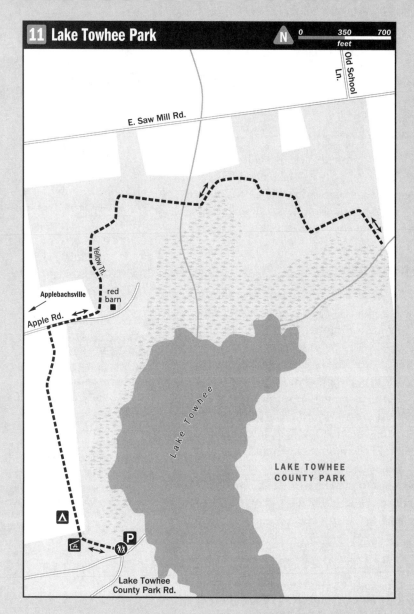

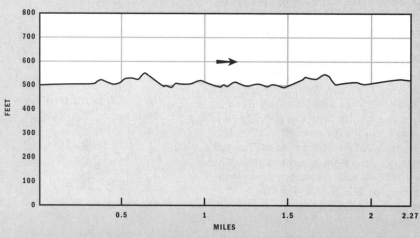

> Because of flooding, this hike is an out-and-back rather than the loop it once was.

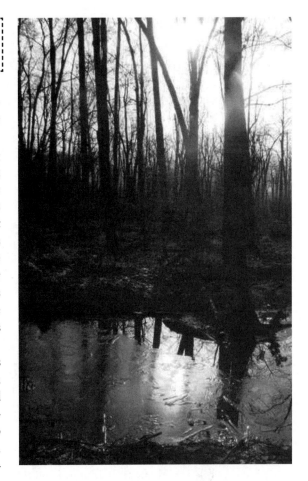

like "drink-your-teaheehee-hee," set it apart from other birds.

Towhees are monogamous. During breeding season, from mid-April to late May, the male arrives at the breeding site first and sings until the females come to listen. The male then chooses his partner and gathers grass and twigs so the female can build the nest. Then the male protects the nest and his territory.

Although these birds were once abundant in eastern Pennsylvania and New England, their numbers are declining, so keep your eyes open as you hike. Find the Yellow Trail trailhead behind a picnic pavilion, just north of the main parking lot; look for the yellow markers. You pass some campgrounds to your left shortly after you begin. In the winter, some residences are also visible at the beginning of the hike to your left, just outside the park. Four or five downed trees scattered along the trail require some interesting maneuvering and a little climbing.

The Yellow Trail zigzags near a house, shifting right to join a dirt road (Apple Road) and then left, back on course just before a big red barn. After about 0.2 miles from that turn, you come to a Y by a small pine forest; stay left and continue east around the northern tip of the lake.

The Moravian Pottery and Tile Works of Doylestown still uses clay dredged from the bottom of the lake almost two decades ago for its hand-crafted tiles. The lake often turns to ice in midwinter, providing a skating rink better than Rockefeller Center's, with far fewer people to bump into. You may come across an occasional ice fisher, but with 50 acres of frozen surface, there is plenty of room for all. Red and green flags at the parking lot indicate ice conditions.

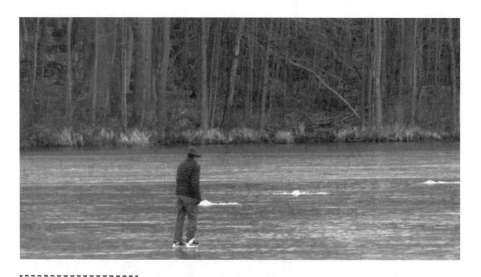

Skate at your own risk.

At almost 1 mile into the hike, the Yellow Trail crosses a brook. In the winter, you can walk on ice. The rest of the year, you must make careful hops from rock to rock. A plank bridge crossing a wider part of the stream indicates that the trail was once tended, but more downed trees across the trail show current neglect.

The downed trees (and those still standing) provide a good representation of Bucks County's native species, including cedars, aspens, sugar maples, pin oaks, and white pines. Elm trees thrived here decades ago but were largely wiped out by Dutch elm disease.

Past the fallen trees, about 0.2 miles from the brook, diabase rocks provide natural stepping-stones. (For more about the diabase rocks of Haycock Township, see page 80.) The trail then bends right and continues to bend eastward until it reaches a stream that is perfect for frog catching and pollywog watching, but not so hot for hiking. So turn around and head back to the parking lot. However, this quiet spot at the trail's end is an ideal location to stop and listen for the eastern towhee. After this hike, you just might find that its subliminal message leads you to head home for a hot cup of "teaheehee."

## NEARBY ACTIVITIES

DIABASE LODGE
*(Art studio; call for hours)*
860 Old Bethlehem Road,
Quakertown
(215) 804-7537

RAVEN'S NEST
*(Pub with blues music on weekends)*
625 Old Bethlehem Road,
Quakertown
(215) 536-5369

# LENAPE AND MENLO PARKS 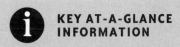 12

## IN BRIEF

This hike spans two parks, from Perkasie to Sellersville Borough, that were one resort in the late 19th and early 20th centuries. The route is part of a planned Liberty Bell Trail that will run for 25 miles in Montgomery and Bucks counties.

## DESCRIPTION

Baseball, hot dogs, apple pie, and Perkasie—if you wanted to take someone from a foreign country to a quintessential American town, Perkasie Borough would certainly make your short list. In some neighborhoods these days, you rarely see anyone out and about. The kids and families sit inside, watching television and playing on their computers. In Perkasie Borough, especially in pleasant weather, residents are at Lenape and Menlo parks.

In the late 19th and early 20th centuries, Philadelphians traveled in droves to Menlo Park, a popular amusement and resort area

### Directions

Take Interstate 76 west from Philadelphia. After 12.6 miles, take Exit 331B to merge onto US 476 toward Plymouth Meeting (partial toll road). After 14.7 miles, take Exit 31 for PA 63 toward Landsdale. After 0.6 miles, turn left at PA 63–Sumneytown Pike, then left at Forty Foot Road. After 2.9 miles, take a slight left at West Broad Street. Take a left at North Main Street and continue on Cowpath Road. Take a right at Bergey Road, then a left at Hatfield–Souderton Pike. After 0.8 miles, take a left at County Line Road and then a slight right at Bethlehem Pike. After 2.5 miles, continue on South Main Street until you see East Walnut Street on your right. Park access is on your left. *298 East Walnut Street, Sellersville, PA 18960.*

### KEY AT-A-GLANCE INFORMATION

**LENGTH: 2.2 miles**

**CONFIGURATION: Balloon**

**DIFFICULTY: Easy–moderate**

**SCENERY: Lake, suspension bridge, covered bridge, antique carousel (when open)**

**EXPOSURE: Full sun–full shade**

**TRAIL TRAFFIC: Light–moderate**

**TRAIL SURFACE: Paved, dirt, gravel**

**HIKING TIME: 1 hour**

**DRIVING DISTANCE FROM CENTER CITY: 40 miles**

**ACCESS: Daily, dawn–dusk, year-round; free admission (carousel 35¢/ride)**

**MAPS: USGS Telford**

**WHEELCHAIR TRAVERSABLE: Partially**

**FACILITIES: No public restrooms; try aquatic center or carousel at Menlo.**

**SPECIAL COMMENTS: If you're interested in seeing the carousel, visit www.perkasieborough.org/historical_landmarks.html for an updated schedule. More information: (215) 257-5065.**

GPS Trailhead Coordinates

UTM Zone (WGS84)  18T

Easting  0474057

Northing  4468097

Latitude  N 40° 21' 46.9"

Longitude  W 75° 18' 20.0"

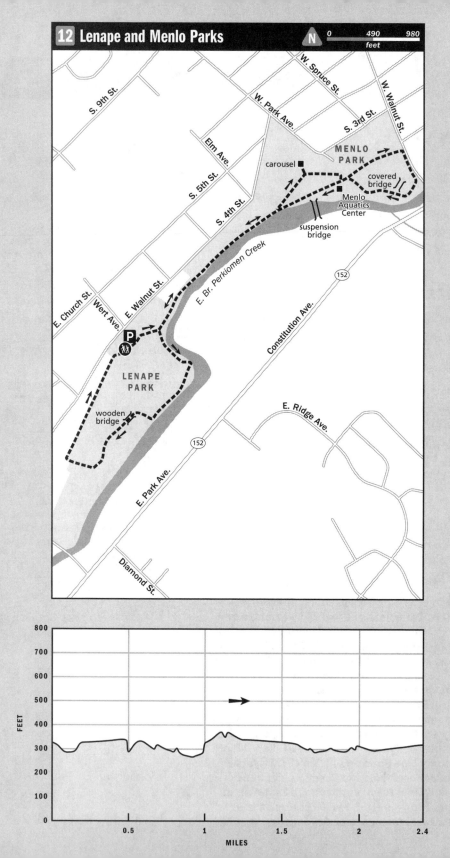

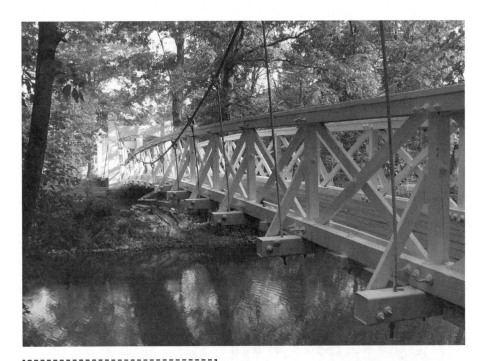

White suspension bridge in Lenape Park

where city slickers could escape for the day or the weekend. They could boat in the nearby stream, enjoy the carousel, or ride the first on-land toboggan down a hillside. Eventually, a trolley service was added, then a swimming pool, a casino, a bowling alley, an ice-cream parlor, and a dance-and-movie hall. In 1955 the park's owner, Henry S. Wilson, put the park up for sale; Perkasie Borough purchased it and made it public. Even though most of the old-timey attractions are now gone, the carousel and swimming pool (now the Menlo Aquatics Center) still attract crowds of Perkasonians.

Adjacent Lenape Park, which was once part of Menlo Park, contains one of the oldest remaining covered bridges in Bucks County. The bridge still contains this inscription: $5 FINE FOR ANY PERSON RIDING OR DRIVING OVER THIS BRIDGE FASTER THAN A WALK OR SMOKING SEGARS ON. So be sure to leave your "segars" at home. The bridge, which was moved in 1958 from nearby Pleasant Spring Creek to its present location, is preserved and protected by the Perkasie Historical Society.

On this hike you will pass the covered bridge and a baseball field. A bike path adjoins Sellersville Borough's bike path on one side and on the other the Perkiomen Path, which subsequently links to East Rockhill Township's bike path. The trails all connect and compose part of what will eventually become the Liberty Bell Trail. This hiking and biking trail will one day run for 25 miles in southeastern Pennsylvania, from East Norriton to Quakertown. The trail will partially follow the line of

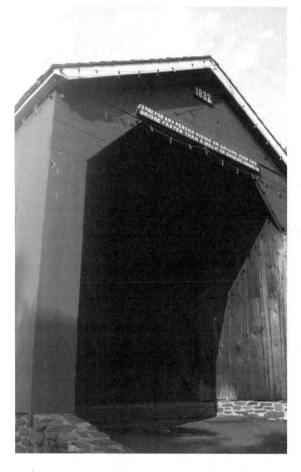

One of the oldest covered bridges in Bucks County stands in Lenape Park.

the long-defunct Liberty Bell Trolley Route, which was so named because it hugged Bethlehem Pike, the road along which the Liberty Bell was transported in October 1777. The bell was moved at that time from Philadelphia to the Allentown area for safekeeping before the British occupation of Philadelphia during the Revolutionary War. The finished trail will pass through 15 municipalities and adjacent countryside, allowing people in the area to reach more places using nonmotorized transportation.

So part of your hike today involves the past and part involves the future. Start the hike from the Sellersville entrance to Lenape Park on East Walnut Street. Walk downhill from the parking lot toward the baseball diamond and join a paved all-purpose trail on your left. Stay left where the trail splits, and keep the East Perkiomen Creek on your right.

Butterfly bushes dot the creek's edge with splashes of violet in early summertime. Bikers, hikers, dog walkers, and skateboarders pass by occasionally, many with a smile and a "hello." Even the rebellious teenagers who hang out here have a warm, nonthreatening demeanor.

Fly anglers wade and wait for trout, stocked in the creek for fishing season, to tug their line. Many anglers fly-fish by the sides of two unique white footbridges, built in 1938 to serve people walking through the park; they were restored in 2000.

Beyond the bridges, continue straight until the creek curves and you approach another baseball field, on the right. Curve past the field and take the sidewalk, then walk toward the large red covered bridge. The Perkasie Historical Society and other volunteers from Perkasie maintain the bridge, which received a new roof in 2000.

Continue to loop the paved trail, but instead of going directly back the way you came, walk uphill on a dirt-and-gravel trail that leads to Menlo Park. This section adds a workout to the walk; those unable or not wishing to negotiate the dirt-and-gravel should continue straight on the paved trail. You may get a treat at the top of the hill—during certain times of the year, the park's carousel is open. Purchased in 1951, it replaced an 1891 model that had hand-carved wooden horses. The carousel building dates from 1895; after a heavy snowfall collapsed the roof in 1995, the community organized a major restoration. A community pool sits next to the carousel.

Descend the hill, bearing right to join the trail that leads back to the fork. Here, go left to view more of the creek, which is now on your left, along with an array of majestic old trees. The route eventually veers left, away from the creek, and crosses a stream via a footbridge. Now follow the trail back to the parking lot to complete the loop.

But first admire some of the homes on the trail's northwest side, complete with gardens and patios reminiscent of a time when people played outside instead of surfing the Internet, a time when if you saw a person walking outside, you didn't feel afraid to smile and say hello—practices that still hold true today in Perkasie and Sellersville.

## NEARBY ACTIVITIES

Olde Towne Restaurant and Tavern
518 West Walnut Street, Perkasie
(215) 258-5668

Pearl S. Buck House
520 Dublin Road, Perkasie
(215) 249-0100
**www.psbi.org**

Tabora Farm and Orchard
1104 Upper Stump Road, Chalfont
(215) 249-3016
**www.taborafarmandorchard.com**

# 13  NESHAMINY STATE PARK: River Walk

**KEY AT-A-GLANCE
INFORMATION**

**LENGTH:** 2.3 miles
**CONFIGURATION:** Loop
**DIFFICULTY:** Medium
**SCENERY:** Woods and freshwater estuary
**EXPOSURE:** Mostly shade
**TRAIL TRAFFIC:** Medium
**TRAIL SURFACE:** Paved, dirt
**HIKING TIME:** 1 hour
**DRIVING DISTANCE FROM CENTER CITY:** 15 miles
**ACCESS:** Year-round, daily, dawn–dusk; free admission
**MAPS:** USGS Beverly
**WHEELCHAIR TRAVERSABLE:** No
**FACILITIES:** Several restrooms and pavilions throughout the park, plus barbecue pits, tot lot, and a public swimming pool accessed for a small fee
**SPECIAL COMMENTS:** This is the only hike in this book that has a view of a freshwater estuary.
**More information:** (215) 639-4538.

## IN BRIEF

This hike combines views of bayside flora and fauna with a hike through forest areas near the Delaware River. Highlights include marine life, sailboats, and a variety of trees, some of them planted by the Philadelphia Eagles football team and the Conservation Fund.

## DESCRIPTION

This unique hike takes you on walkways along the water to enjoy the natural habitats seen along both river and ocean. Access the hike from a gravel path off the first parking lot. You will soon see that the park is a showpiece for environmental protection and conservation of water and forested areas.

In spring of 2008, volunteers and state park staff planted 1,200 trees in the park. The Eagles Forest, a 6.5-acre site at Neshaminy State Park, planted to help offset the Philadelphia Eagles' carbon footprint, is one example of the team's Go Green program to better the planet through responsible business practices. The program, launched in 2003, incorporates green initiatives, sustainable business practices, and educational outreach as core operating principles of the Philadelphia Eagles.

Two of the acres within Eagles Forest were planted in partnership with the Conservation

GPS Trailhead
Coordinates
UTM Zone (WGS84)  18T
Easting   0506758
Northing   4436353
Latitude   N 40° 4' 38.9"
Longitude   W 74° 55' 14.8"

*Directions* ⟶

**Take Interstate 95 north toward Trenton/
Philadelphia. Continue 14.5 miles and take
Exit 37 for Street Road toward PA 132. Turn
right at Street Road. Look for State Road on
your left. The park entrance will be on your
right. Park in the first parking lot on the left.**
*3401 State Road, Bensalem, PA 19020-5930.*

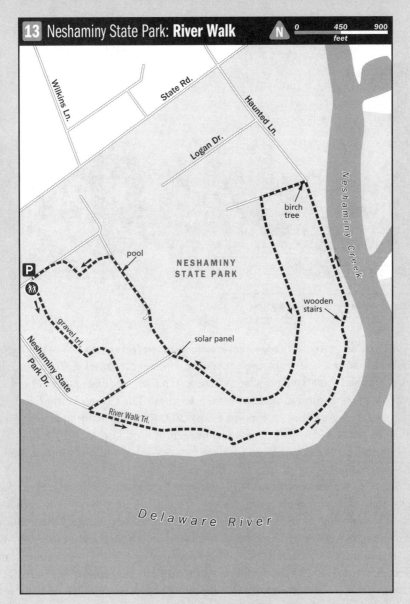

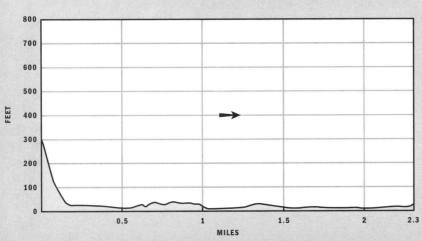

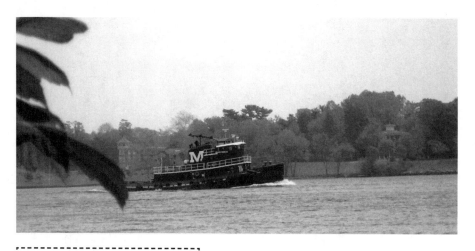

Boat cruising down the Delaware River

Fund's Go Zero program (**www.conservationfund.org/gozero**) to offset the carbon emissions that resulted from the team's away-game air travel during the 2007 season. Dubbed the "Go Zero Grove," the 870 native seedlings planted here will trap 565 tons of carbon dioxide over their lifetime. The Conservation Fund's Go Zero program has restored a total of nearly 20,000 acres, planting almost 6 million native trees, which will trap the equivalent of 8 million tons of carbon dioxide from the earth's atmosphere over the next century and will protect against global warming.

Signs at Neshaminy State Park ask you to assess your own carbon footprint—the amount of carbon dioxide emitted as a result of your daily activities, such as commuting to work or heating and cooling your home. When you use less energy, recycle, and reuse—rather than consume natural resources—you reduce your carbon footprint. Conservation saves the planet. Neshaminy State Park is not just a safe haven for plants and animals; it encompasses part of the freshwater intertidal zone along the shores of the Delaware River and Neshaminy Creek and is protected by the Coastal Management Act.

An estuary is essentially an arm of the sea at the lower end of a river. At this point on the Delaware River, you are 116 miles from the ocean, but the water here is affected by the tide's rise and fall. Follow the trail to the park's waterway and the well-marked River Walk, where the plants and animals include a mix of freshwater and saltwater inhabitants. You will see sea crabs, marsh grass, and cattails just yards from pine forests. The waterway on your right stretches from the bay to the river and from the river to Neshaminy Creek. Oak trees and grassy knolls border your path on the left. Follow the trail about 0.5 miles to a fork just before you reach a giant white birch that shades both land and water. Here, veer left on a gravel path, away from the river, and into a shady forest. In 2008, unfortunately, this park saw a renewed infestation of gypsy moths.

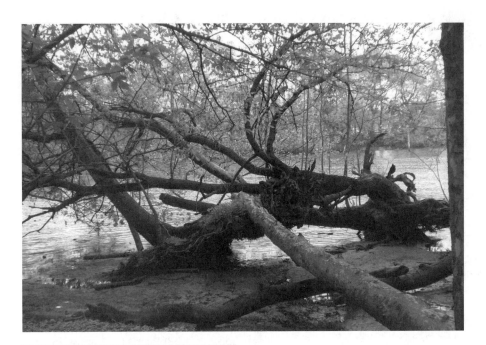

The river rises and falls affected by the tides.

Accidentally introduced to America in the late 1860s by an amateur entomologist, these hungry insects are one of the most destructive forest pests in Pennsylvania, defoliating and even killing host trees, such as oaks, and many shrubs. With forest areas under threat from both humans and insects, forest restoration becomes even more important.

Follow the gravel path until you reach a paved trail near a bright Japanese maple, near the park's many facilities. In addition to boating, fishing, and hiking, the park offers barbecue pits and pavilions and a public swimming pool that can be accessed for a small fee. Continue straight, in the opposite direction of an arrow painted on the pavement. After you pass the pool, turn left to follow the paved trail back to the parking lot. Before you reach the end of this hike, you will pass a tot lot where children play, enjoying the fruits of preservation and fresh air, made possible by forward thinkers who knew enough to preserve and conserve, not just for themselves, but for their children and grandchildren—the movers, shakers, and hikers of tomorrow.

## NEARBY ACTIVITIES

COMMERCE BANK AMPHITHEATER
2400 Byberry Road, Bensalem
(215) 633-3635
www.bcbaevents.com

WINGS OF GOLD BALLOON RIDES
2517 Dunksferry Road, Bensalem
(215) 244-9323

## NOCKAMIXON STATE PARK:
### Lake Nockamixon

**14**

### KEY AT-A-GLANCE INFORMATION

**LENGTH:** 7.1 miles

**CONFIGURATION:** Out-and-back

**DIFFICULTY:** Hard

**SCENERY:** Lake views, pine-tree walks

**EXPOSURE:** Mostly shaded

**TRAIL TRAFFIC:** Medium

**TRAIL SURFACE:** Dirt, partial pavement

**HIKING TIME:** 3 hours

**DRIVING DISTANCE FROM CENTER CITY:** 46.6 miles

**ACCESS:** Daily, dawn–dusk, year-round; free admission

**MAPS:** USGS Bedminster; maps available at main office or online at dcnr.state.pa.us/stateparks/parks/nockamixon/nockamixon_mini.pdf

**WHEELCHAIR TRAVERSABLE:** No

**FACILITIES:** Restrooms on other side of park, next to boat launch

**SPECIAL COMMENTS:** The largest lake in Bucks County; often ices over in January. More information: (215) 528-1340; dcnr.state.pa.us/stateparks/parks/nockamixon.aspx.

### GPS Trailhead Coordinates

UTM Zone (WGS84)  18T

Easting   0478620

Northing   4475310

Latitude   N 40° 25' 41.5"

Longitude   W 75° 15' 7.1"

### IN BRIEF

This hike is accented by stretches of unique lake views, pine groves, and log-cabin walks.

### DESCRIPTION

On almost any given day at Lake Nockamixon, you can watch boats with multicolored sails glide by while anglers stand near the lake's edge vying for more than 25 species of fish, such as channel catfish, striped bass, walleye, and pickerel. Blue herons, Canada geese, and mallards soar overhead, waiting for a throwback. The lake covers over 1,400 acres, which leaves another 4,000 acres for hiking. In winter, it's fun to stroll out to the middle of the lake when it's safely frozen over.

The name *Nockamixon* comes from the Native American phrase *Nocha-miska-ing*, which is Lenni Lenape for "At the place of

### Directions

Take Interstate 76 west from Philadelphia. After 12.7 miles, take Exit 331B for US 476 north (the Blue Route). After 14.8 miles, take Exit 31 toward Lansdale and turn left onto PA 63–Sumneytown Pike; within a block, turn left at PA 63–Forty Foot Road, and stay straight for 2.7 miles. Continue on PA 463–Forty Foot Road–West Broad Street. After 0.7 miles, turn left at North Market Street; quickly take a slight right at Union Street, and continue on Unionville Pike for 1 mile. Turn left at PA 309–Bethlehem Pike–County Line Road. After 5.5 miles, take the exit toward Perkasie/PA 563. After 0.2 miles, turn left at Lawn Avenue and then right at PA 563–Ridge Road. After 6.4 miles, turn left in the town of Elephant onto Elephant Road. The park entrance and parking lot will be on the right in about a half mile (after a farm). *1542 Mountainview Drive, Quakertown, PA 18951.*

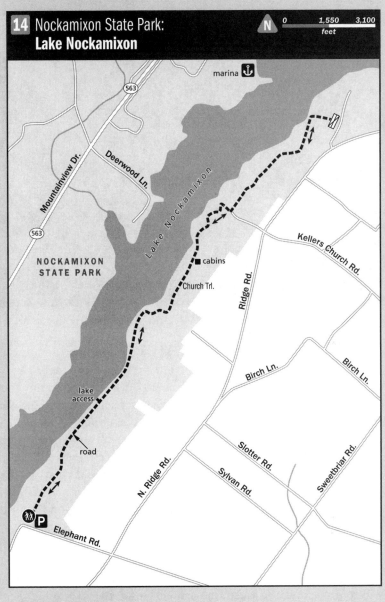

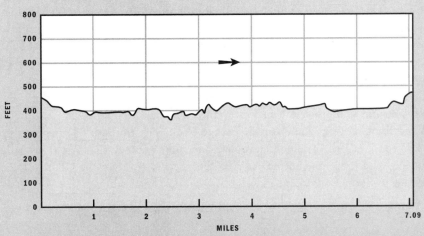

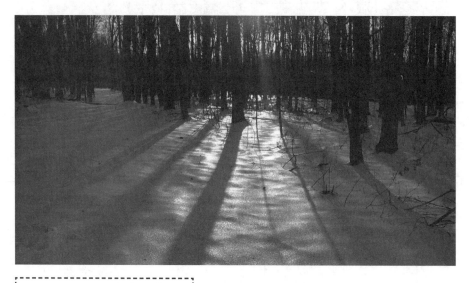

Bare mid-winter trees next to the lake

soft soil." The lake was formed in the early 1970s by damming the Tohickon Creek, Haycock Run, and Three Mile Run waterways. The best hiking is on the south side of the lake; this hike starts from the Elephant Road parking lot.

The direction is northeast for most of the hike and southwest on the way back. The first half mile of the hike goes through the woods with a mix of maples, oaks, and pines. It ends at a road where the hike continues to the right. This road is very close to the river, and in a few spots there are points where the road-trail is only few yards from the lake. Haycock Mountain, on the north side of the lake, is visible from every one of these vantage points. At more than 900 feet tall, Haycock Mountain is the only official mountain in Bucks County (see Hike 15, page 78).

After 1.5 miles, the entrance for the Church Trail appears on the left. The trail will continue down to where the main cabins at the lake reside. These log cabins have electric heat and can be rented even in winter. There are ten cabins in total at Lake Nockamixon, all with eat-in kitchens, toilets, and shower rooms. So one can explore and stay at the lake without having to rough it too much. This is the 2-mile mark for the hike. If you can only handle a 4-mile hike on this day, then turn around at this point.

Just beyond the cabins are some passages through midsized pine trees. Be careful during winter—there may be hunters in this area between December and February, so wear some sort of orange blaze. The trail goes across a main road, through a line of telephone poles, and onto another road. At this road, turn right and look for another parking lot on the left. Here the Church Trail continues and, once again, meanders closer to the lake at many points. The trail does have other turns in the last section, but stay left toward the lake.

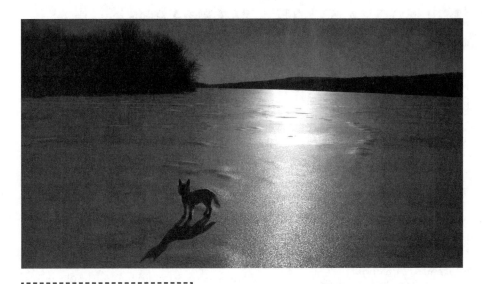

Lake Nockamixon frozen in January

On the last portion of the hike, the marina is clearly visible on the other side of the lake. There are docking facilities here for 648 boats. Rentals are available for canoes, motorboats, rowboats, and paddleboats. Just to the east and out of site is the dam that created the lake. At this point, where the lake is at its widest, the first half of the hike ends about 3.5 miles from the start. There is a short stretch onto a road that ends in a gate to the east. You'll most likely need a rest before heading back on the same 3.5 miles.

On the way back, keep a look out for birds of prey that have made a comeback in Lake Nockamixon. Bald eagles have been seen on the lake, along with osprey. If it's later in the day during the return trip, the large birds may be more likely to venture out with fewer people visible. You may get lucky and see one of these beautiful birds swoop into the lake to catch a fish—the favorite food of bald eagles.

## NEARBY ACTIVITIES

PEARL S. BUCK HOUSE
520 Dublin Road, Perkasie
(215) 249-0100
**www.psbi.org**

PIPERSVILLE INN
*(Restaurant)*
6946 Old Easton Road, Pipersville
(215) 766-7100

TOP ROCK TRAIL AT
HAYCOCK MOUNTAIN
*(See Hike 15, page 78)*
Top Rock Trail Road, Quakertown
(215) 538-1340

# NOCKAMIXON STATE PARK:
## Top Rock Trail at Haycock Mountain

**15**

### KEY AT-A-GLANCE INFORMATION

**LENGTH:** 1.4 miles

**CONFIGURATION:** Out-and-back

**DIFFICULTY:** Hard

**SCENERY:** Wooded hills with boulders, mountaintop view

**EXPOSURE:** Shade

**TRAIL TRAFFIC:** Moderate

**TRAIL SURFACE:** Dirt

**HIKING TIME:** About 1 hour, depending on bouldering ability

**DRIVING DISTANCE FROM CENTER CITY:** 42 miles

**ACCESS:** Daily, dawn–dusk, year-round; free admission

**MAPS:** USGS Bedminster

**WHEELCHAIR TRAVERSABLE:** No

**FACILITIES:** No restrooms here, only in main part of park

**SPECIAL COMMENTS:** Involves some bouldering. Pack a picnic lunch and, if you have them, lightweight binoculars. No restrooms on this hike. More information: (215) 538-1340.

## IN BRIEF

This hike features a shady mountain ascent to a peak with diabase rock formations of various shapes and sizes, plus a view of Lake Nockamixon in the winter and late fall, with glimpses in the summer and spring when the foliage is full.

## DESCRIPTION

Postcard images of mountains usually feature snow-dusted peaks climbing gracefully into a cobalt-blue sky. Haycock Mountain just barely meets these requirements—appearing from the distance, as its name implies, as a simple mound of hay. Upon closer examination, however, the mound offers climbing and hiking enjoyment for amateur and expert alike. In fact, this state gameland bordering the northern side of Lake Nockamixon is the tallest mountain in this part of Bucks County.

Clearly, the best time to travel in state gamelands during hunting season is on Sundays, when hunting is prohibited in Pennsylvania. But Sunday might not be the best day to find parking in the lot near the Top Rock Trail. If the parking lot is full, off-street parking is available, but you should park so as not to obstruct traffic. If you choose to hike this

---

### GPS Trailhead Coordinates

UTM Zone (WGS84) 18T

Easting 0482479

Northing 4482428

Latitude N 40° 29' 32.20"

Longitude W 75° 12' 25.92"

### *Directions* ⟶

From Center City, take PA 611 north. After approximately 28.5 miles, exit onto PA 611–Easton Road. After 11.3 miles, bear left at the fork onto PA 412–Durham Road. After approximately 0.25 miles, at the first light, make a left onto PA 563–Mountainview Drive heading south. Go 1 mile, then make a right on Top Rock Trail Road. The main parking lot will be 1 mile down, on the left. *Top Rock Trail Road, Quakertown, PA 18951.*

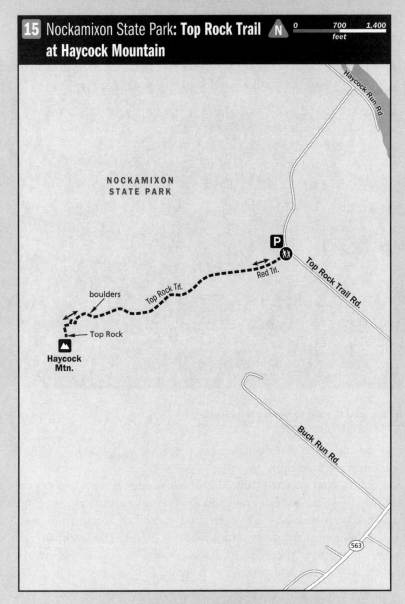

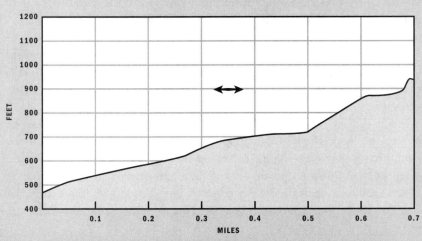

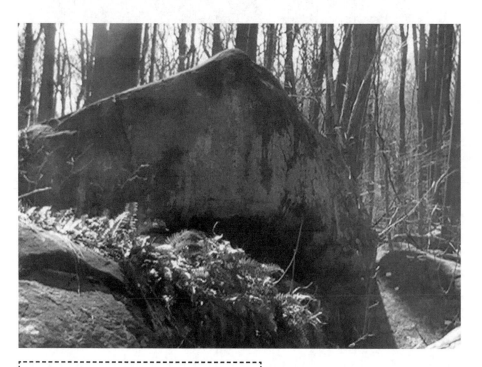

Wild ferns grow abundantly beside a large boulder.

route on any other day during hunting season, be sure to wear bright orange, lest you get mistaken for a deer.

At the parking lot, the trailhead is obvious, and there is no place left to go but up. The Red Trail provides the most direct route to the peak, but other trails can also take you there with less-steep climbing and bouldering. The bouldering is part of the appeal for many and provides a unique and seemingly primeval workout: as you near the ridge of diabase rocks, male climbers emerge from their shelters, shirtless and covered with chalk, as if straight out of *The Clan of the Cave Bear*.

These igneous rocks, formed from molten magma deep within the earth, are more than 200 million years old. They were forced to the surface thanks to the movement of the earth's tectonic plates. Diabase rock consists mostly of feldspar and pyroxene. It ranges in color from dark gray to black, and in texture from medium to fine-grained. Often polished and shaped to make monuments and gravestones, this rock can be found from central New Jersey to Devils Den in Gettysburg.

Legend states that Top Rock, the split monolith at the top of Haycock Mountain, and its neighbor, Table Top, were used for Native American rituals, and rumor has it that a few satanic cults have used the area for animal sacrifice. Some report that glowing eyes or orbs of light can be seen in these woods at night, and local lore labels the area as haunted. Another, less-widespread rumor touts actions by deranged monsters, but the lack of evidence is overwhelming,

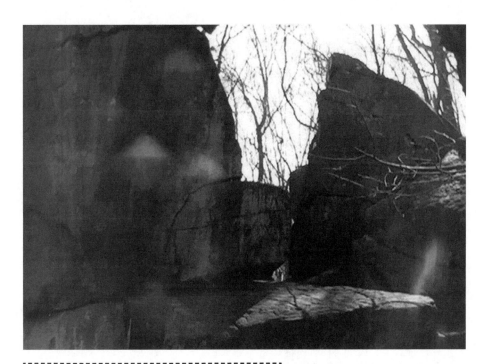

Top Rock offers diabase rocks of many shapes and sizes.

and hikers are in more danger of being tangled in briars or afflicted with poison ivy than being chased by a pistol-wielding ghostly being.

If you tread carefully, you will safely and easily reach your destination. Poor weather and logging practices of the indigenous oak and beech trees have obstructed some of the trails, which need to be re-marked and cleared regularly; still, the current indicators are relatively easy to follow, and where the trails split, markers on trees and larger rocks point you in the correct direction. Soon the smaller rocks give way to small caves and grottoes of collected boulders, with a smattering of white chalk marks from the buffed climbers. If climbing isn't your forte, simply admire the natural beauty and go around the rocks to continue the hike, but be prepared for at least some bouldering, because not all of the upward paths offer an alternative.

You are rewarded for your efforts at the 960-foot summit with views, weather and foliage permitting, of 1,450-acre Nockamixon Lake. Wise hikers pack a lunch to enjoy at Table Top.

Bird-watching is great from this airy perch, and binoculars allow you to zoom in on an array of raptors and vultures that circle the top of the mountain. Intricate rock formations at Top Rock provide a fascinating spectacle for those not interested in avian acrobatics. It's easy to lose track of time while atop the mountain, so be sure to leave enough time to get back to the parking lot before sundown.

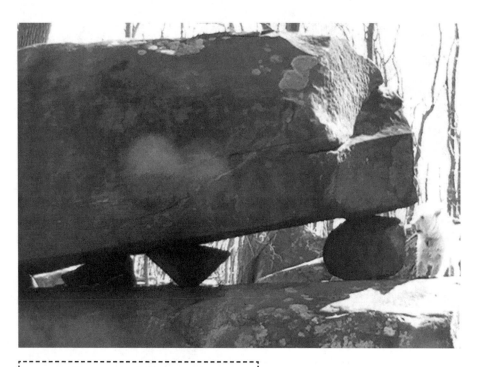

Some rock formations don't seem naturally feasible.

There is so much more of the park to explore, but this mountainous trail provides the perfect day hike and picnicking spot for adventurous hikers. Nockamixon State Park offers other hiking and biking trails, horseback riding, picnicking, and fishing. Canoes, motorboats, rowboats, sailboats, paddleboats, kayaks, and pontoon boats are available for rent during the summer season; cabins and hostels can also be rented.

## NEARBY ACTIVITIES

JOSEPH'S ITALIAN MARKET
2301 North Fifth Street, Perkasie
(215) 258-2828

LOST RIVER CAVERNS
726 Durham Street, Hellertown
(610) 838-8767
www.lostcave.com

PEARL S. BUCK HOUSE
520 Dublin Road, Perkasie
(215) 249-0100
www.psbi.org

# PEACE VALLEY PARK: Lake Galena 16

## IN BRIEF

This 6-mile hike on almost entirely paved trails around an artificial lake sometimes affords views of bald eagles. The highlight is a walk directly over a dam.

## DESCRIPTION

The area now filled by this artificial lake once provided valuable lead with which the Lenni Lenape Indians made their cooking and hunting implements. Later, it is said, nearby creeks provided the ore that was smelted into musket balls for Washington's army during its encampment at Valley Forge. An old frame building labeled a "cannon ball factory" lends further credence to the theory that valuable elements found in this area were used to make cannon balls for the Union Army during the Civil War. This rich valley also once offered zinc, lead, silver, copper, gold, and uranium to miners and prospectors. Where picks and dynamite

 **KEY AT-A-GLANCE INFORMATION**

**LENGTH:** 6 miles

**CONFIGURATION:** Loop

**DIFFICULTY:** Moderate

**SCENERY:** Lake, dam

**EXPOSURE:** Mostly sunny, some shade

**TRAIL TRAFFIC:** Medium

**TRAIL SURFACE:** Paved

**HIKING TIME:** 2 hours

**DRIVING DISTANCE FROM CENTER CITY:** 40 miles

**ACCESS:** Year-round, every day, 8 a.m.–sunset; free admission

**MAPS:** USGS Doylestown

**WHEELCHAIR TRAVERSABLE:** Partially

**FACILITIES:** Restrooms off most parking areas and in the visitor center

**SPECIAL COMMENTS:** You may want to bring binoculars because bald eagles are frequently spotted here. More information: (215) 345-7860 or www.peacevalleynaturecenter.org.

### *Directions* ⟶

Take Exit 331B from Interstate 76 west to merge onto I-476 north toward Plymouth Meeting. Continue approximately 4 miles, then take Exit 20 to merge onto I-276 east/ Pennsylvania Turnpike, toward New Jersey. Take this road 4.7 miles to Exit 339, to merge onto Fort Washington Expressway/PA 309 north toward Ambler. In just under 6 miles, bear right at North Bethlehem Pike. Go 3.5 miles, then turn right at Doylestown Road/ US 202. Turn left off US 202 onto North Main Street, then make a right at Park Avenue, which becomes Callowhill Road. Turn left at Creek Road. Take a right into Pavilion 1 parking area. The trailhead begins on your right at the sign that reads ONE WAY, BIKE AND HIKE PATH. *170 Chapman Road, Doylestown, PA 18901.*

## GPS Trailhead Coordinates

UTM Zone (WGS84)  18T

Easting   0483820

Northing   4463154

Latitude   N 40° 19' 14.3"

Longitude   W 75° 11' 25.3"

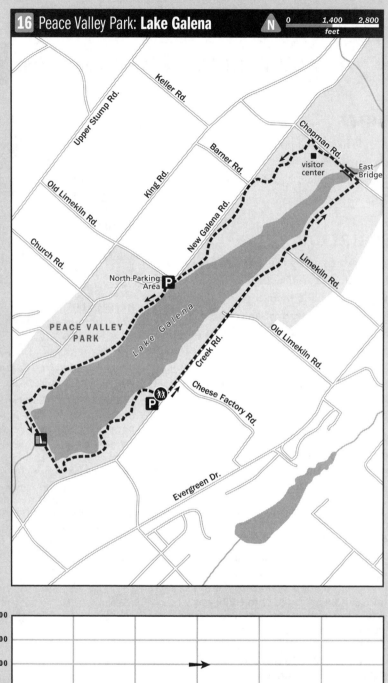

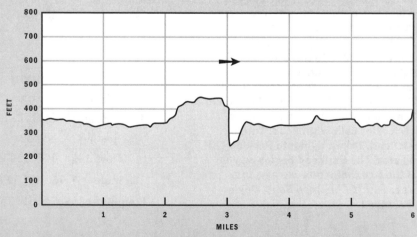

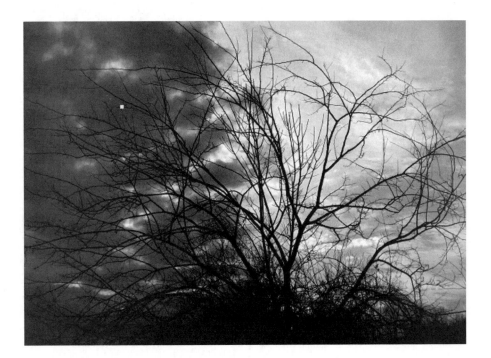

Clouds roll in behind the bracken at Peace Valley.

once rocked this area, Lake Galena and Peace Valley—a 1,500-acre park with 14 miles of nature trails—now provide rich respite for hardworking Philaburbians, and a nature sanctuary alive with gulls and geese.

Instead of a pick and shovel, hikers bring binoculars and backpacks to make the 6-mile trek around the lake, created in the early 1970s by the damming of Neshaminy Creek. Start the hike at the bike-and-hike path near Pavilion 1. A short paved trail on the left leads to the angler's pier, a favorite spot for fishermen and bird-watchers alike. This quiet corner of the park, lined with tall trees, makes a popular nesting spot for the park's birds, including the bald eagle, which began repopulation in the Bucks County area in the 1990s. This regal raptor will often look down over the hundreds of black-backed gulls that swarm the lake waters foraging for fish and nudging aside the local mallards. In spring, elegant tundra swans often pass through, appearing as dots of white along the marshy lake.

The tremolo of the common loon, perhaps agitated by a curious canine, may be heard nearby. Hawk watchers will have their best luck in September. In fact, as fall arrives, warblers, sparrows, tanagers, kinglets, orioles, and flycatchers fill the park's visitors with excitement, and binoculars point skyward from all points along the lake's perimeter. Lucky bird-watchers will spot a great blue heron stopping for refreshment.

After a short interlude with the birds, hikers can trudge through the woods beside the lake. This eventually dead-ends into a paved trail that hugs the lake

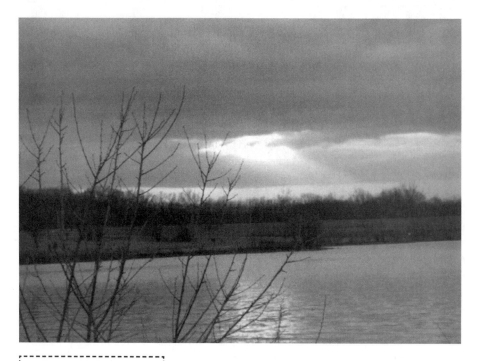

Late afternoon at Lake Galena

and provides ample space for hikers, bird-watchers, and bikers. The marshy lands to the left of the trail are off-limits, providing sanctuary for both flora and fauna. Nests can be observed in the tall trees that line the trail. Along the way, additional paths, on the right, provide options for those who wish to tread the road less traveled. The paved trail continues to the wildlife area at the trail's east end, where hikers can find peace and rest. This is a great spot to stop and look for ducks or find a family of turtles along the rocky inlet.

After this short respite, cross the bridge and follow signs to Peace Valley Nature Center (PVNC). The center's waterside trails sport bird blinds for viewing. A solar-powered building on the grounds features a weather center, maps, lookouts, educational displays, and a gift shop. The original building, built in the early 1980s, had design flaws and structural damage that left it leaky and dilapidated. The PVNC raised funds to upgrade it, completing the project in 2006. The new structure's 4.8-kilowatt array of solar panels demonstrates the modern possibilities of renewable-energy options for heating, cooling, and lighting.

After exploring the nature center, head back to the paved trail and follow it over a rolling course that offers an athletic challenge to hikers and bikers, who, up until this point, have enjoyed a smooth ride. Speaking of easy going, seasonal boat rentals are available at parking Pavilion 2, with nonmotorized water vehicles such as rowboats, paddleboats, sailboats, and kayaks. Fishing can be bountiful in season, with bass, walleye, catfish, bluegill, carp, and other native species biting.

Soon the trail diverges from the lake, and more paths appear in the woodland buffer, both left and right. Benches on this side of the lake provide a perfect spot to rest, have a sip from your water bottle, or enjoy some trail mix. The trail narrows as you head toward the northern parking pavilion, once again enjoying spectacular views of the lake. This open view marks the halfway point of this long trek.

Also near the hike's midpoint is a fishing pier that provides a perch for the many seagulls that inhabit the lake—hardly what a landlubber expects to see in the woodsy Philadelphia suburbs. However the name "seagull" is actually a misnomer, since several species of gulls can be found far from the sea. Once you reach the lake's dam, you are about three-quarters of the way around the loop. Flocks of Canada geese often use this area around the dam as a launching pad for their flight south. You, on the other hand, are heading due north toward the boat-launch pavilion, from where you'll have a remarkable view of the sunset in the early evening. After soaking in this well-deserved sunset, enjoy the last stretch of the hike, knowing that you have nearly completed a peaceful and vibrant 6-mile walk.

## NEARBY ACTIVITIES

BUCKS COUNTY CIVIL WAR MUSEUM
32 North Broad Street, Doylestown
(215) 348-8293

THE COUNTY THEATER
(Artistic and independent films)
20 East State Street, Doylestown
(215) 345-6789
www.countytheater.org

THE DOYLESTOWN INN (LODGING)
18 West State Street, Doylestown
(215) 345-6610
www.doylestowninn.com

THE JAMES A. MICHENER MUSEUM
138 South Pine Street, Doylestown
(215) 340-9800
www.michenermuseum.com

JULES THIN CRUST PIZZA
78 South Main Street, Doylestown
(215) 345-8565
www.julesthincrust.com

MORAVIAN POTTERY AND TILE WORKS
(Pottery and tile museum)
130 Swamp Road, Doylestown
(215) 345-6722
moravianpotteryandtileworks@
co.bucks.pa.us

# 17 POINT PLEASANT COMMUNITY PARK

## KEY AT-A-GLANCE INFORMATION

**LENGTH:** 2.41 miles

**CONFIGURATION:** Out-and-back

**DIFFICULTY:** Moderate

**SCENERY:** Creek, small waterfalls

**EXPOSURE:** Full shade

**TRAIL TRAFFIC:** Light

**TRAIL SURFACE:** Dirt, rocks

**HIKING TIME:** 50 minutes

**DRIVING DISTANCE FROM CENTER CITY:** 35.7 miles

**ACCESS:** Year-round, daily, dawn–dusk; free admission

**MAPS:** USGS Lumberville; no maps at park

**WHEELCHAIR TRAVERSABLE:** No

**FACILITIES:** No restrooms available

**SPECIAL COMMENTS:** Trail can be treacherous in winter.

## IN BRIEF

This hike is easier than the High Rocks hike up the river and still affords a glimpse of the Tohickon Creek.

## DESCRIPTION

Point Pleasant Community Park features a short hike up Tohickon Creek. It is easy to overlook this small park among the many surrounding attractions, such as tubing on the nearby Delaware River and the numerous activities at Tohickon Valley Park farther up the creek. Point Pleasant, known today for antiques shops and inns, once served canalmen and rafters who labored on the Delaware Canal, which passes between Tohickon Creek and the Delaware River. The town was also a way station for the Doylestown–Frenchtown–New York stage line.

The park is off Tohickon Hill Road. Entering the small parking lot, you will see a small veterans' memorial and a bridge on your right—one of several interesting old bridges crossing the creek in this area. To start the hike, take the path on the left (the only path available). On your right, several old buildings overlook the creek. In winter, large clumps of ice pile up and form shapes on the banks. The creek is not deep here, and

## GPS Trailhead Coordinates

UTM Zone (WGS84)  18T

Easting   0494303

Northing   4474697

Latitude   N 40° 25' 22.3"

Longitude   W 75° 4' 1.9"

## *Directions*

From Philadelphia, take PA 611 north 13.8 miles. At the fork in Willow Grove, take a right onto PA 263. After 13.1 miles, turn left onto PA 413. Drive 4.3 miles and turn right onto Ferry Road–Point Pleasant Pike. Continue 4.3 miles, then turn left onto Tohickon Hill Road in Point Pleasant, just before PA 32. Park in the lot immediately on the right. *Tohickon Hill Road, Pipersville, PA 18947.*

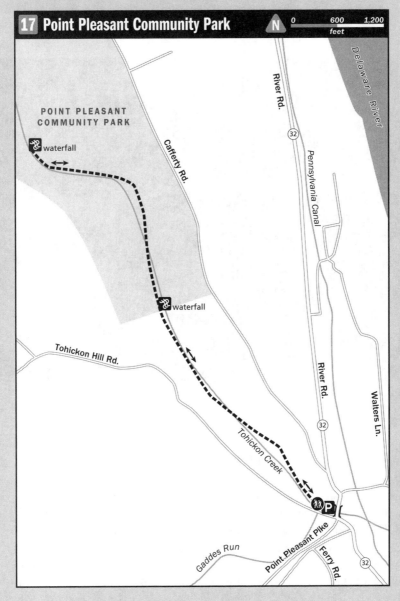

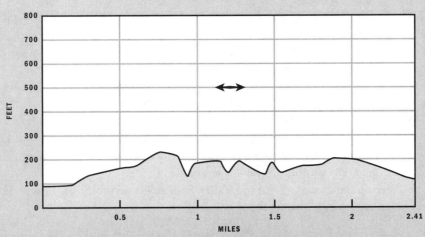

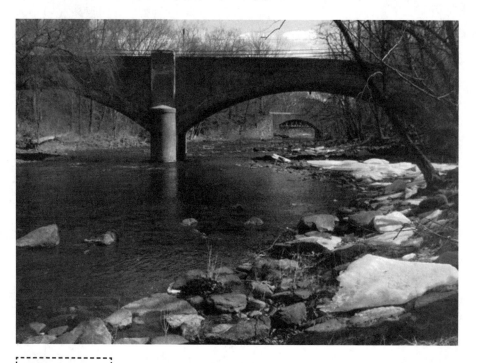

River Road bridge

you can see the rapids running over large stones. The sound of rushing water accompanies you the length of this hike.

Point Pleasant Community Park is near the end of Tohickon Creek, which begins at the Lake Nockamixon dam. When the dam releases excess lake water into the creek, it creates perfect conditions for kayaking. Because of its constant flow, Tohickon Creek is one of the cleanest streams in Pennsylvania and is full of carp, pickerel, bass, and, reputedly, freshwater mussels. *Tohickon* is a Lenape name meaning "Deer Bone Creek," indicating that the area was a robust hunting ground. The diverse array of plant life includes toothwort, bloodroot, wild ginger, and bishop's cap.

After 0.25 miles, the path starts to ascend and get rockier. You'll see rock formations on the left. Water runs down these rocky slopes into the creek at several points on this hike. In winter, ice decorates the cliffs. The rocks can be slippery, especially after snow or rain. Occasionally, a large tree blocks the trail.

After 0.5 miles, the trail climbs more steeply, and you walk on what appears to be a stone wall, perhaps once marking a property line.

Nearly a mile into the hike, and across the creek, is a stone foundation that may be from a mill. Mills were common along the creek during the 18th century. In fact, gristmills here ground grain during the Revolutionary War. Earlier, the Lenape quarried argillite to fashion weapons.

Farther up the creek, a Tohickon Valley Park cabin is visible, one of several rustic rental cabins near the creek.

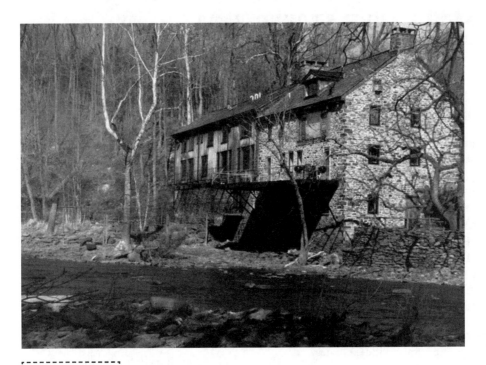

Old Village House

The path ends at a large rock formation. From its top you can see the porch of a private house. You can also sit here and relax as you watch a waterfall pour from a cliff into the valley below. To finish the hike, retrace your steps.

The landscape can change dramatically along Tohickon Creek. Parts of the valley are relatively level; others feature steep cliffs and rocky terrain that can challenge even the most experienced hiker. For example, at the High Rocks farther up the creek, vertical walls of stone reach heights of 200 feet. In comparison, the area around Point Pleasant seems relatively level—perfect for those who want to see the area but aren't ready for a more advanced hike.

## NEARBY ACTIVITIES

BUCKS COUNTY RIVER COUNTRY
*(Tube and canoe rentals)*
2 Walters Lane, Point Pleasant
(215) 297-5000
**www.rivercountry.net/august/index.html**

SAND CASTLE WINERY
255 River Road, Erwinna
(610) 294-918
**www.sandcastlewinery.com**

# RALPH STOVER STATE PARK:
## 18 High Rocks

## KEY AT-A-GLANCE INFORMATION

**LENGTH:** 1.43 miles

**CONFIGURATION:** Loop

**DIFFICULTY:** Moderate, with 1 strenuous descent

**SCENERY:** Canyon view and creek

**EXPOSURE:** Sunny, some shade

**TRAIL TRAFFIC:** Light

**TRAIL SURFACE:** Dirt, shale

**HIKING TIME:** 1 hour

**DRIVING DISTANCE FROM CENTER CITY:** 53 miles

**ACCESS:** Daily, dawn–dusk, year-round; free admission

**MAPS:** USGS Lumberville; no maps at park

**WHEELCHAIR TRAVERSABLE:** No

**FACILITIES:** Outhouse in parking lot

**SPECIAL COMMENTS:** One outhouse available at parking area. There are some great views and some steep drops. More information: (610) 982-5560; dcnr.state.pa.us/stateparks/parks/ralphstover.aspx.

## GPS Trailhead Coordinates

UTM Zone (WGS84) 18T

Easting 0491437

Northing 4476714

Latitude N 40° 26' 27.64"

Longitude W 75° 6' 3.51"

## IN BRIEF

This challenging hike features some of the best vistas near the Delaware River.

## DESCRIPTION

The High Rocks vista area is part of Ralph Stover State Park at Point Pleasant, Pennsylvania. The canyon cut by the Tohickon Creek, more than 300 feet deep in some spots, defines the park. The cliffs create beautiful vistas from many vantage points. For this adventurous hike, you should be in reasonable physical condition in order to handle the steep pathways in the middle section.

After entering High Rocks from the parking lot across the road, you can enjoy the views from behind the black safety fence along the cliff's edge. The hike starts to the right (west). To begin, start following the fence line to the right. Where the fence line ends, there will be small pathways leading down to the middle trail. These pathways descend only

--------------------------------------------

## Directions ⟶

Take Interstate 95 north from Philadelphia. After 29 miles, take Exit 51 and turn left at the end of the ramp. Take the first right onto Woodside Road, then the first left onto PA 32–River Road. Follow PA 32 a scenic 20 miles north along the Delaware River to Point Pleasant. At Point Pleasant, take a left at the fork onto Cafferty Road (there's a church at the fork). After almost 2 miles, turn left onto Tory Road, a dirt road. After 1.5 miles, stay left on Tory Road, which will turn into a dirt-and-gravel road (do not take Wormansville Road on the right). After 1,000 feet, the small parking lot is on the right. After parking, cross the street to High Rocks. *6011 State Park Road, Pipersville, PA 18947.*

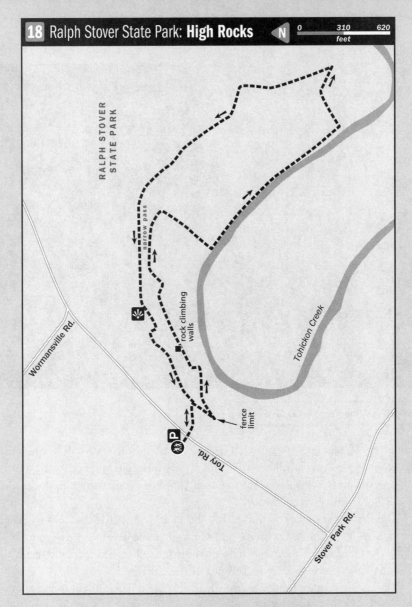

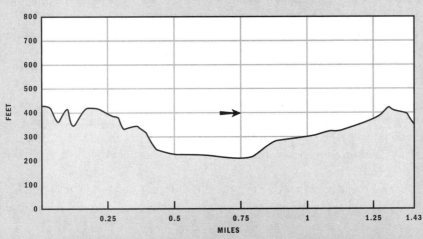

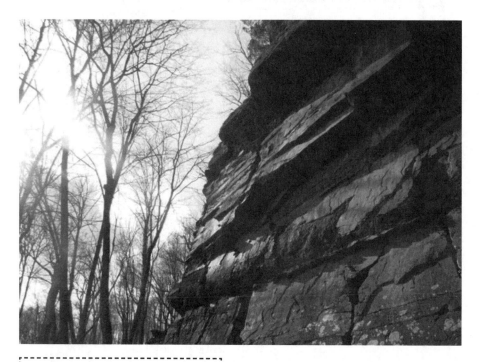

The don't call them High Rocks for nothing.

some 30 or 40 feet and are not well defined. The middle trail will become more defined once you reach a large cliff face to the left. This middle trail, which is sometimes quite narrow, is a natural trail that runs along the cliff faces about 100 feet up from the creek below.

The first sight is the top half of the sheer, 200-foot cliff face. On weekends, it attracts rock climbers. Farther along the trail, some overhangs are too dangerous for the climbers. The only inhabitants of these cliffs are turkey vultures and red-tailed hawks, which soar in and out of the canyon.

The creek sounds louder as the trail descends. Toward the bottom of the cliff, there is a 20-foot pass less than a foot wide, with a 50-foot drop below. Fortunately, a safety rope was recently attached to the cliff.

Soon after the narrow pass, the middle trail ends (more or less). Take a sharp right turn along the side of a short, east-facing cliff that leads to the creek. This is not a well-defined path, but rather one of many ways to get down to the creek's edge. If the path at first seems too steep, walk farther along the middle trail and look for an easier way down to the creek. Either way, it's best to walk sideways as you descend, because loose shale makes the footing treacherous. If the creek sounds especially loud, then extra water has been released from the Lake Nockamixon dam a few miles northwest, to the delight of kayakers farther down the creek.

Once you reach the creek's edge, the difficult part of the hike is over. This is a good time to have lunch on one of the many boulders on or in the creek. The cliffs you just hiked can be seen from the middle of the creek. Water runs in this spot even during a dry August.

Follow the creek downstream for almost a quarter mile. This may seem strange since downstream is a northwesterly direction—against the direction in which the Delaware River flows—but the creek takes a dramatic hairpin turn to the northwest for a half mile before it flows southeasterly and eventually drains into the Delaware. It's this hairpin turn that carved out the dramatic landscape over many thousands of years. If the creek is not too high, it's fun to jump from boulder to boulder. Otherwise, use the trail on the bank. When you see a Boy Scout camp clearing across the stream on the right (it may have archery targets), start looking for the returning trail entrance on the left. This entrance has no signage of any kind but can be clearly seen, just a few yards after the Boy Scout camp.

The quarter-mile climb up is not as steep as the climb down, and pine trees shade the trail. The trail eventually intersects the black safety fence. This is the best spot for pictures of the Tohickon canyon.

Walk along the black fence line (going west) and stop at any of the designated vista points. After a couple hundred yards, a small red pedestrian bridge on the right will lead you back to the parking lot.

## NEARBY ACTIVITIES

BUCKS COUNTY RIVER COUNTRY
*(Tube and canoe rentals)*
2 Walters Lane, Point Pleasant
(215) 297-5000
www.rivercountry.net/august/index.html

SAND CASTLE WINERY
255 River Road, Erwinna
(610) 294-918
www.sandcastlewinery.com

# 19  RINGING ROCKS COUNTY PARK

### KEY AT-A-GLANCE INFORMATION

**LENGTH:** 1 mile

**CONFIGURATION:** Balloon

**DIFFICULTY:** Difficult

**SCENERY:** Boulders and waterfall walk (in wetter months)

**EXPOSURE:** Full sun–full shade

**TRAIL TRAFFIC:** Moderate

**TRAIL SURFACE:** Rocky

**HIKING TIME:** 1 hour or less

**DRIVING DISTANCE FROM CENTER CITY:** 60 miles

**ACCESS:** Year-round, every day, dawn–dusk; free admission

**FACILITIES:** Restroom off the parking lot

**MAPS:** USGS Rieglesville

**WHEELCHAIR TRAVERSABLE:** No

**SPECIAL COMMENTS:** Dogs and small children may have trouble negotiating this landscape. Bring a small hammer or other blunt object to produce ringing tones with the rocks. To hit some virtual rocks before you go, visit www.unmuseum.org/ringrock.htm.

- - - - - - - - - - - - - - - - - - - - - - - - - - - -

GPS Trailhead
Coordinates

UTM Zone (WGS84)  18T

Easting   0489099

Northing   4489963

Latitude   N 40° 33' 37.27"

Longitude   W 75° 7' 43.54"

## IN BRIEF

Bring a hammer and hold your own rock concert at this park where many of the rocks in its seven-acre boulder field produce distinct musical notes and tones. Visit the nearby High Falls for more privacy and geological wonders.

## DESCRIPTION

*"No one knows who they were, or what they were doing. But their legacy remains hewn into the living rock."*

—Christopher Guest speaking of Stonehenge in *This Is Spinal Tap*, 1984

Like Stonehenge, Ringing Rocks in Upper Black Eddy, Pennsylvania, has been shrouded in its own lore and local mystery, but the seven-acre boulder field in the park is actually 100 percent natural.

The rock found in the park was formed from volcanic magma during the Pleistocene epoch. This part of Pennsylvania, although not glaciated at that time, contained frozen ground, and the bedrock progressively broke

- - - - - - - - - - - - - - - - - - - - - - - - - - - - - - - -

*Directions* ———————————————➤

**From Philadelphia, follow US 95 north 30 miles. Take Exit 1 to reach PA 29 north toward Lambertville, and merge onto PA 29, continuing 9 miles. This road becomes 165/PA 165. After a few blocks, look for Bridge Street/PA 179 on your left. Make the left here to head over the bridge to New Hope. Right after you cross the bridge, make a right onto PA 32, then travel 11 miles north along the river on a scenic drive. Turn left at Bridgeton Hill Road. After 1.5 miles, turn right at Ringing Rocks Road. The park entrance is a few blocks down on the right. The trail starts just behind the parking lot, on the north side. *Ringing Rocks Road, Upper Black Eddy, PA 18972.***

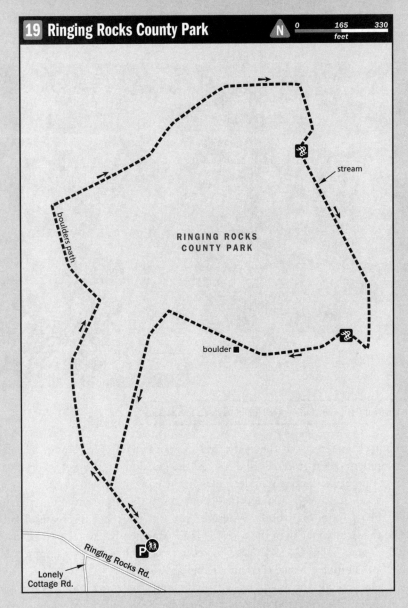

N

0    165    330
feet

RINGING ROCKS
COUNTY PARK

stream

boulders path

boulder ■

P

Ringing Rocks Rd.

Lonely
Cottage Rd.

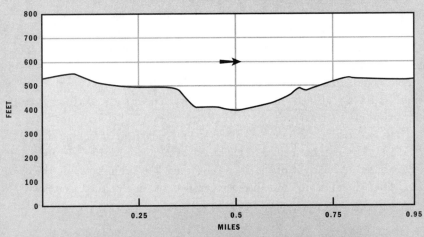

FEET

800
700
600
500
400
300
200
100
0

0.25        0.5        0.75        0.95
MILES

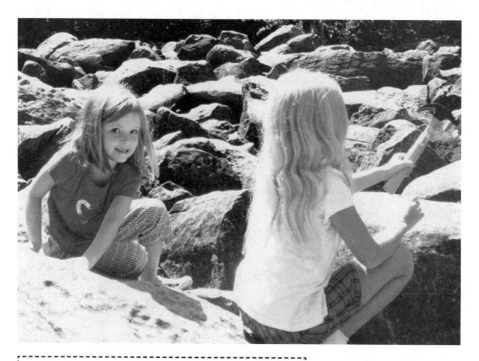

Kaelyn Kear (left) and Clarissa Kear (right) having a jam session

apart into boulders from the cyclic freezing and thawing of water. The large rock fragments then gradually slid toward the meadow on the wet, slippery soil, creating one of the largest boulder fields in the eastern United States.

The ten-foot-deep boulder field contains little flora and limited fauna, unlike the surrounding woods. When the sun hits the rocks, it creates a microclimate that is warmer than the forested landscape nearby. What attracts people to this 65-acre Bucks County park, however, is not the landscape so much as its musical possibilities; hence the name Ringing Rocks.

When you hit the boulders with a hammer or other blunt object, they produce a unique tone and note. Geologists have studied this phenomenon for decades, conducting laboratory experiments with sophisticated equipment to determine the cause of the sounds. They believe that the high content of metals such as iron and aluminum, combined with the size of the boulders, their internal pressure, and their spatial relationship with surrounding boulders give them each their own distinct sound. Folks joke that these diabase rocks are the perfect instruments for a real heavy-metal rock concert. These sorts of ringing rocks, though found in other parts of the world, too, are especially abundant here.

Locals like to give the rock field more of a mystical bent, attaching a curse to the field and claiming that compasses spin out of control toward their midpoints and that animals steer clear of the area altogether. You cannot dispute the eerie feel of the place, and its mystique has been argued and analyzed ad nauseam.

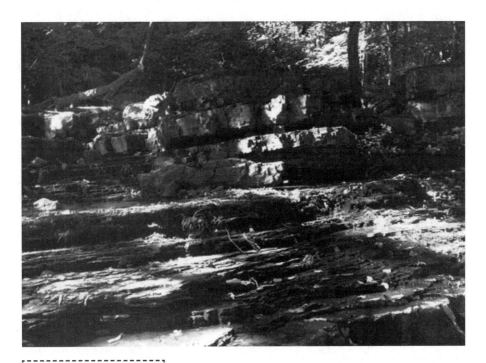

Flat rocks near the waterfall

Despite the supernatural myths and scientific explanations, the best reason to visit is the fun—scampering from rock to rock, noticing the patterns from hammer indentations and erosion, and finding a rock that makes your own personal joyful noise. But the park offers more than just a bunch of boulders.

The trailhead is at the northern corner of the parking lot. The trail, lined with oak and sassafras, soon forks. Bear left and head northeast to the rocks. After you have clanged to your heart's content, climb through the boulder field and find the trail's continuation on your right, heading north.

The trail, although not blazed, is easy to follow. However, downed trees sometimes obstruct the path. The ringing in the distance is soon drowned out by the sound of water flowing and birds chirping, with no signs of civilization save the occasional plane overhead.

Continue north until you come to more boulders by a stream. Climb along the right side of the boulder field and then walk toward the flat rock in the middle. This is a nice spot to sit and enjoy the surroundings, but steer clear of the edge—a 20-foot drop can be fatal.

After your rest, continue uphill until you see cliffs above and the trickle of a waterfall ahead. Despite the height of the cliffs, the High Falls rarely gushes and usually spouts a mere shower at best, meaning you won't get wet unless you really want to.

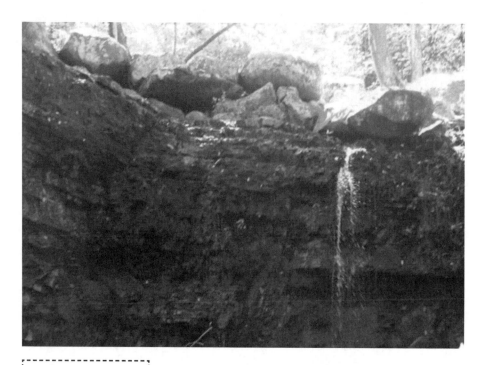

The "Falls" on a dry day

This romantic spot—secluded on weekdays—is cool in midsummer and provides a natural backdrop for photographs. When you are ready, continue up the boulders to the top of the cliff to pick up a trail on the eastern side of the boulder field, for more harmonious banging.

The park is nature's playground; no jungle gym could ever duplicate what God has placed in these seven acres. You can bring a sample back to a lab for examination or search local literature for folkloric explanations. Or you can just accept the great mystery and enjoy the music, one note and one rock at a time.

## NEARBY ACTIVITIES

THE BAKER
*(All-natural baked goods and coffee)*
60 Bridge Street, Milford
(908) 995-4040
(908) 995-9669 (fax)

CHESTNUT HILL ON THE DELAWARE
*(Bed-and-breakfast)*
63 Church Street, Milford
(888) 333-2242 or (908) 995-9761
**www.milfordonthedelaware.com**

THE MILFORD OYSTER HOUSE
*(Fresh-seafood restaurant and tavern)*
92 Water Street, Milford
(908) 995-9411
**www.milfordoysterhouse.com**

# TAMANEND PARK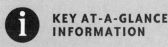

## IN BRIEF

This hike offers well-designed trails and a slice of history, with a classic farmhouse and barn listed in the National Registry of Historic Places. This part of Bucks County also saw dealings between the Native Americans and William Penn during the first settlement period.

## DESCRIPTION

The park office–visitor center offers plenty of literature to introduce hikers and visitors to the park's natural sites and other amenities. Old buildings on the property date back to the 18th century. The farmhouse, carriage house, and white barn offer glimpses into a simpler time, and the stone springhouse reminds visitors of the refrigeration techniques used for centuries before the icebox and well before electric refrigerators.

But the name, *Tamanend,* provides the best hint about the history of this park and its nearby land. Chief Tamanend (Tammany), along with other Lenni Lenape leaders, worked with William Penn and his settlers to established peace between the Native Americans and the colonists when Philadelphia was first founded. The part of Bucks County where

### KEY AT-A-GLANCE INFORMATION

**LENGTH: 1.4 Miles**

**CONFIGURATION: Double loop**

**DIFFICULTY: Easy–moderate**

**SCENERY: Old trees and historic farm buildings**

**EXPOSURE: Some full sun, but mostly shade**

**TRAIL TRAFFIC: Light on weekdays, medium on weekends**

**TRAIL SURFACE: Dirt, mowed grass**

**HIKING TIME: 30 minutes**

**DRIVING DISTANCE FROM CENTER CITY: 25 miles**

**ACCESS: Year-round, every day, dawn–dusk; free admission**

**MAPS: USGS Hatboro**

**FACILITIES: Restrooms off the parking lot near tot lot; picnic areas with pavilions, tennis courts, a tot lot, a gazebo, gardens, and softball fields**

**WHEELCHAIR TRAVERSABLE: No**

**SPECIAL COMMENTS: The property has some historic buildings from the early 1800s. The Tribute Rocks are toward the northeastern end of the parking lot.**

## Directions

Take Interstate 95 north from Center City. Take Exit 37 for Street Road toward PA 132. Turn left at Street Road. Turn right on Second Street Pike. The park is less than 1 mile farther, on the right. Once you enter the park, find a parking space toward the back of the long driveway, beside the park office and carriage house. *1255 Second Street Pike, Southampton, PA 18966.*

### GPS Trailhead Coordinates

UTM Zone (WGS84) 18T

Easting 0497282

Northing 4447738

Latitude N 40° 10' 48.04"

Longitude W 75° 1' 54.93"

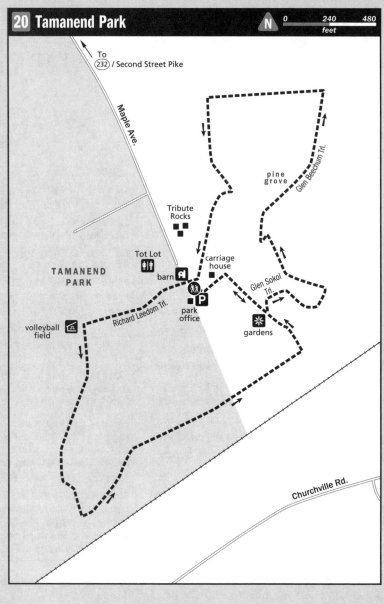

N

0    240    480
**feet**

To
(232) / Second Street Pike

Maple Ave.

pine
grove

Glen Beechum Trl.

Tribute
Rocks

Tot Lot

carriage
house

barn

**TAMANEND
PARK**

Glen Sokol
Trl.

volleyball
field

Richard Leedom Trl.

park
office

gardens

Churchville Rd.

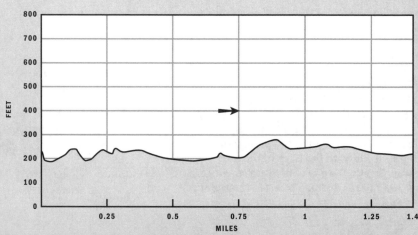

800

700

600

500

400

300

200

100

0

FEET

0.25    0.5    0.75    1    1.25    1.4

MILES

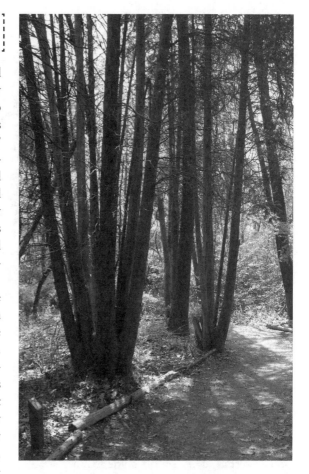

The trails at Tamanend are well maintained.

Tamanend Park is located was sold to Penn in "a treaty of friendship" intended to endure "as long as the grass is green and the rivers flow." Chief Tamanend later became somewhat of a legend because of his service and kindness to the area's early settlers, and St. Tammany's Day, May 1, was observed for many years with a joyous festival.

Clearly, not everyone had peaceful relations with the Native Americans in the 17th and 18th centuries. Some early settlers considered the Native Americans savages and pagans. But Penn himself had personally experienced persecution for his beliefs. As a young man, he rebelled against the Anglican Church by joining the Quakers (The Religious Society of Friends) and was arrested and jailed several times for his writings and religious practices.

King Charles II of England owed a large sum of money to Penn's father, Admiral Sir William Penn. The king settled the note by granting a large area west and south of New Jersey to Penn after Admiral Penn's death. Charles also honored Sir William by naming the area Pennsylvania. Penn maintained Pennsylvania as an area where freedom of religion could thrive. He befriended the local Native Americans and ensured that they were paid fairly for their lands, gave them the right to fair trial, and learned some of their languages to promote communication.

Penn had to return to England in 1701, however, because his financial advisor, Philip Ford, had cheated him out of thousands of pounds. In England he tried to resolve his case in court, a case that dragged on for more than a decade. In 1712 Penn suffered a stroke, which left him feeble and unable to communicate or argue his case. He died penniless in 1718. His family retained ownership of the colony of Pennsylvania. Unfortunately, his son James, who inherited the family property, did not share his father's love of peace, democracy, and religious freedom.

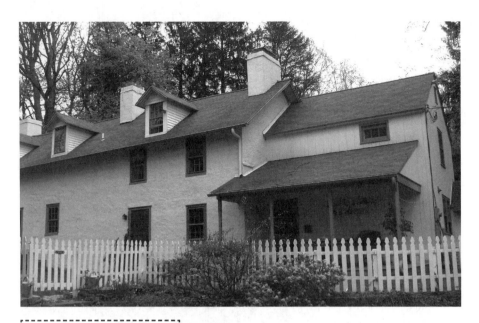

Old farmhouse at Tamanend Park

Penn's descendants told the local tribes that, according to a document in the Penn family's possession, the Lenni Lenape had promised to sell a tract of land beginning at Wrightstown, Bucks County, and extending back "as far as a man could go in a day and a half." The legal veracity of this document has never been proven, but, if true, the "day and a half" would translate into about 40 to 50 miles. But the colonists hired their fastest runners to run the distance on a prepared trail. They set off on September 19, 1737, to cover as much ground as possible, stopping only to sleep. The pace was so intense that only one of the men continued the full day and a half. But on that marathon, he had reached the town of John Thorpe, more than 70 miles away. This trick permitted the Penns to inherit 1.2 million acres of land (approximately the size of Rhode Island). The event went down in history as "The Walking Purchase." Most of the Lenape were eventually driven toward the Ohio River Valley and beyond.

In 1975 a contest was held by Southampton Township to name the park. The winning entry was "Tamanend," which reminds residents of Chief Tamanend and what occurred when settlers first came to this area.

Despite the land's history, the park certainly has its share of harmonious landscapes and peaceful corners for quiet meditation. In addition to the trails, the park offers picnic areas with pavilions, tennis courts, a tot lot, a gazebo, gardens, and softball fields. As you walk past the visitor center and farmhouse and into a clearing, you come to a grove of trees that includes oaks, maples, and pines, each labeled by species. These labels will help you become familiar with some of the common native trees found in this part of Pennsylvania. Bear left to reach an herb garden, which scents the air with spice in late spring and summer.

Head past a magnificent pine, and then continue straight to the start of the Glen Sokol Trail. There are park benches and picnic tables here, a perfect lunch spot for later in the day.

Continue along the trail, and listen for the sound of the many birds that make this park their year-round residence, including Carolina chickadees, tufted titmice, American robins, cedar waxwings, eastern towhees, house finches, brown-headed cowbirds, mourning doves, and various sparrows.

Continue to follow signs for the Glen Sokol Trail, ignoring various side trails that depart left and right. Follow the trail back to the farmhouse and visitor center, and then join the Glen Beecham Trail. Maps at the visitor center will ensure you find your way back to the main trail should you decide to explore an unmarked trail among the 5 miles or so of trails in the park's 100 wooded acres.

As you stroll along, white birch peak through the green forest; a beech magnolia glade and butterfly garden lie to the right. Continue to a shady stand of pines. This quiet spot is dedicated to Jesse Dyer, an Eagle Scout who loved Tamanend Park and helped maintain its trails. Jesse died at age 20. "Do as many things as you can, if not more," he said. "The memories will last forever."

Continue along Glen Sokol Trail until you come to a **T**-junction. Turn left and then left again when you glimpse a school on your right. Now, with a brook to your right, continue until you arrive back at the farmhouse. Next to the visitor center, find the bird blind for a closer look at the resident birds. Afterward, pick up Richard Leedom Trail, which is 25 feet or less from the visitor center. This trail wanders beside colorful wildflowers and blooming trees in spring and summer. Continue straight, then make a left at the volleyball field onto a wide trail that leads to an open field. Here, bear right and amble through a pine grove. Continue straight at the junction ahead. Descend and bear left, with old railroad tracks on your right. After about 0.25 miles, find a tree with a red mark near a junction. Turn left here to make the scenic stroll back to the trailhead.

Before you leave the park, you may want to stop by the Tamanend Tribute Rocks. These river boulders honor the Lenni Lenape Indians, who made peace with this area's first European settlers and with William Penn, who said, "I desire to enjoy [this land] with your love, and consent that we may always live together as neighbors and friends."

## NEARBY ACTIVITIES

This hike is near the Churchville Nature Center hike, which is described in this book on page 21.

THE BLUE SAGE VEGETARIAN GRILLE
772 Second Street Pike, Southampton
(215) 942-8888
**www.bluesagegrille.com**

# 21 | TINICUM COUNTY PARK

## KEY AT-A-GLANCE INFORMATION

**LENGTH: 1.8 miles**

**CONFIGURATION: Loop**

**DIFFICULTY: Easy**

**SCENERY: Canal, open field, historic home and barn**

**EXPOSURE: Full shade–full sun**

**TRAIL TRAFFIC: Light**

**TRAIL SURFACE: Gravel, paved, grass**

**HIKING TIME: 45 minutes**

**DRIVING DISTANCE FROM CENTER CITY: 42 miles**

**ACCESS: Year-round, every day, dawn–dusk; free but a fee applies for the Erwin–Stover Tour.**

**MAPS: USGS Frenchtown**

**WHEELCHAIR TRAVERSABLE: Not this hike, but the park contains paved paths to the fields and historic homes**

**FACILITIES: Outhouse near the barn**

**SPECIAL COMMENTS: Kid friendly; seasonal art shows and tours from June–September, Friday and Saturday, noon–4 p.m. Visit the Bucks County Parks and Recreation Web site at www.buckscounty.org/ government/departments/Parks andRec/Parks/TinicumPrograms. aspx or call (908) 996-3321 to learn about events such as symphonies and antique shows within the park.**

## IN BRIEF

A breathtaking river drive takes you to this park that sits near quaint, historic Frenchtown; weekend fairs and activities abound at the park and in the town. Take a lazy walk along a strip of the canal, admire the wildlife, then shoot into town for dinner and window-shopping.

## DESCRIPTION

When townies think of Tinicum County Park, they often think of colorful polo matches, with helmet-clad jockeys raising their whips as they fly cross the field, bouncing on their saddles and swinging their mallets. Tinicum County Park has become a favorite day trip for Philadelphians who want to make the scenic drive up River Road, take in some sport, and then wind down in nearby Frenchtown at one of its gourmet restaurants or cafés.

Tinicum County Park has more to offer, and much of this gets lost in the hustle and bustle of the park's Saturday afternoon polo match. Access the trailhead from the back parking lot (the farthest from the entrance), where a small playground offers swings and monkey bars for children. Walk westward until you reach the entrance to the Delaware Canal towpath; here, turn right and head north along the gravel path.

GPS Trailhead
Coordinates

UTM Zone (WGS84) 18T

Easting 0493800

Northing 4483920

Latitude N 40° 30' 21.4"

Longitude W 75° 4' 23.3"

## *Directions*

**From US 95 north, take Exit 51 toward New Hope. Keep right at the fork, following signs for Yardley, and merge onto Taylorsville Road. Make a U-turn at Highland Drive, and turn left to stay on Taylorsville Road. Turn left at River Road (PA 32). Continue north 15 miles on this famous scenic drive, then look for Tinicum County Park on your left. *963 River Road, Erwinna, PA 18972.***

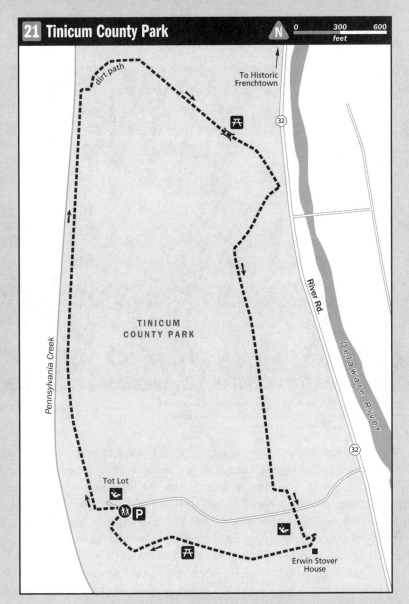

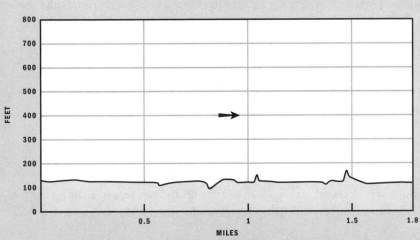

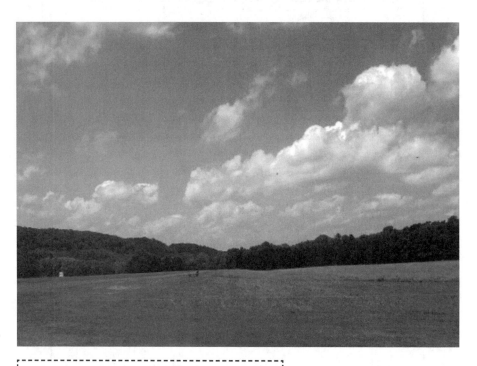

The grassy fields forefront to hills at Tinicum County Park.

The park borders a 0.25-mile stretch of the canal, where lowlands climb toward rolling hills. Along the canal, painted turtles meander along fallen trees, and white-tailed deer roam to the water's edge for food and drink. Butterflies flutter and dragonflies buzz back and forth. Frogs and bunnies hop from the canal area to the park and back. Woodchucks, skunks, mice, voles, squirrels, foxes, and more than 90 species of birds are among the other animals seen along the canal. As the sun dips, so do the nocturnal bats that come to dine on flying insects.

In midsummer, canal waters fall below a foot in some places and almost disappear in the swampy growth. Residential development along the Delaware River has encroached upon many areas along the canal, affecting runoff and water levels. The canal rises and falls, depending on the time of year and the weather.

After a leisurely stroll, and with a few private residences in the distance, turn right on a dirt path and walk eastward across a grassy slope toward open fields. Be careful not to slip, especially when the ground is damp, while descending into the grassland below. Walk along the trees and listen for the sparrows, blue jays, and cardinals as they flit through the forest.

Soon you can take advantage of a break in the trees on your right to cross via a small bridge. Once you're across, a picnic table offers the perfect spot to stop for a packed snack and a sip of cool water from your bottle. Although this is a relatively short hike, the sun can become oppressive in midsummer.

Once you've rested, cross back over the bridge and continue along the tree line until you see a baseball field on your right. Turn right (southward) behind the ball field while you admire the rolling hills, now on your right. Pass behind some red outbuildings and find the paved trail, which takes you to the road that originally brought you into the park. Cross over this road and enter a gravel parking lot close to River Road. The Erwin–Stover house and barn stand to the left of the lot.

William Erwin built this home in 1810. His father, Colonel Arthur Erwin, bought the land after serving in the Revolutionary War. In 1849 Henry S. Stover, a gristmill and sawmill businessman, purchased the farm. Stover doubled the size of the original house and built the enormous red barn that now welcomes visitors to the park and also hosts seasonal art shows and tours.

Stover's grandson John donated the house, barn, and 126 acres to the county. This land became Tinicum County Park in 1957. In addition to touring the federal-style home, visitors can use the park's playgrounds, pavilions, and picnic areas; hike, boat, and fish; and even reserve an overnight campsite.

Once you have toured the home and barn, take the gravel path that leads west from the Erwin–Stover parking lot through an open field. Across the field, turn right, toward a clearing that offers picnicking under the pines and a shaded path back to the canal and the parking lot where you started this loop.

Families with children can enjoy the playground or play a round of disc golf, but before ending your day, spend some time in nearby Frenchtown. This historic river town hosts a Wine and Arts Weekend, the locally renowned Bastille Day, River Fest, and Dogs on the Delaware (with silhouettes of painted pooch statues). Frenchtown's artsy boutiques, bike shops, and cafés make a visit here a perfect ending to a day along the scenic Delaware River drive.

## NEARBY ACTIVITIES

BUCKS COUNTY RIVER COUNTRY
*(Canoe and tube rentals)*
2 Walters Lane, Point Pleasant
(215) 297-5000
**www.rivercountry.net**

HISTORIC FRENCHTOWN
*(Boutiques, antiques, and lots of shopping without mall crowds)*
**www.frenchtown.com**

## FRENCHTOWN RESTAURANTS

BRIDGE CAFÉ
*(Ken and Lisa Miller, proprietors)*
8 Bridge Street
(908) 996-6040

COCINA DEL SOL 10
Bridge Street
(908) 996-0900

CORNERSTONE CAFÉ
Twelfth and Harrison Streets
(908) 996-2885

FRENCHTOWN CAFÉ
44 Bridge Street
(908) 996-0663

FRENCHTOWN INN
7 Bridge Street
(908) 996-3300

## 22 TOHICKON VALLEY PARK:
### Tohickon Creek Gorge

### KEY AT-A-GLANCE INFORMATION

**LENGTH: 5 miles**

**CONFIGURATION: Loop**

**DIFFICULTY: Difficult**

**SCENERY: Forest, old stone walls, cliffs overlooking a creek**

**EXPOSURE: Mostly shaded**

**TRAIL TRAFFIC: Light**

**TRAIL SURFACE: Dirt, gravel**

**HIKING TIME: 2 hours**

**DRIVING DISTANCE FROM CENTER CITY: 50 miles**

**ACCESS: Year-round, every day, dawn–dusk; free admission**

**MAPS: USGS Lumberville; maps available at park in summer**

**FACILITIES: Restrooms near the pool and playground when open**

**WHEELCHAIR TRAVERSABLE: No**

**SPECIAL COMMENTS: If you continue on Cafferty Road to the Ralph Stover State Park Lookout Point parking lot, you can walk approximately 50 feet down to the lookout with its views of the wide-open gorge—one of the best views in Bucks County; see www .buckscounty.org/government/ departments/parksandrec/Parks/ Tohickon.aspx or call (215) 297-0754 for more information.**

### GPS Trailhead Coordinates

UTM Zone (WGS84)  18T

Easting   0493490

Northing   4476370

Latitude   N 40° 26' 16.7"

Longitude   W 75° 4' 35.9"

### IN BRIEF

This hike may well be the most scenic hiking experiences in eastern Pennsylvania, and it is certainly one of the best. After weaving through old logging areas and farm country and up a cliff walk to a vast scenic peak, it dips down to the crystal-clear creek below.

### DESCRIPTION

If no one has ever told you about Tohickon Valley Park, it is because nobody wants to give away the secret. This 612-acre park weaves through dry-stack walls of natural stone and old logging communities. White-tailed deer wander through forests of tulip poplar, oak, hickory, and hemlock. In the fall, these trees look as if someone has plugged them in. At the end of the cliff, walk to the High Rocks vista, where you're rewarded with a view of the snakelike southern course of Tohickon Creek some 200 feet below.

Tohickon Valley Park and the adjacent Ralph Stover Park are not only among the best hiking spots in eastern Pennsylvania, but one of the best vacations spots as well. You could pay thousands of dollars to fly your

### *Directions*

Follow Interstate 95 north 29 miles from Philadelphia and then take Exit 51. Turn left at the end of the ramp. Make the first right onto Woodside Road, then the first left onto PA 32 (River Road). Follow PA 32 a scenic 20 miles north along the Delaware River to Point Pleasant. At Point Pleasant, take the left fork, onto Cafferty Road (there's a church between the forks). Tohickon Valley Park is on the left after about 1 mile. A wooden post marks the trailhead, to the right of the parking lot. *127 Cafferty Road, Point Pleasant, PA 18950.*

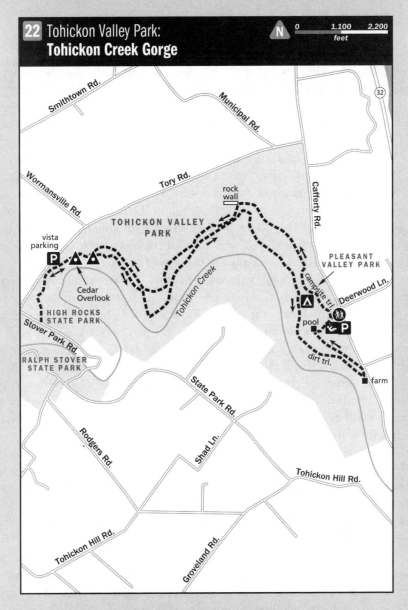

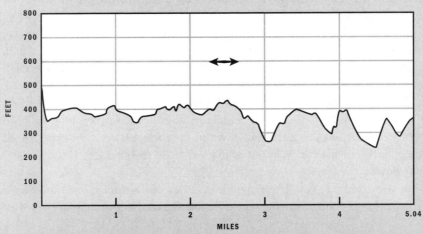

family to some exotic tourist trap, or you could rent a cabin 20 feet from the soothing sounds of a flowing creek and listen to the crickets while watching the stars illuminate the sky. Then you could retire to your cabin, make s'mores in the fireplace, wake up to hike the cliffs the next morning, and enjoy one of the best views in Pennsylvania.

After your hike, take a dip in the pool (if you visit in summer), or go fishing, paddle a canoe, or simply lie on a warm, flat rock in the middle of the creek and watch the leaves rustle in the wind while bursts of dappled sunshine warm your cheeks. If this sounds too relaxing, hop in the car and enjoy some of the nearby attractions of the Upper Bucks County river country, such as tubing, antiquing, or wine tasting. And why not visit the historic Stover Mill (now an art gallery) or go bike riding along the Delaware Canal?

Your morning hike is all mapped out before you arrive. The hike starts at the parking lot, but the trail can also be picked up from the tent-camping area. Looking into the park from the parking lot, less than 50 feet ahead, to the right, take the asphalt walkway to the wooden TRAILS sign, where the path leads you north. At the next TRAIL sign, turn left and head west. Continue along the well-maintained path through the tent-camping area, heading northwest.

At the end of the tent-camping area, the trail descends slightly, then crosses a stream lined with slate. This is just an introduction to some of the rock formations you will encounter. The creek banks contain Triassic shale, argillite, and sandstone in many shapes and sizes.

After the stream, you start to see the hills ahead, especially when winter has opened the view by stripping the trees of leaves. Soon the hardwoods combine with white pines as the trail meanders through the forest and comes to the first in a long series of stone walls, which once marked property lines. You can almost imagine farmers and loggers of a long-gone era, sleeves rolled up, stacking the stones one by one.

The trail bends and twists, continuing southwest. Look for a new path on your right, heading due west, and turn there. You will then come to a fork; these two trails parallel each other. The right-hand path takes you higher up the hillside, and the left-hand one runs closer to the creek. Turn right for now, and return on the lower trail.

As you continue northwest on the upper trail, you will start to glimpse, through the trees, more of the creek below and the hills on the other side. Watch for a rocky gorge. Keep to the right of this deep gully unless you like the challenge of skipping from rock to rock.

The ultimate payoff lies only a few hundred feet before the gorge. The first lookout point, used mainly by rock climbers, does not have retaining walls, so be *extremely* cautious. Do not climb down to the rocks below; even experienced climbers have fallen here. Without going too close to the edge, you can see a near-oxbow in the creek.

As you continue, you are treated to a series of overlooks, each offering a different vantage point above the creek. Follow the trail into a cool forest, which

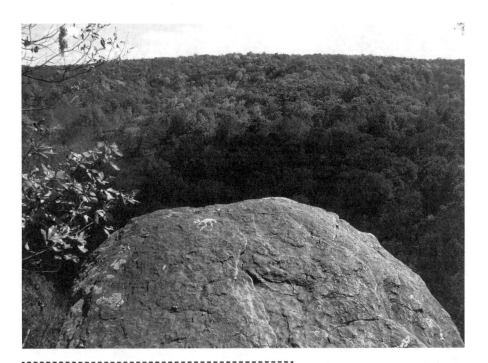

One of a handful of lookout points at Tohickon Valley Park

leads to the end of the road, where you turn around and head back. This time, when you reach the fork, try the lower trail for a different perspective.

Toward the end of the lower trail, you will begin to see red and white trail markers. Follow these markers and continue east, past the campsite, now on your left. Turn right at the park road, and walk downhill (southwest) to get a close view of the cabins and creek.

After you see two cabins close together on your left, the road takes a sharp southward turn (right) toward the clear creek below. Tohickon Creek has a reputation as one of the cleanest streams in the state, providing prime habitat for riverweed, freshwater mussels, fish, turtles, and other wildlife.

You may see an angler or two bidding for trout from one of the dry, flat boulders in the middle of the creek, or you might occasionally notice an overworked writer lying there, gazing up at the sky, wondering how she's going to make her next deadline.

You could literally stay here all day, and many people do, renting one of the four cabins close to the creek. But eventually you'll have to hoist that backpack, go back up to where the road curved near the cabins, and pick up another dirt trail heading south for one last, butt-busting loop.

Follow this trail to the top of a hill where it curves 90 degrees to the left, turning north and eventually leading you behind a pool and playground—past these lies the parking lot from which you entered. Turn right at the pool and head east; you will see the lot straight ahead. But this hike is not really over.

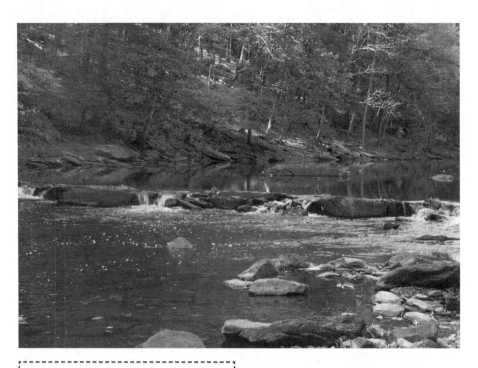

The crystal-clear waters of the Tohickon Creek

Once the joys of this park make their way into your heart, you will want to return again and again. You are simply closing the door temporarily on the first in a series of pleasant memories.

## NEARBY ACTIVITIES

STOVER MILL
*(19th-century river mill,*
*now an art gallery)*
852 River Road, Erwinna
**www.pennridge.org/works/**
**wheatflour.html**

CANAL BAR
*(Bar and restaurant)*
River Road, Upper Black Eddy

HOMESTEAD GENERAL STORE
*(Old-fashioned deli, ice cream,*
*convenience items)*
1650 Bridgeton Hill Road,
Upper Black Eddy
(610) 982-5121

# TYLER STATE PARK: Covered Bridge   23

## IN BRIEF

This hike displays a unique combination of tree-lined, rolling hills along with large, undisturbed agricultural fields, wide-open vistas, sun-dappled pine forests, and some classic Pennsylvania stone houses, not to mention the historic Schofield Ford Covered Bridge, which spans the width of Neshaminy Creek.

## DESCRIPTION

From the parking lot, locate the trailhead marker and take the stairway to begin the hike. Once down the log steps, keep left, following a winding 0.25-mile path toward the historic Schofield Ford Covered Bridge. The bridge, originally built in 1873, survived in its initial form until 1991, when vandals burned it. In 1997 it was rebuilt to its original specifications.

At 170 feet, Schofield Ford, also known as Twining Ford Bridge, is the longest covered

### KEY AT-A-GLANCE INFORMATION

**LENGTH:** 3.7 miles

**CONFIGURATION:** Loop

**DIFFICULTY:** Moderate

**SCENERY:** Agricultural, combined with tree-lined hills, covered bridge, and stone homes

**EXPOSURE:** Full shade–full sun

**TRAIL TRAFFIC:** Light traffic; some horseback riders, a few joggers

**TRAIL SURFACE:** Combined; both paved and unpaved surfaces

**HIKING TIME:** Approximately 1.5 hours

**DRIVING DISTANCE FROM CENTER CITY:** 34 miles; approximately 40–45 minutes from Center City

**ACCESS:** Year-round, every day, dawn–dusk; free admission

**MAPS:** USGS Langhorne

**WHEELCHAIR TRAVERSABLE:** No

**FACILITIES:** Outhouse near water fountains just before White Pines Trail

**SPECIAL COMMENTS:** Trails can be muddy after heavy rains. Call (215) 968-2021 for more information.

## *Directions* ⟶

From US 95 in Philadelphia, go north 26.4 miles to Exit 49, then turn left and take PA 332 toward Newtown/Yardley. After 1.4 miles, turn right at Newtown Yardley Road/Silver Lake Road/Yardley Newtown Pike. Continue to follow Newtown Yardley Road/Yardley Newtown Pike 2.5 miles; stay right to continue on Swamp Road. At the next light, you will see the main entrance for Tyler State Park on the left—do *not* take this entrance. Instead, continue straight, through the light, remaining on Swamp Road. Look for the Schofield Ford Covered Bridge entrance on the left just over a mile ahead. If you reach a stop sign, you have gone too far. Steps to the trailhead are on the southwest side of the parking lot as you drive in. *Swamp Road (Covered Bridge entrance), Newtown, PA 18940.*

### GPS Trailhead Coordinates

UTM Zone (WGS84)  18T

Easting  0501838.8

Northing  4455027.2

Latitude  N 40° 14' 44.32"

Longitude  W 74° 58' 43.04"

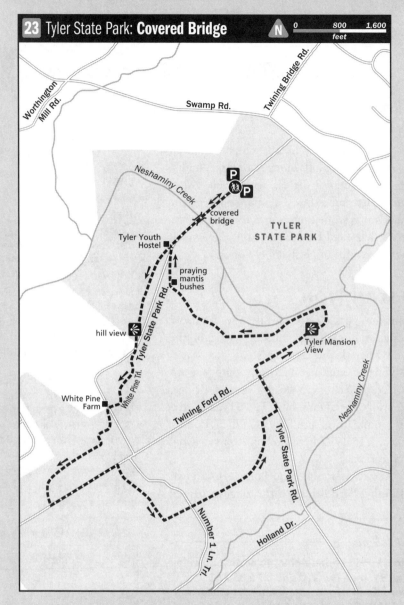

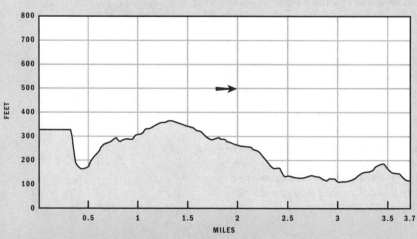

bridge of the 11 covered bridges in Bucks County. Spanning Neshaminy Creek, which meanders through part of the park's 1,711 acres, the bridge is open to hikers, horses, and bicycles. Information regarding the bridge's history and restoration, posted near the bridge, describes a concerted community effort to restore this unique landmark. Newcomers can't help but tarry at the bridge and peek through its diamond-shaped windows to spy on the wild ducks or catch a beaver building its dam near the large stone pillar that supports the extensive span of this oak-and-hemlock structure. The creek serves as home to a wide variety of creatures, such as snapping turtles, eels, frogs, water snakes, and muskrats, in addition to several species of warm-water fish. Occasionally, a horseback rider will trot across the bridge; a boarding stable and horse rental facility are only a short distance north on Swamp Road.

Continue past the bridge, then onto the gravel trail to a large youth hostel with English ivy creeping up its cream-colored stone walls. This hostel, known as the Solly House and Annex, are available for overnight and weekend stays through Hostelling International Inc. George Tyler, a banker, purchased this homestead in 1919 and lived here until the completion of his family mansion, also located within the park.

Just past the hostel, the trail splits into a paved equestrian trail and a meadow trail, which run parallel to each other. Hikers may choose either trail but should keep an eye out for horseback riders while on the equestrian trail. From here the route leads to a hilltop, where you can have a drink and enjoy the country vista, ablaze with color in the fall.

When you've taken in the view, continue up the hill on the horse trail until it joins a paved walkway. Turn right and look for the entrance to a pine forest on your left, just off the paved path. The forest smells like Christmas and provides a cool alternative route on a summer hike. Deer scamper in the vicinity as you trod upon the pine needles and admire the towering trees. Where the trail splits, keep right to wind through the forest until you reach a clearing and rejoin the paved trail.

Wave hello to the horses at White Pine Farm, on the right, an equine boarding facility adjacent to the park, then continue straight, soon crossing a road that hugs the nearby agricultural fields. Keep straight on the dirt path along the fields.

Among the trees found along this part of the route are oak, maple, pine, white birch, and walnut. In this arboreal area, look and listen for song sparrows, northern cardinals, mourning doves, and, of course, the American crows that come to clean up after the harvest. Bright-colored warblers and tanagers decorate the tree branches in early spring, along with thrushes and vireos. These spring and summer visitors are all but gone by October, when wild Canada geese migrate overhead, loudly announcing their passage.

The trail continues to Twining Ford Road, where you turn sharply left. From here, the agricultural fields slope downward, providing a serene landscape of rolling, tree-lined fields. This is an excellent place to break out the binoculars and spot a hawk flying overhead, circling around with its lifetime mate. As the sun falls, you may hear a horned owl's hoot as it awakes for its nightly hunt.

The trail now zigzags through the fields of corn and soy, eventually coming to a spot where you have a view of the Tyler mansion, with its 60 rooms. The French–Norman style mansion, located on the campus of the Bucks County Community College, houses a display of gardens, fountains, and sculptures, which makes this nearby attraction a worthwhile stop year-round.

A short distance beyond the mansion, your route curves left, joining a brush-lined trail in an area that is home to foxes and cottontails. But this is no ordinary hedgerow; from spring to fall, if you look closely you may find a rare praying mantis, camouflaged in the thicket. The word *mantis* comes from the Greek word for "prophet" or "fortune teller," and in the ancient world this insect was believed to possess supernatural powers. So make a wish as you walk by, but take care where the trail turns right and descends through the brush, because the path can be muddy and slippery after heavy rains.

Once you have braved this last, possibly slick, section, look right and enjoy a view of the wetlands; occasionally, a great blue heron gracefully soars by, casting its shadow on the waters below. You soon reach the paved trail that brought you to this loop. If you are staying the night, you can walk directly to the hostel, find your cot, and call it a night. If not, turn right to take another stroll through time toward the covered bridge and Neshaminy Creek. Once across, leave the sparkling waters behind and retrace your route to the parking lot.

## NEARBY ATTRACTIONS

CAROUSEL VILLAGE AT INDIAN WALK
591 Durham Road (PA 413),
Wrightstown
(215) 598-7165

THE OCTAGONAL SCHOOLHOUSE
Swamp Road and Route 232
(Second Street Pike), Newtown
(215) 598-3313
(Call ahead for hours of operation)

THE SUMMER KITCHEN
2310 Second Street Pike, Penns Park
(215) 598-9210
**www.thesummerkitchen.net**

TYLER MANSION AND FORMAL GARDENS
275 Swamp Road, Newtown
(215) 968-8000

TYLER PARK STABLES
451 Swamp Road, Newtown
(215) 860-1791

TYLER YOUTH HOSTEL AT
TYLER STATE PARK
P.O. Box 94, Newtown
(215) 968-0927

# TYLER STATE PARK: East Side 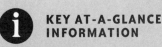 24

## IN BRIEF

This hike displays a unique combination of rolling tree-lined hills, large agricultural fields, wide-open vistas, and classic Pennsylvania stone houses; there is also a springhouse at the hike's midpoint.

## DESCRIPTION

*This hike is dedicated to Dee the flower lady, who lived in one of the park homes and passed away unexpectedly in 2008.*

This hike begins along the pedestrian causeway that spans Neshaminy Creek; anglers stand to the side of the causeway, hoping to catch smallmouth bass or sunfish, dogs splash in the cool waters, and children examine the river stones for the perfect skimmer. To the north the dam's falls glimmer and flow. Snapping turtles, muskrats, frogs, and even some beavers can be found along the banks.

Once across the concrete causeway, turn right on the paved trail. After several hundred yards, you may see chickens grazing near an old stucco farmhouse on the right. From here,

## KEY AT-A-GLANCE INFORMATION

**LENGTH: 4 miles**

**CONFIGURATION: Loop**

**DIFFICULTY: Intermediate**

**SCENERY: Agricultural, tree-lined hills, stone homes**

**EXPOSURE: Full shade–full sun**

**TRAIL TRAFFIC: Medium; some equestrians, a few joggers**

**TRAIL SURFACE: Both paved and unpaved**

**HIKING TIME: Approximately 1.5 hours**

**DRIVING DISTANCE FROM CENTER CITY: 33 miles**

**ACCESS: Year-round, every day, dawn–dusk; free admission**

**MAPS: USGS Langhorne, or download at www.dcnr.state.pa.us/state parks/parks/tyler/tyler_maps.aspx**

**WHEELCHAIR TRAVERSABLE: No**

**FACILITIES: Restrooms near start of hike, at boathouse**

**SPECIAL COMMENTS: Picnic area near dam and boat launch; canoe rental for trips to the Schofield Ford Covered Bridge; trails can be muddy after heavy rains. Call (215) 968-2021 for more information.**

## *Directions* ⟶

From Interstate 95 north, take PA 332, Exit 49, toward Newtown/Yardley. Make a left off the exit ramp toward PA 413 (Newtown bypass). Stay left on 413, which turns into Swamp Road. Immediately on the left (at the light) will be a turn into the main entrance at Tyler Park. Once in the park, you will reach a stop sign. Take a right here and drive 0.5 miles to the parking lot next to the dam and creek. From the parking lot, walk north to the trailhead at the pedestrian causeway, which spans Neshaminy Creek. *101 Swamp Road, Newtown, PA 18940.*

## GPS Trailhead Coordinates

UTM Zone (WGS84)  18T

Easting   0502329

Northing   4453547

Latitude   N 40° 13' 56.88"

Longitude   W 74° 58' 21.60"

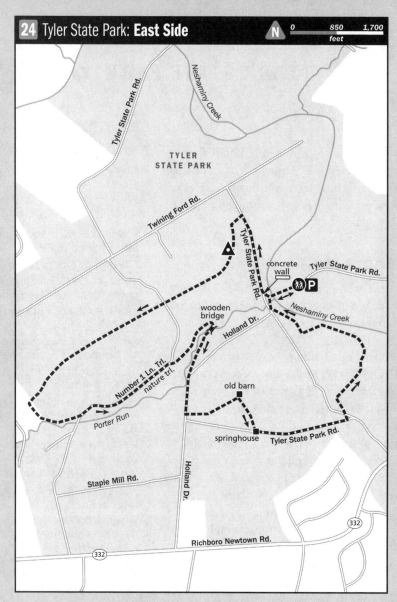

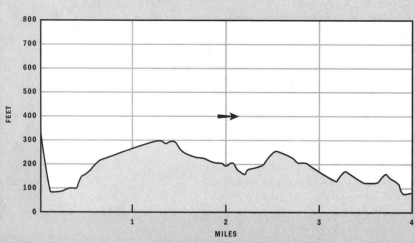

turn left, cross a road, and find an entrance to a dirt trail. This trail-less-traveled wanders through a pastoral field that may be planted with corn or soy. In summertime, stalks bend in the wind. The farmers who lease the land from the park service keep a small trail cleared for hikers and equestrians. Overhead, you can often spot the red-tailed hawk. If it's early morning, foxes and deer scamper in the fields.

Continue about 1.5 miles to a view of rolling hills, made possible when trees were cleared for a natural-gas pipeline. Soon you cross a paved road lined with old pin oaks. In the summertime, walkers on the road may look surprised to see you appear, seemingly out of nowhere, from among the tall corn. Once across the road, continue straight through another agricultural field, alone except for the company of an occasional equestrian.

Eventually the field ends and you meet another paved road, where you turn left. You may hear babbling Porter Run, which drains into Neshaminy Creek, on your right. Farther down the road is a white stucco house and a restored barn. Make sure *not* to take the equestrian trail (marked with a horseback-rider emblem) just before the little stream bridge on the right. The trail you want is unmarked and just past the little stream bridge on the right. Make a right turn onto this nature trail.

Now you are in a cool, dense forest. Warblers and thrushes can be heard, and perhaps seen, in spring. After about 100 yards, the trail forks. To shorten the hike by 1.5 miles, turn left and return to the parking area. To complete the full hike, keep right. As the trail nears Porter Run, the stream's burbling grows louder. Stay straight on the trail, which hugs the north side of the stream. You will soon cross Porter Run via a Boy Scout–built bridge; there, turn right and take the trail that hugs the south side of the river. This trail climbs to about 20 feet above the stream, providing a view of the lush riparian vegetation in spring and summer. Now the trail veers away from the stream to meet a paved trail.

Here, turn right and climb a short, steep pitch. At the top of the hill, turn left on an equestrian field that enters an agricultural field with fine views of distant hills. The trail turns sharply right, toward another white stucco house, an old barn, and remnants of an even older structure. The ruins are the foundation of a 200-year-old barn.

Just behind the white stucco house is a springhouse that looks like it emerged from the ground—like one of those hobbit houses from *Lord of the Rings*. The original settlers used springhouses to keep food and drink cool in the times before refrigeration. The natural spring that bubbles up into this springhouse is still working and keeps the temperature inside at a steady 57°F— even in August. Former residents of this private home chilled their beer in the springhouse as recently at the 1990s. And because of the lack of development in Tyler State Park, the springhouse may continue to work for decades to come.

Just past the springhouse, turn left on a paved, tree-lined road. After about 0.25 miles, turn left on another paved road and, almost immediately, veer right

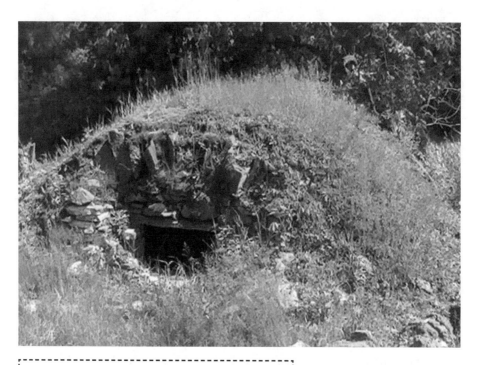

Springhouse near a private residence within Tyler State Park

on a trail with exercise stations. Because you have now gone more than 3 miles, be content to simply observe the stations, unless you want a more intense workout. After turning sharply right, you descend to the concrete pedestrian causeway. From here, cross the bridge and retrace your route to the parking area. Be it spring, summer, or fall, you might want to visit that ice-cream truck you may have only glanced at toward the beginning of this rigorous hike.

## NEARBY ATTRACTIONS

CAROUSEL VILLAGE AT INDIAN WALK
591 Durham Road (PA 413),
Wrightstown
(215) 598-7165

THE OCTAGONAL SCHOOLHOUSE
Swamp Road and Route 232
(Second Street Pike), Newtown
(215) 598-3313
(Call ahead for hours of operation)

THE SUMMER KITCHEN
2310 Second Street Pike, Penns Park
(215) 598-9210
www.thesummerkitchen.net

TYLER MANSION AND FORMAL GARDENS
275 Swamp Road, Newtown
(215) 968-8000

TYLER PARK STABLES
451 Swamp Road, Newtown
(215) 860-1791

TYLER YOUTH HOSTEL AT
TYLER STATE PARK
P.O. Box 94, Newtown
(215) 968-0927

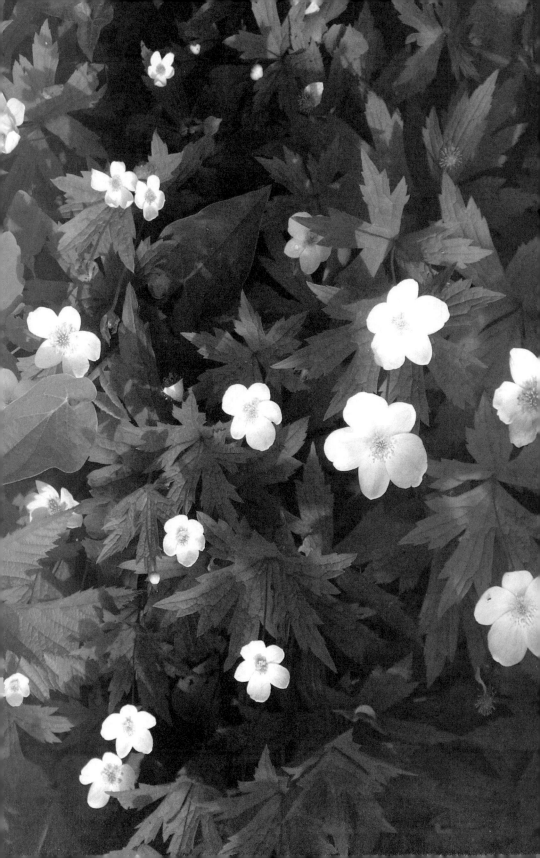

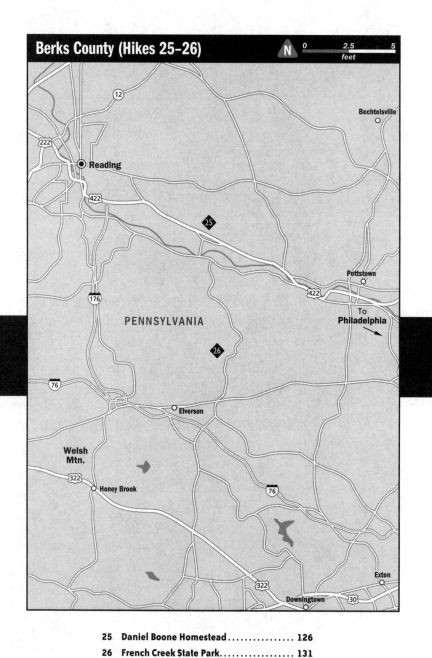

# Berks County (Hikes 25-26)

N    0       2.5       5
feet

12

222

⦿ Reading

422

◈ 25

176

PENNSYLVANIA

◈ 26

Bechtelsville ○

Pottstown ○

422

To
Philadelphia
→

76

○ Elverson

Welsh
Mtn.

322 ○ Honey Brook

76

322

Downingtown ○

30

Exton ○

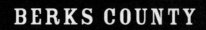

# BERKS COUNTY

# 25 DANIEL BOONE HOMESTEAD

## KEY AT-A-GLANCE INFORMATION

**LENGTH:** 3.23 miles

**CONFIGURATION:** Balloon

**DIFFICULTY:** Easy

**SCENERY:** Wildflower meadows with a background of rolling hills, woods, horses, and historic homes and outbuildings

**EXPOSURE:** Full sun–full shade

**TRAIL TRAFFIC:** Light

**TRAIL SURFACE:** Grass, gravel, asphalt

**HIKING TIME:** 1.5 hours

**DRIVING DISTANCE FROM CENTER CITY:** 50 miles

**ACCESS:** Tuesday–Saturday, 9 a.m.–5 p.m.; Sunday, noon–5 p.m. (reduced schedule during January and February). Admission for house tour: $6 ages 12–64; $5.50 motor/travel-club members, the military, and seniors; $4 kids ages 3–11

**MAPS:** USGS Birdsboro; maps at visitor center and Web site (see below)

**WHEELCHAIR TRAVERSABLE:** No

**FACILITIES:** Restrooms in gift shop at Homestead

**SPECIAL COMMENTS:** Hike is on bridle trails; house tours start at the visitor center; watch for groundhog holes on the trails. More information: (610) 582-4900; www.daniel boonehomestead.org.

## GPS Trailhead Coordinates

UTM Zone (WGS84)  18T

Easting    0432135

Northing   4460703

Latitude   N 40° 17' 39.0"

Longitude  W 75° 47' 54.6"

## IN BRIEF

Trek through the meadows, forests, and valleys in which the young Daniel Boone learned to hunt and survive. Bring a picnic to eat by Daniel Boone Lake, and then take a tour through Boone's childhood home, now a historic site.

## DESCRIPTION

Imagine if the survival of your family largely depended on your skill as a hunter, angler, and farmer. For early American settlers, it most certainly did. Boys were trained quite young in these skills. In fact, when Daniel Boone was just 12 years old, his father gave him his first rifle.

Legends far outweigh reality regarding this 18th-century icon, but Daniel Boone was certainly a brave outdoorsman who helped blaze the way into the Kentucky frontier, fighting for the settlers and defending them

## *Directions*

Take Interstate 76 west from Philadelphia. After 17 miles, take Exit 328A-B for US 202 toward West Chester/US 422/King of Prussia/Pottstown. Keep left at the fork, and pick up US 422 at King of Prussia. Take Exit 328A to merge onto US 422 west toward Pottstown. Stay on US 422 for 30 miles. After Pottstown look for these landmarks: Merritt's Doll Museum on the right and then C&J Tires on the right. After C&J Tires, look for a brown sign with white letters—DANIEL BOONE HOMESTEAD—with an arrow pointing to the right. Make the first right after the sign at the traffic light, onto Daniel Boone Road. Travel 0.5 miles to the site. Take a left down the main road near the visitor center. This will bring you to the bridle-trail entrance. If needed, there will be someone at the visitor center to help you. *400 Daniel Boone Road, Birdsboro, PA 19508.*

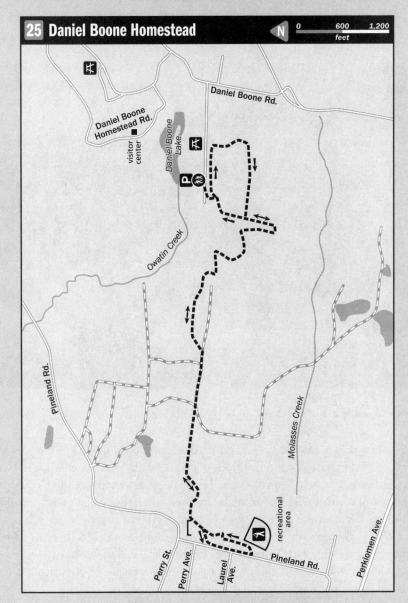

N

0        600      1,200
_feet_

Daniel Boone Rd.

Daniel Boone
Homestead Rd.

Daniel Boone Lake

visitor center

Owatin Creek

Pineland Rd.

Molasses Creek

recreational area

Perry St.

Perry Ave.

Laurel Ave.

Pineland Rd.

Perkiomen Ave.

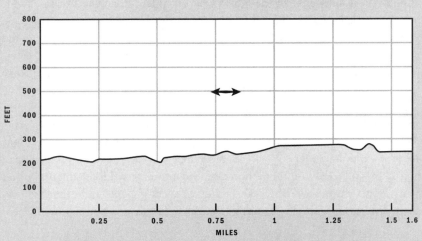

FEET

800
700
600
500
400
300
200
100
0

0.25    0.5    0.75    1    1.25    1.5  1.6

MILES

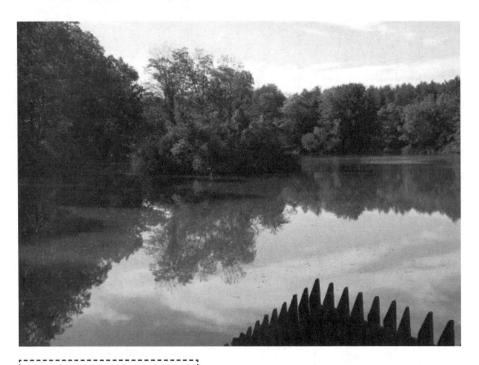

View overlooking Daniel Boone Lake

against attack. He also explored and lived in parts of North Carolina and Missouri, but his first explorations started in an area called the Oley Valley in southeastern Berks County, Pennsylvania. Here, in what is today called Birdsboro, Boone hunted, tended farm animals, assisted his father's blacksmith business, and formed friendships with the nearby Native Americans.

When you visit the Daniel Boone Homestead, with its 579 acres of open space, you will see why this part of the country sparked the curiosity of a young man who became one of the most famous frontiersmen in American history. Tours of the homestead are available at the visitor center.

On the tour you can visit the house where Daniel Boone was born in 1734. It's been extended over the years, from a one-story log house to a picturesque two-story stone dwelling. The original spring flows through a trough in the basement of the home. This cool cellar served as food storage long before refrigeration. Meats were preserved in the nearby smokehouse, where a fire of hickory and apple wood smoked the pork that hung from overhead joists.

The tour also includes a visit to a blacksmith shop. Daniel's father, Squire Boone, worked as a blacksmith, creating tools and hardware for nearby farms and homes. Other buildings, not originally located on the homestead, represent life in early colonial America: a log cabin (circa 1737), a bake house with clay roofing tiles, and a sawmill. The homestead contains a wildlife sanctuary and sponsors events throughout the year, including encampments and other history-oriented programs. Camping facilities on the grounds are popular with local

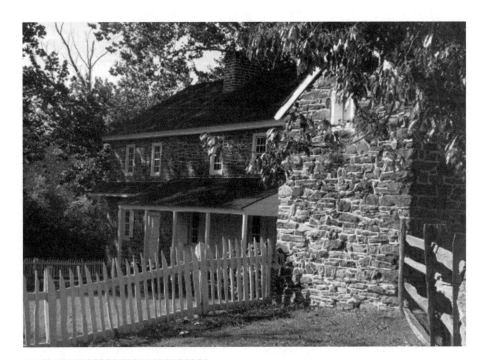

The original Daniel Boone Homestead

Scouts. (Incidentally, one of the precursors to the Boy Scouts of America was called the Sons of Daniel Boone.)

The hike starts at the bridle trails, which are next to the picnic area on the south side of Daniel Boone Lake. To get there, take the first left-hand turn from the south entrance of Daniel Boone Road. Go just past the picnic area and park in the gravel parking area on your right. A large sign welcomes you to the bridle trailhead. Equestrian trail maps should be in a box attached to the sign. If not, you can get a map at the visitor center.

From the trailhead, walk west on asphalt to a junction marked by an orange arrow leading to a dirt path. Turn left and look for trail marker No. 1. From here, head east toward a mountain range and a nearby meadow, ablaze with goldenrod and teeming with butterflies in the late summer. About 0.25 miles from the trailhead, you reach a junction and trail marker No. 2. Here turn right and head south. Look for the hawks flying overhead and the steam clouds rising from the Limerick Nuclear Power Plant in the distance.

When you reach trail marker No. 3, turn right and head west through a sunny meadow. The gnats may get somewhat bothersome at this point, but the next trail markers—5, 6, and 7—are within a cool woodland, where the insects soon disperse, and your greatest annoyance may be mounds of horse poop.

When you reach marker No. 8, two trails branch left, one parallel to the other. There is an outer loop that does not contain trail markers but is easy to follow. If you choose the outer loop, be sure to take a right when you reach a

**T**-junction and head west. From here on, the numbered markers on the inner loop are harder to find because of the underbrush, but this is a great spot to look for rabbits or listen to the sparrows singing as they fly from bush to bush. You soon cross a gravel road and then reach a small recreational park on the southwest end of the open space. This small park, with its skateboarders and basketball players, stands in stark contrast to the recreational opportunities in Boone's day.

Your trail is now concrete, but look for a dirt path on your left where the trailhead continues. A wooden bench on the left provides a convenient rest stop at about the halfway point.

Once you resume your hike, the surroundings soon become familiar as you merge with the trail on which you came. Follow this path all the way back to the first meadow, or take a short cut north from marker No. 4 back to the trailhead.

Tonight after you take a warm soak in your cozy bathtub, put on your clean night clothes, and lay down your head on a soft, billowy pillow, you can think of the early settlers, or better yet of Daniel Boone, who, after a day of exploring the same meadows and forest through which you trekked today, would return home to his little log cabin to sleep in a room, with his ten brothers and sisters, on a paltry straw mat.

## NEARBY ACTIVITIES

BROOKE MANSION
*(Victorian bed-and-breakfast)*
301 Washington Street, Birdsboro
(610) 582-9775
**www.brookemansion.com**

FRENCH CREEK STATE PARK
*(See Hike 26, page 131)*
843 Park Road, Elverson
(610) 582-9680

POTTSGROVE MANOR
*(Museum and circa-1752 home of Pottstown founder John Potts)*
100 West King Street, Pottstown
(610) 326-49014
**www.montcopa.org**

# FRENCH CREEK STATE PARK

## IN BRIEF

This heavily wooded hike has a steep climb in the beginning and lake views in the second half.

## DESCRIPTION

The Boone Trail is part of 7,475-acre French Creek State Park's 35-mile trail system. Its mountainous terrain presents a challenge. Most of the time, you seem to be either climbing or descending. The footing can be tricky in winter. The beginning is the most demanding part because of a 950-foot hill.

Delineated by blue markers, the trail starts on the north side of Park Road, 100 yards from the parking lot. The trail follows what looks like a streambed where water rushes during and after rainfall. Within the first mile, you pass a small group of cabins exposed to the elements. Farther up the path, a green water tower collects rainwater. In these thick woods, it would have been easy to

### KEY AT-A-GLANCE INFORMATION

**LENGTH:** 6.16 miles

**CONFIGURATION:** Loop

**DIFFICULTY:** Moderate

**SCENERY:** Woods, pines, lake

**EXPOSURE:** Full shade–full sun

**TRAIL TRAFFIC:** Medium

**TRAIL SURFACE:** Dirt, grass, some asphalt and rocks

**HIKING TIME:** 2.5 hours

**DRIVING DISTANCE FROM CENTER CITY:** 54.5 miles

**ACCESS:** Daily, dawn–dusk, year-round; free admission

**MAPS:** USGS Elverson; maps available at park stations and at the park Web site (see below)

**WHEELCHAIR TRAVERSABLE:** No

**FACILITIES:** Restrooms by the south entrance, near Scotts Run Lake, and near Hopewell Lake

**SPECIAL COMMENTS:** For more information, call (610) 582-9680 or visit dcnr.state.pa.us/stateparks/parks/frenchcreek.aspx.

## Directions

Take Interstate 76 west from Philadelphia. After 18.1 miles, take the ramp at the Pennsylvania Turnpike interchange to stay on I-76. After another 28 miles, take Exit 298 to merge onto Interstate 176 heading north, then immediately take Exit 1A and merge onto PA 10–Morgantown Road–Reading Road. After 0.7 miles, turn right onto Joanna Road. After almost a mile, turn right at the T-intersection onto Elverson Road. After 0.6 miles, take a slight left onto Hopewell Road. This becomes Park Road after 2.4 miles. Once in the park, take the fourth right into the parking lot next to Hopewell Lake. The Boone Trail starts across Park Road on the north side. Look for blue markers and a BOONE TRAIL sign. *843 Park Road, Elverson, PA 19520.*

### GPS Trailhead Coordinates

UTM Zone (WGS84) 18T

Easting 0432690

Northing 4450210

Latitude N 40° 11' 58.8"

Longitude W 75° 47' 26.7"

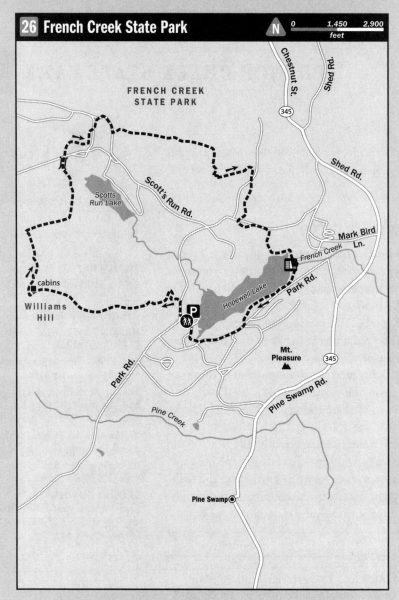

FRENCH CREEK
STATE PARK

Scotts
Run Lake

Scott's Run Rd.

Chestnut St.

Shed Rd.

345

Shed Rd.

Mark Bird
Ln.

French Creek

cabins

Williams
Hill

Hopewell Lake

Park Rd.

P

Park Rd.

Mt.
Pleasure

345

Pine Swamp Rd.

Pine Creek

Pine Swamp

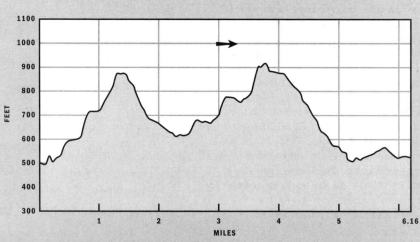

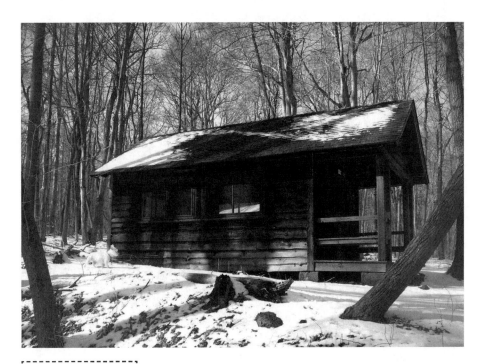

Rustic cabin on hilltop

lose one's way during the frontier days. Without a clearly marked path, the area would seem an endless forest.

These woods were once quite barren. Trees were cut to supply charcoal for the nearby Hopewell Furnace, which smelted iron from 1771 to 1883. The original growth of American chestnuts and mixed oaks was almost completely cleared. The forest's recovery got a boost in the 1930s, when the federal government purchased the land for recreation. The forest now looks more like it did during frontier days than it did in the early 19th century.

In slightly more than a mile, you reach the top of the first hill. The descent is quite steep and it is wise to watch your step, especially after snow or rain. Around the 2-mile mark, pine trees surround the path. This is one of the hike's most dramatic changes in landscape. The trail continues through the forest and crosses a small bridge spanning a creek. Just past the bridge, the trail crosses Fire Tower Road, then loops back to follow the same road. You continue to follow the road until you see the trail marker on the left. This is where the trail continues back into a wooded area, traveling east

If you look carefully through the trees and other plants, you might see white-tailed deer, raccoons, and an occasional chipmunk. Scarlet tanagers flit through the treetops. Tulip poplars soar above the mushrooms decorating the forest floor.

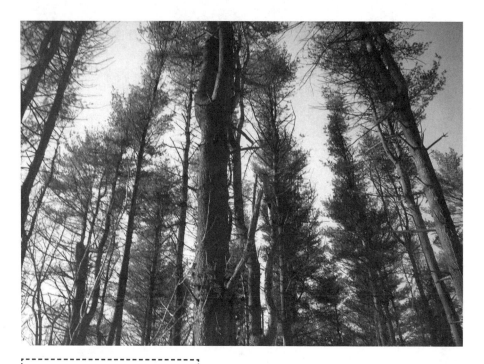

Pine grove at French Creek State Park

The section of the hike after you leave Fire Tower Road leads to the main campground area, which is just over the 3-mile mark. As you pass the campsites, you cross the main road leading to the campground. On the other side of the road, the trail drops dramatically, and its rocky surface can be treacherous. The path then stops at Scott's Run Road. Turn left for about 100 yards until you see the blue marker on your right marking the trail's continuation. On your right you will eventually see Hopewell Lake.

This 68-acre lake is popular for fishing in the spring and summer and ice fishing in the winter. As you cross a bridge you will see a dam on your right, built by the Civilian Conservation Corps in the 1930s. Hopewell Lake provided much of the water needed to run the Hopewell Furnace; behind the dam and bridge is the Hopewell Furnace National Historic Site. Because French Creek State Park and the Hopewell Furnace site share so much history, it's interesting to visit both on the same day. A path on your left just before you cross the bridge leads to the historic site, as does Scott's Run Road.

After you pass the dam, continue around the lake. You will pass the main swimming area on your right, and a fishing pier is visible in the distance. As you reach the road to finish the hike, an old stone springhouse is on the left. More than a century ago, people cut ice on Hopewell Lake and stored it there to preserve food. The hike ends in the main parking lot facing Hopewell Lake.

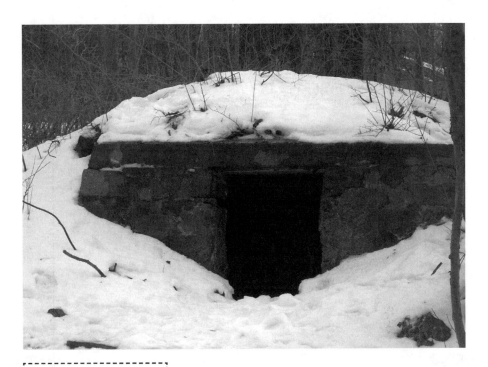

Old springhouse in the snow

## NEARBY ACTIVITIES

CROW'S NEST PRESERVE
201 Piersol Road, Elverson
(610) 286-7955
www.natlands.org

HOPEWELL FURNACE
NATIONAL HISTORIC SITE
2 Mark Bird Lane, Elverson
(610) 582-8773
www.nps.gov/hofu

MARSH CREEK STATE PARK
*(See Hike 29, page 148)*
675 Park Road, Downingtown
(610) 458-5119

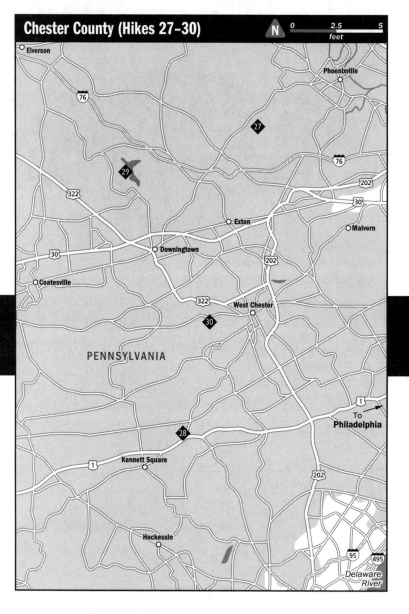

# Chester County (Hikes 27–30)

Elverson

Phoenixville

76

27

76

202

29

30

322

Exton

Malvern

Downingtown

30

202

Coatesville

322

West Chester

30

PENNSYLVANIA

1

To
Philadelphia

28

Kennett Square

202

1

Hockessin

95   495

Delaware
River

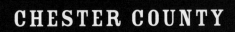

CHESTER COUNTY

# 27  BINKY LEE PRESERVE

## KEY AT-A-GLANCE INFORMATION

**LENGTH:** 2 miles

**CONFIGURATION:** Balloon

**DIFFICULTY:** Moderate

**SCENERY:** Meadows, young and old forests, stone barn

**EXPOSURE:** Full sun–full shade

**TRAIL TRAFFIC:** Light

**TRAIL SURFACE:** Dirt and grass

**HIKING TIME:** 45 minutes

**DRIVING DISTANCE FROM CENTER CITY:** 33.6 miles

**ACCESS:** Daily, dawn–dusk; free admission

**MAPS:** USGS Malvern; maps at kiosk; see also www.natlands.org/uploads/preserve_4252007122810.pdf

**WHEELCHAIR TRAVERSABLE:** No

**FACILITIES:** No public restrooms

**SPECIAL COMMENTS:** For more information, call (610) 827-0156 or visit www.natlands.org (search for "Binky Lee").

## IN BRIEF

Binky Lee and the Natural Lands Trust counterbalance the recent development in this area with the beauty of rolling hills, young floodplain forests, cool- and warm-season grasslands, pine plantations, and mature native woodlands.

## DESCRIPTION

A 1999 report in the *Philadelphia Inquirer* estimated that uncontrolled development in the greater Philadelphia area consumed 1 acre of open land per hour. Urban sprawl, or uncontrolled development, not only destroys open space, habitats, and ecosystems but also destroys watersheds, exacerbating flooding and lessening water quality. Law-enforcement and fire-department needs soar; roadways require more maintenance; traffic and pollution increase. Scenic landscapes are lost and, in some cases, tourism decreases.

The Philadelphia suburbs have certainly experienced urban sprawl over the past 10 to 20 years. The U.S. Census Bureau estimates that between April 2000 and July 2007,

## GPS Trailhead Coordinates

UTM Zone (WGS84)  18T

Easting   0448664

Northing   4438685

Latitude   N 40° 5' 48.69"

Longitude   W 75° 36' 8.17"

## Directions ——→

From Philadelphia, take Interstate 76 west 16.8 miles to Exit 328A and merge onto US 202 south, toward West Chester. After 9.6 miles, take the Frazer exit and merge right onto PA 401–Conestoga Road. After 1.9 miles, turn right onto Valley Hill Road. After 0.2 miles, continue straight as the road becomes Bodine Road; then, 1.4 miles farther, turn right to stay on Bodine. After 1.1 miles, turn left onto Pikeland Road. Drive a half mile to the Binky Lee Preserve entrance, on the right. Look for the trail to the right of the preserve's kiosk. *1445 Pikeland Road, Chester Springs, PA 19425.*

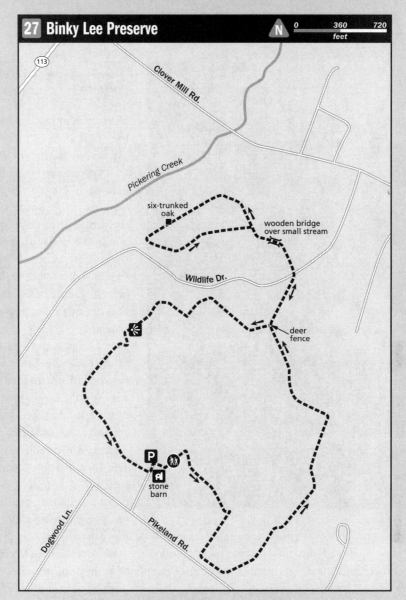

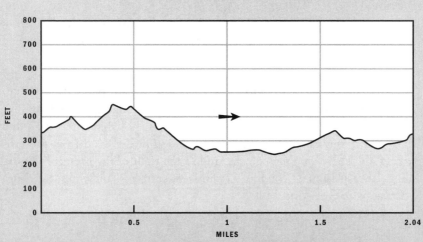

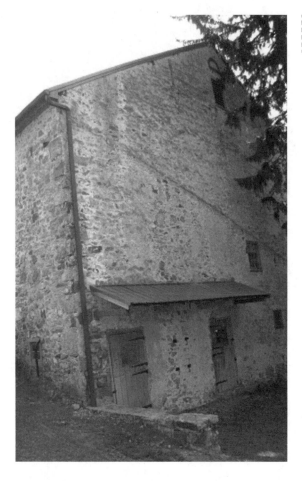

Chester County, site of the Binky Lee Preserve, saw a population increase of approximately 52,844, making it one of the fastest-growing counties in the United States. This is where the need for institutions such as the Natural Lands Trust, the region's largest nonprofit conservation organization, becomes crucial.

The trust protects land in the Delaware Valley via a network of open space and what it calls "green growth," a process that helps burgeoning municipalities save important natural resources. The organization acquires land through purchases or donations, then maintains the preserved land and restores it as needed to ensure long-term ecological health. The trust also may buy the development rights to a specific property through a conservation easement. A landowner sells the development rights but can continue to live on, maintain, and even sell the land. Any new owner, however, would be prohibited from building on the property.

Founded by a group of bird-watchers in 1953, the trust has helped preserve 100,000 acres of land, including 50 nature preserves in the Delaware Valley. The Binky Lee Preserve constitutes only 89 acres of that property.

As small as it is, the preserve was voted the 2008 Neighbors' Choice Award for Chester County by the *Inquirer*. The trust has planted more than 10,000 trees within Binky Lee to change open fields to woodland. Former agricultural land is being converted to natural grassland to provide habitats for birds and small mammals. You can see the tall grass bending in the wind from the visitor parking lot. There, you pick up the trail to the right of the preserve's kiosk, heading northeast. Soon all you hear are birds and crickets, and you see dragonflies buzzing by in every direction.

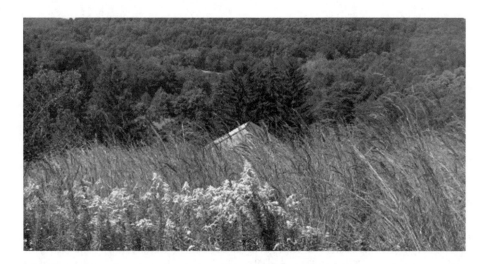

A private resident peaks through the preserved landscape.

The trails are not marked but are well groomed. In 0.1 mile, take your second right turn, where dappled sun penetrates the newly forested area, alive with greenery. At the end of this grove, turn left and head east into a mature woodland spotted with boulders. At the NO HORSES sign, take a left. Continue east and uphill until the trail turns north. Natural stone walls line the trail as you cross a wide bridle trail and pick up the hiking trail on the right, heading northeast.

You are sandwiched between new and old reforested areas, providing a glimpse of both what was and what shall be. This preserve showcases a variety of landscapes, such as young floodplain forests, grassy floodplain areas, cool- and warm-season grasslands, old fields becoming naturalized, pine plantations, mixed plantations, and mature native woodlands with sizable oaks and other hardwoods.

The trail weaves northwest and downhill, then turns to the right, heading north; horse droppings alert you to the fact that many of these trails are shared with your equine friends. The trail bends left, heading north-northwest. The dirt path turns to grass, and the fresh green meadow ahead indicates a right turn, so when you come to a split in the trail, stay right, heading north until deer fencing stands to your right. The path along the fence continues but then drops off; after you cross over a dirt driveway, take a dirt path on your left, heading northwest, away from the fencing and into a loop that circles mature woodland, perfect for bird-watching.

You may see the yellow-bellied Eastern meadowlark as it forages for seeds and berries, or you may hear its calming song. The fresh air and the sounds of nature make you feel thankful for preserves such as Binky Lee that remove the stress from your body, and carbon pollution from the atmosphere. The Eastern bluebird and other thrushes also frequent the preserve. This bluebird reached critical conservation status by the mid–20th century because of habitat destruction, competition from nonnative sparrows and starlings, and pesticide use. However, because of conservation efforts, it is no longer considered threatened.

After about 300 feet, you come upon a bridge over a small stream, along with a wooden bench. Continue west along the loop. Soon, 600 feet from the bench, the trail curves left and you reach a large six-trunked oak. There are several ways to estimate the age of a tree, and one way for oak trees is to measure the circumference of the trunk about 1.5 meters off the ground. You would measure in centimeters and then divide by 2.5. Unless you carry a tape measure in your backpack, you cannot make this educated estimation, but generally, the larger the trunk, the older the tree—and this one is very old indeed.

Two hundred fifty feet from the six-trunked oak, stay to the left with the trail, heading southeast. The trail turns again 250 feet later, and eventually you will see the bench. Turn right and walk until you see the deer fencing. At the end of the fencing, turn right and follow the trail down until it swoops back up into a grassy area. There you will stay to the right, heading west.

Your path turns southwest at the end, where you stay on the outer portion of the trail. Hawks fly over the mountains to the west, while a pine forest lines the eastern perimeter of the trail. Turn left at the end of the pines, where the grassy trail turns due south and leads you back to the 18th-century stone barn that stands beside the parking lot. But first enjoy a scenic vista, which offers a look at rolling hills and woodlands in all directions with only a few homes to obstruct the view. This Binky Lee vista demonstrates what's possible when building and nature are in balance.

*The Natural Lands Trust has a wealth of hikes in the Delaware Valley. Check its Web site, **www.natlands.org**, where you can click on a county and find out which trust lands offer trails.*

## NEARBY ACTIVITIES

HISTORIC YELLOW SPRINGS
*(Village of historic homes and villages)*
1685 Art School Road,
Chester Springs
(610) 827-7414, x10
**www.yellowsprings.org/about/
mission.html**

THE INN AT HISTORIC YELLOW SPRINGS
*(Fine dining)*
1701 Art School Road,
Chester Springs
(610) 827-7477
**www.innathistoricyellowsprings.com**

THE MILL AT ANSELMA
*(1747 mill and National Historic Landmark)*
1730 Conestoga Road,
Chester Springs
(610) 827-1906
**www.anselmamill.org**

# LONGWOOD GARDENS  28

## IN BRIEF

This trail loops through a renowned botanical complex showcasing a European water garden, historic Pennsylvania meadows, historic homes, breathtaking conservatories, mature plantings, a musical tower, and topiary wonders.

## DESCRIPTION

Longwood Gardens is a prime example of the positive contributions made possible by people with mega-money. Pierre S. du Pont turned his family business, the DuPont chemical company, into a corporate empire. He used some of his resulting fortune to develop the Longwood property, an arboretum that he purchased in 1906 to prevent the trees from being cut for lumber. Over the next 30 years, du Pont created a breathtaking oasis with a massive conservatory, spectacular gardens, dancing fountains, and verdant meadows. Du Pont himself traveled the world over and researched horticulture extensively to aid in the gardens' design.

After his death in 1954, Longwood became known as one of the premier botanical gardens in the United States. The mission of the Longwood Foundation, established in 1937, was to maintain the gardens "for the sole use of the public for purposes of exhibition, instruction, education, and enjoyment."

### KEY AT-A-GLANCE INFORMATION

**LENGTH: 2 miles**

**CONFIGURATION: Loop**

**DIFFICULTY: Moderate**

**SCENERY: Expert landscaping and mature horticulture**

**EXPOSURE: Full sun–full shade**

**TRAIL TRAFFIC: Moderate**

**TRAIL SURFACE: Concrete, brick and asphalt pavement, dirt**

**HIKING TIME: 1 hour**

**DRIVING DISTANCE FROM CENTER CITY: 34 miles**

**ACCESS: $16 adults, $14 ages 62+, $6 ages 5–18 and students with ID; free for children age 4 or younger. For detailed hours, go to the Web site (see below) and click on "Hours" at the top of the home page.**

**MAPS: USGS Kennett Square (part of Unionville); maps available at visitor center; see www.longwoodgardens .org/docs/MapOutdoor2009.pdf**

**WHEELCHAIR TRAVERSABLE: Yes, except the meadow**

**FACILITIES: Restrooms in visitor center and at restaurant**

**SPECIAL COMMENTS: Bring a camera. Bring a bag lunch, or enjoy the buffet at the restaurant. More information: (610) 388-1000; www.longwoodgardens.org.**

---

*Directions* ———————————➤

**Take Interstate 95 south from Philadelphia. After 14 miles, take Exit 3A and merge onto US 322. After 7.5 miles, turn left onto US 1–Baltimore Pike. After 8 miles, take the Long-wood Gardens exit and follow the signs to the visitor center. *1001 Longwood Road, Kennett Square, PA 19348.***

GPS Trailhead
Coordinates
UTM Zone (WGS84)  18S
Easting  0442351
Northing  4413742
Latitude  N 39° 52' 18.3"
Longitude  W 75° 40' 26.9"

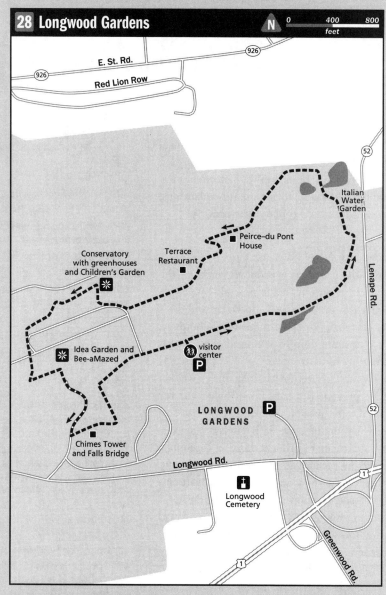

N

0   400   800
feet

E. St. Rd.

926

926

Red Lion Row

52

Italian
Water
Garden

Peirce–du Pont
House

Terrace
Restaurant

Conservatory
with greenhouses
and Children's Garden

Lenape Rd.

Idea Garden and
Bee-aMazed

visitor
center

P

52

LONGWOOD
GARDENS

P

Chimes Tower
and Falls Bridge

Longwood Rd.

Longwood
Cemetery

1

Greenwood Rd.

1

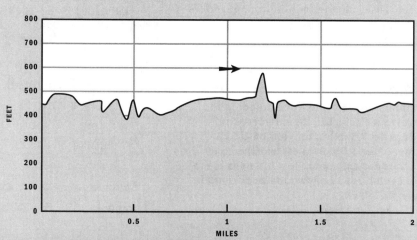

| | | | |
|---|---|---|---|
| 800 | | | |
| 700 | | | |
| 600 | | | |
| 500 | | | |
| 400 | | | |
| 300 | | | |
| 200 | | | |
| 100 | | | |
| 0 | 0.5 | 1 | 1.5 | 2 |

FEET

MILES

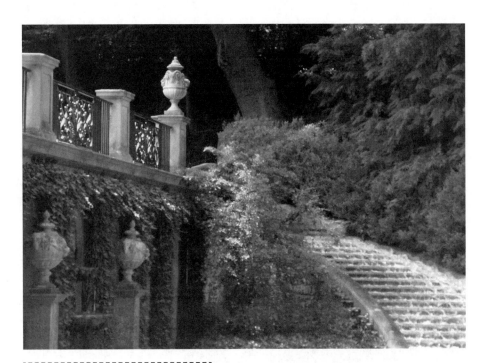

The Italian Water Garden at Longwood

The enjoyment begins as soon as you enter Longwood Road, with its floral arbors. The visitor center, visible from the parking lot, provides a visual hors d'oeuvre to the exquisite main course that lies just through its doors. After grabbing a map, turn right onto the path that circles the perimeter of the gardens. To map out a hike with a seasonal flavor, visit **www.longwoodgardens.org** to see which flowers will be blooming when you visit. Even Christmastime can be breathtaking with masses of myrrh, holly, and poinsettias, and a seemingly nonstop chorus of carols. You will see something different every time you come; this particular hike highlights early summer, but the horticultural experts at Longwood have assured Philadelphians a special experience no matter what month, no matter what season.

As you start, there's a small pond on your right and a larger pond on your left. Some of the trees you'll see are nearly 200 years old, and all have identification tags. Among the trees you can expect to see are the Canada hemlock, the cucumber magnolia, the tulip tree, and the London plane.

Follow the signs for the Italian Water Garden, where you'll feel as if you have stepped from the Pennsylvania woodlands directly into Florence, Italy. Lush, green lawns, precisely manicured littleleaf linden trees, and classical statues surround fountains dancing in symmetrical pools. Water gracefully cascades down concrete steps. Cast-iron fencing and English ivy finish the look. After the sound of the water has sufficiently slowed your heartbeat, leave the water garden and follow the signs for the meadow.

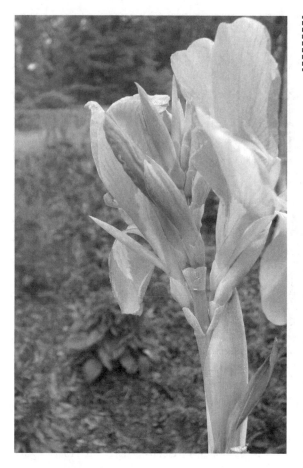

> Visit the Garden's Web site to find
> out what will be in bloom during
> your visit.

Fish, turtles, frogs, and dragonflies thrive in the natural meadow environment. Butterflies weave among goldenrod and black-eyed Susans in the summer. Stay on the dirt path, since the tall grass might harbor Lyme disease–carrying ticks.

At the end of the path, turn right, back onto the concrete pavement, and continue to the driveway of the Peirce–du Pont House. It's the oldest building at Longwood, dating back to 1730. Pierre du Pont added to the structure and used it as his weekend residence from 1906 until his death in 1954.

Follow the driveway to the house, then continue straight where the driveway merges with the main path that leads toward the Conservatory. Use the east entrance to the Conservatory, then veer right and move through the greenhouse into the Exhibition Hall. Hikers with children might detour left to the indoor Children's Garden, with its mystical sculptures, fountains, paintings, and stained-glass art. Children can sit in the tree-lined cove, find a secret room with a drooling dragon, explore the fog-filled grotto, and even weave through a bamboo maze.

In the Exhibition Hall, a few inches of water covers a sunken marble flooring to create a pool that reflects the overhanging floral arrangements. This room's displays often rotate with flower shows from the national rose, lily, rhododendron, orchid, and bonsai societies throughout the year. Next walk into the Outdoor Waterlily Display (June 1 through mid-October). In addition to colorful water lilies, you will notice the giant hybrid water platter in the center pool, which was first successfully hybridized at Longwood from the two South American parent species on display in the smaller side pools. Apparently, each full-grown leaf can support 80 to 100 pounds of evenly distributed weight.

Once you've experienced your little slice of rain forest, continue straight back into the Conservatory and take a right through the floral exhibit to the Orchid Room, featuring exotic varieties in every size, shape, and color. Continue west in the Conservatory, where you will see insect-catching specimens such as pitcher plants and Venus flytraps. Continue westward until you see a door at the westernmost side of the conservatory. Before you exit, take a short jog to the left to see the hibiscuses and roses, You may also want to see the bonsai collection, banana trees, and whatever else interests you—the Conservatory offers much more than can be effectively covered in one day.

When you exit at the west end of the Conservatory, follow the signs to the Idea Garden, a creative collection of plant varieties that grow well in southeastern Pennsylvania. From there, follow the signs to the Bee-aMazed Children's Garden, then turn right toward the Chimes Tower, where a waterfall cascades near the castlelike stone tower. Turn left after you pass the waterfall, climb the hill past the tower entrance, and cross the fall's bridge, where you can see the water up close while sometimes being serenaded by the tower's 62-bell carillon. Descend the path, pick up the main trail at the bottom, and follow the signs back to the visitor center.

On the way, don't miss the Topiary Garden on the left. Yews clipped into 50 different shapes make for a whimsical end to a magical hike. And you'll undoubtedly want to linger, exploring the gardens you missed to top off what is one of the most colorful and creative hikes in the Philadelphia area, and maybe even the world.

## NEARBY ACTIVITIES

BRANDYWINE BATTLEFIELD
HISTORIC SITE
1491 Baltimore Pike, Chadds Ford
(610) 459-3342
www.ushistory.org/brandywine

BRANDYWINE RIVER MUSEUM
US Route 1, Chadds Ford
(610) 388-2700
www.brandywinemuseum.org

CHADDSFORD WINERY
632 Baltimore Pike, Chadds Ford
(610) 388-6221
www.chaddsfordwinery.com

# MARSH CREEK STATE PARK

**KEY AT-A-GLANCE INFORMATION**

**LENGTH:** 6.5 miles
**CONFIGURATION:** Balloon
**DIFFICULTY:** Difficult
**SCENERY:** Tree-covered hills, forest
**EXPOSURE:** Partial shade–full sun
**TRAIL TRAFFIC:** Heavy
**TRAIL SURFACE:** Dirt
**HIKING TIME:** 2.5 hours
**DRIVING DISTANCE FROM CENTER CITY:** 42 miles
**ACCESS:** Year-round, daily, dawn–dusk; free admission
**MAPS:** USGS Downingtown. Maps at main office, some kiosks, and at dcnr.state.pa.us/stateparks/parks/marshcreek/marshcreek_mini.pdf
**FACILITIES:** Restrooms near east boat launch
**WHEELCHAIR TRAVERSABLE:** No
**SPECIAL COMMENTS:** Call (610) 458-5119 or visit dcnr.state.pa.us/stateParks/parks/marshcreek.aspx for more information.

## GPS Trailhead Coordinates

UTM Zone (WGS84)  18T
Easting   0437756
Northing  4435139
Latitude  N 40° 3' 51.23"
Longitude  W 75° 43' 47.57"

## IN BRIEF

This hike features a lake with sailboats, tree-covered hills and valleys, and green fields. The trails within this park are of varying degrees of difficulty.

## DESCRIPTION

At first, the 535-acre lake may appear to be the only attraction in this park. It is certainly a draw for sail boating, fishing, and even winter ice-skating. However, hikers will want to explore the remaining 1,200 acres of diverse trails and, especially on the Blue Trail, check out the beautiful vistas. A hike that includes most of the trails begins at the West Launch parking lot on the west side of the park. The White Trail trailhead near the parking lot is clearly marked behind a kiosk.

The trail will fork near the beginning, so turn right and stay right on the White Trail until you reach a small parking lot (on Chalfont Road). There the trail joins Chalfont Road for a few hundred yards. Then the

## Directions

From Philadelphia, drive 32.7 miles on Interstate 76 west. Take Exit 312 and merge onto PA 100 (Pottstown Pike). After 2 miles, turn left on Park Road, and then take the next right onto Little Conestoga Road. After 2.6 miles, turn left to stay on Little Conestoga Road, then 1.1 miles later (after the name changes to Marshall Road), turn left onto PA 282. After 1.6 miles, turn sharply left onto Lyndell Road, then, 0.6 miles later, turn right onto North Reeds Road. Take the next left onto Marsh Creek Road, drive to the lake's edge, and park. Look for the White Trail trailhead behind the kiosk. *675 Park Road, Downingtown, PA 19335.*

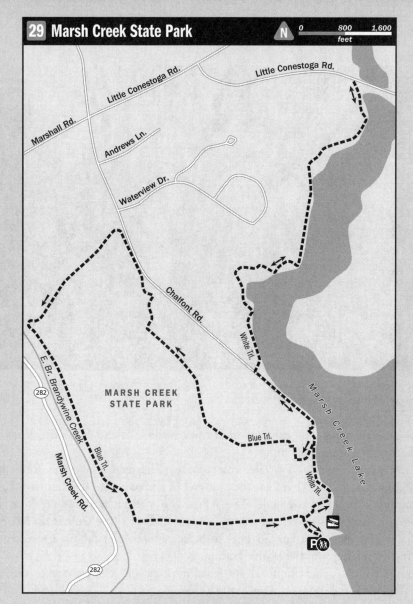

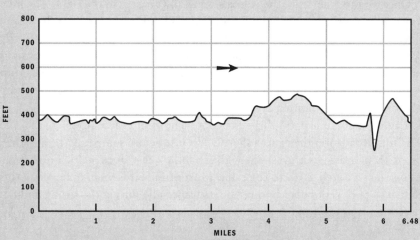

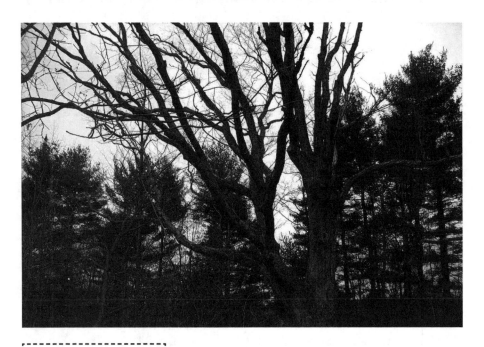

Very old tree on wood's edge

White Trail turns right and downhill toward the lake and continues along the lakefront for almost 1.5 miles.

The lake, a drinking-water reservoir for Chester County, was formed by a dam across Marsh Creek on the east end of the park. It's stocked with large-mouth bass and black crappie. The White Trail continues alongside the water, running through stretches of woods, until it ends at Little Conestoga Road. A rock near the road's edge just begs to be sat upon. After taking a rest, simply retrace your steps on the White Trail.

When you reach the Chalfont Road parking lot, turn right onto the Blue Trail. This is the most scenic part of the hike.

Once on the Blue Trail, the rule is simple: always stay to the right. The hike becomes a bit steep, but the whole northwest-bound portion of the Blue Trail compensates with many beautiful vistas of tree-covered hills that are especially striking in autumn. The wind sweeping across the fields creates a real sense of escape. Many locals will likely be enjoying the same views while hiking, running, or biking. One vista shows the lake and a green area on the other shore that's designated as a hunting area, off-limits to nonhunters.

Stay right to go around the outer loop. The trail eventually hugs the side of Chalfont Road, and then turns sharply left just before some PRIVATE PROPERTY signs. It then heads southwest through the hike's last open field. Look for a giant oak just a dozen yards to the right. Most of the birds seem to be along this stretch. The park is popular among birders, especially during the spring and fall waterfowl migrations.

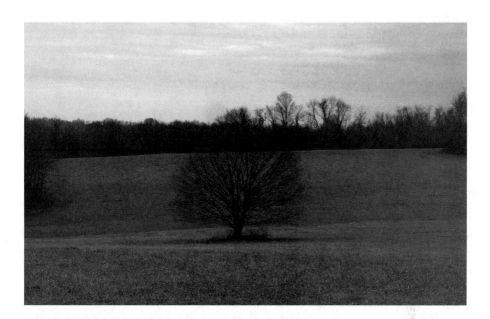

Lone maple in west field

Woods characterize the last part of the hike, with large oaks dominating the forest and keeping hikers cool in summer. The trail for the next 3,000 feet is wide and easy to follow. In the late 19th and early 20th centuries, it was a railroad bed; watch for old ties still in the ground.

The East Branch of Brandywine Creek creeps up on the right. It may be swollen in winter or spring. Some pleasant spots along the creek invite picnicking or just sitting and pondering. Watch on the left for two different Blue Trail turns. A double blue marker indicates turn the first; the marker for the other is on a tall pole. Each marker goes to the same short last leg of the Blue Trail. There is one more beautiful vista of a valley on the right, and then, after about 100 yards, a trail intersects your path from the right; take it back to the kiosk at the beginning of the hike.

## NEARBY ACTIVITIES

DOWNINGTOWN GOLF CLUB
85 Country Club Drive, Downingtown
(610) 269 2000

VICTORY BREWING COMPANY
420 Acorn Lane, Downingtown
(610) 873-0881

WEGMANS FOOD MARKETS
1056 East Lancaster Avenue,
Downingtown
(610) 873-4127

# 30 STROUD PRESERVE

## KEY AT-A-GLANCE INFORMATION

**LENGTH:** 3.88 miles

**CONFIGURATION:** Balloon

**DIFFICULTY:** Moderate

**SCENERY:** Rolling hills, natural grasslands, wetlands, stone houses, barns

**EXPOSURE:** Full shade–full sun

**TRAIL TRAFFIC:** Light

**TRAIL SURFACE:** Dirt, gravel

**HIKING TIME:** 3 hours

**DRIVING DISTANCE FROM CENTER CITY:** 35 miles

**ACCESS:** Year-round, daily, dawn–dusk; free admission

**MAPS:** USGS Unionville and www.natlands.org/uploads/preserve_4252007124645.pdf

**FACILITIES:** No public restrooms

**WHEELCHAIR TRAVERSABLE:** No

**SPECIAL COMMENTS:** For more information about the preserve, visit www.natlands.org/preserves/preserve.asp?fldPreserveId=44; for more information on the Natural Lands Trust, see www.natlands.org; for more information on the Stroud Water Research Center, see www.stroudcenter.org.

### GPS Trailhead Coordinates

UTM Zone (WGS84)  18S

Easting   0444681

Northing  4422749

Latitude   N 39° 57' 10.9"

Longitude  W 75° 38' 51.4"

## IN BRIEF

Deep within the rolling hills of West Chester, the Stroud Preserve, surrounded by historic architecture, represents a model preservation effort for the 21st century with its sustainable agriculture, forest creation, native grasslands, and well-maintained watershed.

## DESCRIPTION

This hike harks back to a simpler and slower time. A renowned geriatrics physician, Dr. Morris Stroud, bequeathed his 332-acre Georgia Farm in Chester County to the Natural Lands Trust in 1990. Other bequests and purchases were made, and the trust today manages 574 acres encompassing a creek, grasslands, farmlands, and forests, which comprise the Stroud Preserve.

The trailhead begins immediately at the preserve's small parking lot and leads you straight to a pedestrian bridge over the East Branch of Brandywine Creek. Its water eventually flows into the Christina River on its way to Delaware Bay, making the preserve an ideal site for the Stroud Water Research

## *Directions*

Take Interstate 95 south from Philadelphia 14 miles to Exit 3A. Merge onto US 322. Stay on US 322 as it turns left to join US 1 in 7.5 miles, then make a right after another mile to join US 202. After 5.7 more miles, turn left in West Chester onto Price Street (PA 100–PA 52). Drive 0.9 miles, then bear left as the road becomes West Miner Street. Continue 1.3 more miles, then turn right onto North Creek Road. The park entrance is slightly more than a mile ahead, on the left. The trail starts next to the parking lot, just over a pedestrian bridge. *454 North Creek Road, West Chester, PA 19382.*

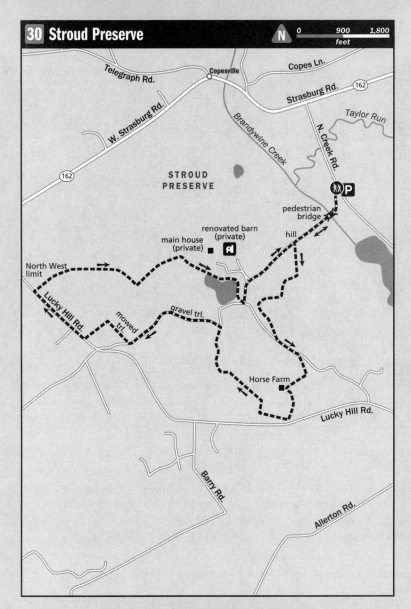

Telegraph Rd.    Copesville    Copes Ln.

Strasburg Rd.    162

W. Strasburg Rd.    Taylor Run

162    Brandywine Creek    N. Creek Rd.

STROUD PRESERVE    P

pedestrian bridge

renovated barn (private)    hill

main house (private)

North West limit

Lucky Hill Rd.    mowed trl.    gravel trl.

Horse Farm    Lucky Hill Rd.

Barry Rd.

Allerton Rd.

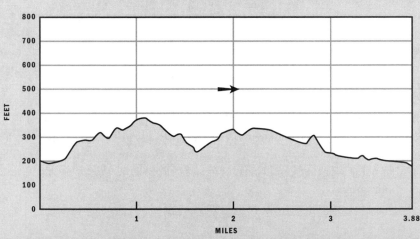

800
700
600
500
400
300
200
100
0

FEET

1    2    3    3.88

MILES

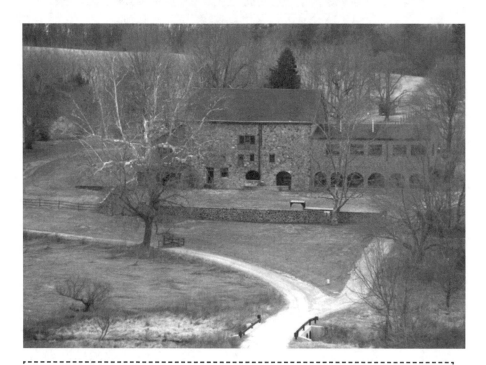

Original stone buildings within the Stroud Preserve have been converted into private residences.

Center, a lab that conducts scientific studies and provides education regarding streams and rivers. Plantings and trees help filter the water that flows into the river and provide food for the fish, river otters, and other riparian animals.

On the bridge, the view opens to hills and rolling fields. This hike starts on a flat gravel pathway, but soon you take a left onto the less traveled dirt trail. At the **T**-intersection at the top of the hill, turn right and head west toward the pond. The 19th-century main house and renovated barn complex in the meadow below are now private residences listed on the National Register of Historic Places.

Native grasslands, carefully maintained by the trust, provide a home for sparrows, bluebirds, meadowlarks, and bobolinks. With pastures disappearing because of rapid development, populations of many of these birds have declined in recent years. Seeds from native and naturalized grasses and wildflowers also provide food for other small mammals, which in turn attract hawks and other birds of prey.

The trail hugs agricultural fields often planted with corn, soybeans, or hay. Active farmland makes up about 100 acres of the preserve and most of it is leased to local farmers. The fields reflect "sustainable agriculture," which seeks to raise healthy food with minimal harm to the environment or wildlife, provide fair and humane working conditions, and support preservation, open space, and rural communities.

Follow the trail as it turns, proceeding through a small grove of trees to head southeast. A private home and horse farm can be seen in the distance. Follow the trail as it bears left to continue around the northern end of this homestead. After this, the trail hugs Lucky Hill Road for about 0.1 mile. (It is the only trail in this part of the park, so you cannot get lost.) Homes, many of then hundreds of years old, can be seen on Lucky Hill Road, and complement the pastoral scenes within the park.

When the trail splits, head left (north) into a forested area, much of which is a prime example of forest creation. In 1992 the trust began planting several fields with seedlings of trees such as sugar maple, ash, red and white oak, poplar, and black walnut. The trust has planted about 5,000 trees and shrubs since then. They continue to grow, protecting slopes from erosion and providing critical wildlife habitat. Green plastic tubes keep deer from eating the young trees and also reduce weed competition and create a greenhouse-like environment.

Some areas within the preserve have been fenced to deter deer and encourage tree growth. You will see one of these fenced-in areas on the right as you take a left turn at a fork and head west. The trail passes wetlands and continues back to the gravel path, where you turn left to continue heading west. Just before the end of the gravel path, make a right, follow a mowed path north to its end, and turn left. Here the hike hugs another section of Lucky Hill Road; more historic homes, such as a stone farmhouse and colonial log cabin, come into view as the preserve connects seamlessly with the surrounding area.

The trail turns right just before another forested area, hugging meadows and heading west. When the private, main farmhouse and barn are in view, the trail turns left and heads northeast, providing an up-close view of Eastern Pennsylvania stone architecture. Stay on the trail to avoid trespassing onto private grounds, but admire the majestic sycamore in front of the barn complex as you walk past the large pond to your right.

A hop over a stream by the pond takes you back to the gravel trail that leads back to the parking lot. You have completed a hike that took you not only back in time, but also forward to a new holistic trend in preservation that balances a healthy and diverse natural environment with the need for food, shelter, health, and well-being.

## NEARBY ACTIVITIES

AMERICAN HELICOPTER MUSEUM
1220 American Boulevard, West Chester
(610) 436-9600
**www.helicoptermuseum.org**

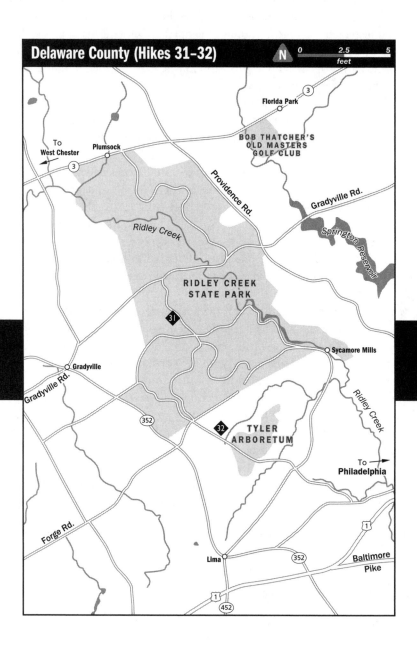

Delaware County (Hikes 31–32)

N

0    2.5    5
feet

Florida Park

BOB THATCHER'S
OLD MASTERS
GOLF CLUB

To
West Chester    Plumsock

Providence Rd.

Gradyville Rd.

Ridley Creek

Springton Reservoir

RIDLEY CREEK
STATE PARK

31

Sycamore Mills

Gradyville

Gradyville Rd.

Ridley Creek

352

32  TYLER
ARBORETUM

To
Philadelphia

Forge Rd.

1

Lima    352

Baltimore
Pike

1

452

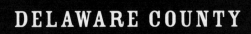

DELAWARE COUNTY

# 31 RIDLEY CREEK STATE PARK

## KEY AT-A-GLANCE INFORMATION

**LENGTH:** 5.16 miles

**CONFIGURATION:** Balloon

**DIFFICULTY:** Moderate

**SCENERY:** Mature woodland, Ridley Creek, historic mill village, ruins

**EXPOSURE:** Mostly shade

**TRAIL TRAFFIC:** Moderate

**TRAIL SURFACE:** Mostly paved, some dirt

**HIKING TIME:** 1.5 hours

**DRIVING DISTANCE FROM CENTER CITY:** 12.2 miles

**ACCESS:** Year-round, daily, dawn–dusk; free admission

**MAPS:** USGS Media; maps at kiosk and at www.friendsofrcsp.org/trailmap.html

**WHEELCHAIR TRAVERSABLE:** Yes, with access from Sandy Flash Drive South (park at the stables)

**FACILITIES:** Restrooms near park office and near exercise court; additional restrooms throughout park; see park map at www.dcnr .state.pa.us/stateParks/parks/ridleycreek/ridleycreek_mini.pdf

**SPECIAL COMMENTS:** Visit the park's Web site at .dcnr.state.pa.us/stateparks/parks/ridleycreek.aspx or call (610) 892-3900 for more information.

- - - - - - - - - - - - - - - - - - - - - - - - - - -

### GPS Trailhead Coordinates

UTM Zone (WGS84)  18S

Easting   0461560

Northing   4422310

Latitude   N 39° 57' 0.2"

Longitude   W 75° 27' 0.0"

## IN BRIEF

Ridley Creek meanders through an 18th-century mill village surrounded by outstanding trees, some of them hundreds of years old, on this hike that makes you feel you've been transported to a different time and place.

## DESCRIPTION

This hike, so close to Philadelphia, feels far, far away from busy, 21st-century city life. Although only 12 miles from downtown, this journey takes you into 2,606 acres that include a pastoral colonial plantation, the shimmering Ridley Creek, an 18th-century mill village, and the Hunting Hill mansion, which was built around a 1789 stone farmhouse.

The park offers an array of recreational opportunities. Have a picnic, fish for fresh-stocked trout, bike along paved trails, take a horse trail ride from Hidden Valley Farms, go cross-country skiing, or camp out. Most important, be sure to enjoy a variety of the park's half dozen trails.

- - - - - - - - - - - - - - - - - - - - - - - - - - - - - - - - -

## *Directions* ⟶

Take PA 3 west from Philadelphia and continue 1.8 miles before turning left onto US 1. Drive 5.8 miles, take the PA 252 exit, and merge right onto PA 252 toward Media. After 0.5 miles, turn left at North Providence Road, and then quickly make another right to remain on it. Drive 2.4 miles, then turn left at Gradyville Road. Continue 0.5 miles and bear left to remain on Gradyville Road, proceeding another 0.7 miles. After turning left into the park, drive 0.5 miles, then turn right into the main parking area. Park in the first parking lot (on the left) and walk downhill toward Trailhead 1E. There is handicapped parking at the stables off Sandy Flash Drive South. *1023 Sycamore Mills Road, Media, PA 19063.*

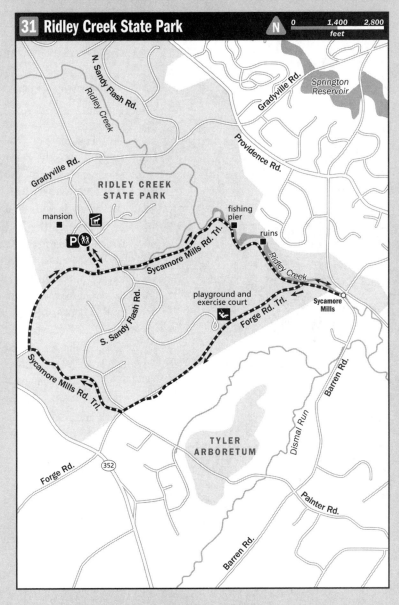

N

0    1,400    2,800
feet

N. Sandy Flash Rd.

Ridley Creek

Gradyville Rd.

Springton
Reservoir

Providence Rd.

Gradyville Rd.

**RIDLEY CREEK
STATE PARK**

mansion

fishing
pier

ruins

P

Ridley Creek

Sycamore Mills Rd. Trl.

playground and
exercise court

Sycamore
Mills

Forge Rd. Trl.

S. Sandy Flash Rd.

Sycamore Mills Rd. Trl.

Barren Rd.

Dismal Run

**TYLER
ARBORETUM**

Forge Rd.

352

Painter Rd.

Barren Rd.

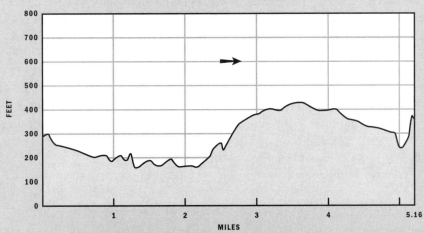

800

700

600

500

400

300

200

100

0

**FEET**

1          2          3          4     5.16

**MILES**

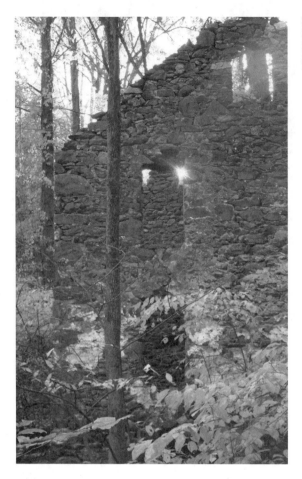

Haunts from an 18th-century milling village peek through stone ruins.

The park's trees are exceptional. The Pennsylvania Department of Conservation and Natural Resources (DCNR) includes several of them in its Big Tree List, which recognizes various specimens of extraordinary height, circumference, and crown spread. If these trees could speak—the sycamores, ashes, cedars, walnuts, and oaks, some of them hundreds of years old—would tell of a different time, one in which millers walked to work and used water power to refine resources into useful goods.

The hike begins at the parking lot in *front* of the mansion. If you reach the second lot, nearer the mansion, you have gone too far. Toward the far end of this first lot, a kiosk welcomes you to Trailhead 1E. Follow the dirt path through woods that include giant, bulbous sycamores until an arched bridge brings you onto the concrete, multipurpose Sycamore Mills Road Trail. Here you will turn left onto the trail, at the DCNR mailbox. A kiosk and bench stand on your right. The trail heads east, then turns southward to follow Ridley Creek, with its many scenic bends and straits. Soon, birches and beeches are mirrored in a vast, rippling reflecting pool—a former millpond.

A short distance on, old mill homes and stone ruins dot the trail. The second site of stone rubble is the remains of a house that burned down in 1974 but was once home to workers from the nearby Sycamore Mills. The house had two entrances, but three exits—one being the funeral door on the second floor, which allowed caskets to be maneuvered out of the building. The narrow, twisting indoor stairs did not allow the departed to easily depart.

Sycamore Mills, a small town previously called Bishop's Mill and Providence Mill, was an industrial site for almost 300 years. A gristmill used millstones to

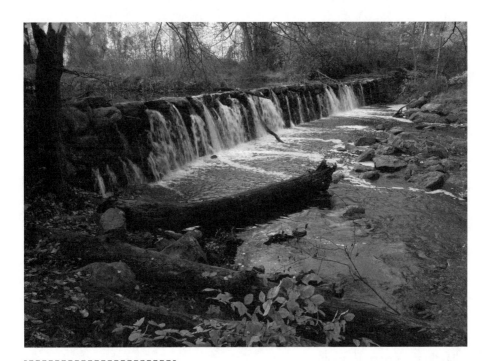

Water roaring over Ridley Dam

grind wheat, rye, barley, and corn, and served as the hub of the community for centuries before burning down in 1901. The long-gone, adjacent sawmill, erected in 1748, buzzed with activity along the banks whenever the gristmill was idle, ensuring that the precious water-generated energy was always put to use.

Water roars over the Ridley Dam past this second set of stone ruins, with more old homes across the creek. Here and farther along on this hike, you will see numbered wooden stakes marking the sites of the gristmill, the sawmill, a blacksmith and wheelwright shop, the mill office and union library, a rolling and slitting mill, a nail factory, a farmhouse, a bridge, a wagon shed, a barn, a springhouse, and a bake house. A kiosk map at the Sycamore Mills site shows the locations of these landmarks and details their historical significance.

At the end of the trail is a gate; turn around here to retrace your steps along the creek until the trail meets Forge Road Trail. Turn left onto this path, hiking uphill and leaving the creek (and the leisurely stroll) behind. The steep hill before you will certainly get your blood flowing and your heart pumping. If you are not up for the challenge, you should return the way you came. Otherwise, take it slow and enjoy the sights of still more historic ruins and stone homes amid mature woodland.

At the top of the hill is an exercise court and playground. If you are a true glutton for punishment, you can do a few pushups and sit-ups on the bars and benches. If not, continue along Forge Road Trail, which parallels another

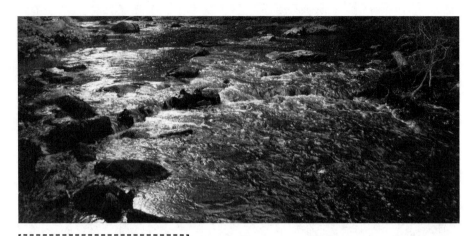

Whooshing waters of Ridley Creek

popular hiking area profiled in this book, Tyler Arboretum (see page 163). The trail levels off next to a pastoral cornfield, where, after the harvest, fawns forage for fallen kernels of corn. In the fall, migrating Canada geese honk overhead. As the trail turns right and heads west, the fields give way to woods and another abandoned stone farmhouse.

Forge Road Trail turns north and intersects Sycamore Mills Road Trail, where you turn right to finish the loop. You are now in the southwest section of the park and on the last leg of the hike. A sign on your left points toward the State Champion Black Oak, which is 140 feet tall, has a circumference of 18 feet, and spreads its crown 101 feet. Take a detour to give that tree a hug, then continue on Sycamore Mills Road Trail to where you started, while thinking of all the people and events that this oak tree and this part of Pennsylvania have seen throughout the last two centuries.

## NEARBY ACTIVITIES

BRANDYWINE RIVER MUSEUM
*(Regional and American art
in a 19th-century gristmill)*
US 1, Chadds Ford
(610) 388-2700
**www.brandywinemuseum.org**

CRIER IN THE COUNTRY
*(Haunted restaurant)*
1 Crier in the Country Lane,
Glen Mills
(610) 358-2411
**www.crierinthecountry.com**

ROSE TREE PARK
*(Scenic park with many activities
and concerts)*
1671 North Providence Road, Media
(610) 891-4663
**www.co.delaware.pa.us/depts/
rosetree.html**

# TYLER ARBORETUM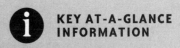

## IN BRIEF

The arboretum offers something for every season—shady hiking paths for warm summers, an explosion of flowers in the spring, stunning foliage in the fall, and seasonal exhibits year-round. But most of all, it renews your appreciation for the many species of trees that may hold the key to the future of the planet.

## DESCRIPTION

*I think that I shall never see*
*A poem lovely as a tree.*
*A tree whose hungry mouth is prest*
*Against the earth's sweet flowing breast;*
*A tree that looks at God all day,*
*And lifts her leafy arms to pray;*
*A tree that may in summer wear*
*A nest of robins in her hair;*
*Upon whose bosom snow has lain;*
*Who intimately lives with rain.*
*Poems are made by fools like me,*
*But only God can make a tree.*
　　　　　　　—Alfred Joyce Kilmer

Many climate experts believe that planting trees may help fight global warming because trees absorb carbon dioxide, a by-product of burning fossil fuels, through the natural

### KEY AT-A-GLANCE INFORMATION

**LENGTH: 6 miles**

**CONFIGURATION: Balloon**

**DIFFICULTY: Moderate–difficult**

**SCENERY: Woodland with state champion trees, meadows**

**EXPOSURE: Mostly shaded, some full sun**

**TRAIL TRAFFIC: Light**

**TRAIL SURFACE: Dirt, mowed grass**

**HIKING TIME: 5 miles**

**DRIVING DISTANCE FROM CENTER CITY: 25 miles**

**ACCESS: Free for members; non-member fees are $7 per adult, $6 for seniors (age 65+), and $4 for children (ages 3–15)**

**MAPS: USGS Media**

**WHEELCHAIR TRAVERSABLE: The described route is not accessible, but there are accessible trails within the park.**

**FACILITIES: Restrooms in barn/ education center**

**SPECIAL COMMENTS: Maps available at visitor center at the hike's start; pets and bikes not permitted on the arboretum grounds. More information: (610) 566-9134; www.tylerarboretum.org.**

## Directions

Take US 1 about 5 miles west from Philadelphia, exiting at PA 252 toward Media. Turn right on PA 252/North Providence Road. Within a few hundred feet, turn left at Lima and Rose Tree Road/West Rose Tree Road. After 1.5 miles, bear right at Painter Road. Drive 1.6 miles; the entrance is on the right. *515 Painter Road, Media, PA 19063.*

### GPS Trailhead Coordinates

UTM Zone (WGS84)  18S

Easting  0462317

Northing  4420617

Latitude  N 39° 56' 5.4"

Longitude  W 75° 26' 27.8"

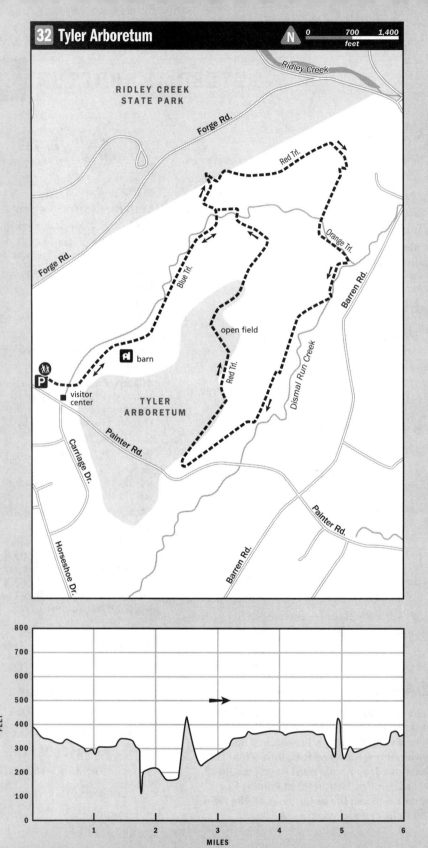

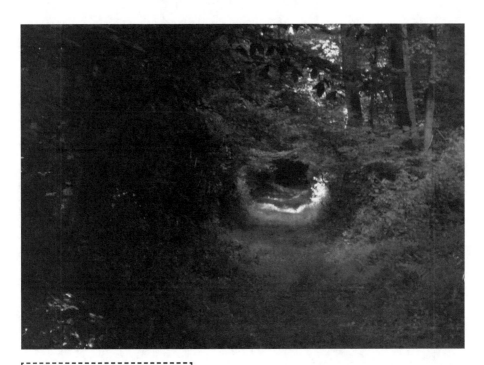

Shaded trails waiting to take you in

process of photosynthesis and then store the carbon and emit fresh, pure oxygen. In this way, trees prevent an important greenhouse gas from reaching the upper atmosphere and trapping heat near the earth's surface.

A single tree can absorb one ton of carbon dioxide over its lifetime; that being the case, Tyler Arboretum, which boasts 650 acres of towering trees, has likely absorbed at least 100,000 tons of carbon. In addition to trees, the arboretum includes blossoming shrubs and seasonal exhibits, woody trails that hug creeks and ponds, meadows and mazes. Twenty miles of trails of varying lengths and configurations wind through this protected forest park.

The Tyler Arboretum trail map, available at the visitor center, shows seven different trails—Green, Yellow, Blue, Pink, Orange, Red, and White—that can be variously combined. The longest is the White Trail, at 8.5 miles; the rest are between 0.9 and 3.1 miles. Be sure to bring this map with you on your hike; with so many choices, it is easy to get lost. Arboretum staff can provide you with brochures and advise you on which route to take, based on your particular interests and the time of year. The trails are well constructed and clearly marked. The arboretum offers about 100 different programs and field trips per year, such as guided nature walks, bird walks, wildflower walks, and horticultural workshops.

Special events include a Maple Sugaring Celebration in February and the Pumpkin Days Festival in October. The knowledgeable volunteers in seasonal butterfly house and garden can show you molting caterpillars, protected pupae

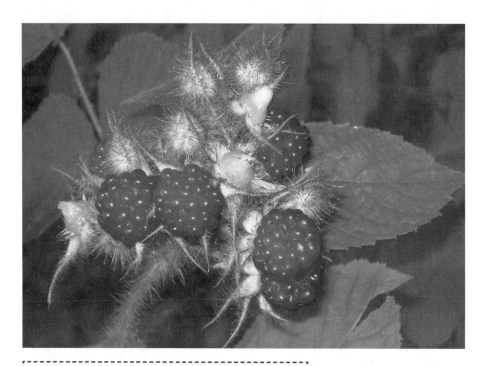

Wild raspberries burst forth in midsummer at the Arboretum.

inside their chrysalides, and mating adult butterflies—some of which live for only about two weeks. Many of the seasonal exhibits are in the area near the visitor center. Save some time after the hike to see the exhibits.

All the forest hikes start at a common trailhead. To find it, descend the trail from the visitor center to the barn, where you'll find an education center and restrooms. This barn is one of the largest still standing in the Delaware Valley. Walk to the front of the barn and continue downhill to a wooden footbridge. The trailhead is across the bridge; follow the trail to Gate 1.

Once through the gate, follow the Blue Trail, which hugs Rocky Run and ascends a steep hill cloaked with brush and fern. Continue on the Blue Trail until you join the Red Trail by turning right. This trail, which leads to the northern edge of the park, provides a cool shady walk, with red raspberries ripe to eat during the midsummer. Keep hiking the Red Trail until you reach a fork. Here, the left branch leads to Ridley Creek State Park, a hike for another day (see page 158). Bear right on the Red Trail, which joins the White Trail here, and admire the various species of trees found within the park.

The arboretum classifies its trees as either canopy or understory. Canopy trees include tulip, pignut hickory, sweet birch, white oak, and black walnut. Among the understory trees are sourwood, American holly, sassafras, redbud, pawpaw, and flowering dogwood. Plumleaf azalea, blueberry, Cumberland azalea, mountain-laurel, and Virginia sweetspire are a few of the shrubs you'll encounter.

If you visit in early spring and early summer, you will also be treated to a show of butterflies, as these insects are attracted to the blue wood aster, creeping phlox, Jacob's ladder, wild ginger, and other herbaceous plants in the arboretum.

The Painter Heritage Tour listed in the visitor's brochure takes in the park's historic structures and features 20 plants that were planted in the early to mid-19th century by the Painter brothers. The Painter brothers were direct descendants of the Quaker Thomas Minshall, who purchased this land from William Penn. The brothers systematically planted over 1,100 plant specimens, of which 20 remain. Five of these 20 are state champions: the cedar of Lebanon, the Yulan magnolia, the giant sequoia, the Corsican pine, and the oriental spruce.

So move forward with your hike, anticipating the many unique features that the park holds. Pick up the Orange Trail where you see markers beside Dismal Run Creek (be careful to watch for the markers and not end up on the White Trail, toward the road). Climb the Orange Trail until you see a gate, which is not the gate from which you entered. Continue through a meadow on this path, which soon joins the Red Trail, then turn right. Follow the Red Trail to its junction with the Blue Trail, and turn left, returning on the Red Trail and back to the Blue Trail, heading northwest until you see Gate 1. After passing through the gate, you enter the area of the Painter Heritage Tour, and the many labeled trees closer to the arboretum's main entrance.

As you view these trees on your way back to the visitor center and parking lot, remember that trees not only store carbon, protecting the world from global warming, but also provide shade from oppressive summer heat. They protect the soil from erosion and provide homes and habitats for countless animals. Some trees provide nuts and fruit—others are used to make medicines. As you look around, appreciate the benefits that trees provide.

For a comprehensive list on ways to combat global warming, see **www.global warming-facts.info/50-tips.html.**

## NEARBY ACTIVITIES

AUNTIE E'S ICE CREAM & CANDIES
1176 North Middletown Road, Media
(610) 558–9176

LONGWOOD GARDENS
1001 Longwood Road, Kennett Square
(610) 388-1000
**www.longwoodgardens.org**

RIDLEY CREEK STATE PARK
1023 Sycamore Mills Road, Media
(610) 892-3900
**www.dcnr.state.pa.us/stateParks/ parks/ridleycreek.aspx**

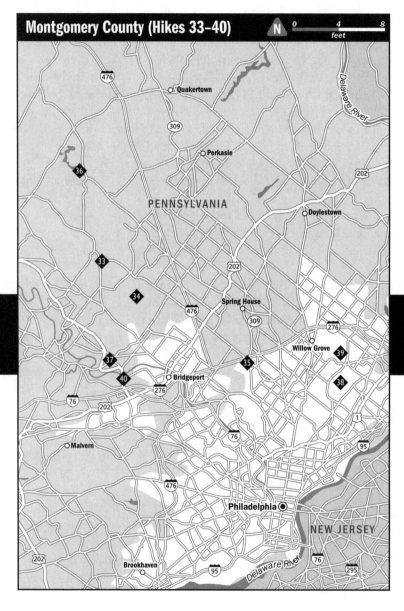

Montgomery County (Hikes 33–40)

N    0    4    8
          feet

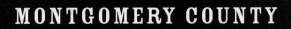

MONTGOMERY COUNTY

# 33  CENTRAL PERKIOMEN VALLEY PARK

## KEY AT-A-GLANCE INFORMATION

**LENGTH:** 4.21 miles

**CONFIGURATION:** Out-and-back with detours

**DIFFICULTY:** Moderate

**SCENERY:** Perkiomen Creek, meadows, woods

**EXPOSURE:** Mostly shade

**TRAIL TRAFFIC:** Light–moderate

**TRAIL SURFACE:** Gravel, asphalt, dirt

**HIKING TIME:** 1.5 hours

**DRIVING DISTANCE FROM CENTER CITY:** 34 miles

**ACCESS:** Daily, 8 a.m.–dusk, year-round; free admission

**MAPS:** USGS Collegeville; maps available at kiosk

**WHEELCHAIR TRAVERSABLE:** Not officially, but there are several flat and paved areas on the trail

**FACILITIES:** Restrooms near playground

**SPECIAL COMMENTS:** Stay on the trail because it sometimes borders private property; watch for horse waste. More information: (610) 287-6970; parks.montcopa.org (click the link for this park in the list on the left).

GPS Trailhead
Coordinates
UTM Zone (WGS84)  18T
Easting   0461313
Northing  4454531
Latitude  N 40° 14' 25.20"
Longitude  W 75° 27' 17.34"

## IN BRIEF

This rails-to-trails hike of the central portion of the Perkiomen Creek offers quiet views of what once was the rolling Perkiomen branch of the Reading Railroad. It also features restored meadows and woodlands along its outskirts.

## DESCRIPTION

Aside from being a veritable cash cow in the game Monopoly, the Reading Railroad was once one of the most prosperous corporations in the United States. The railroad hauled what was then deemed "clean" anthracite from the Pennsylvania coal region to Philadelphia and points south for heating houses and buildings. After World War II, the country shifted toward oil and gas, and the Reading Railroad was forced into bankruptcy by the 1970s.

The Perkiomen Trail, completed in 2003, was once the Perkiomen branch of the railroad. Montgomery County purchased the abandoned rail corridor for a greenway and trail system in 1978, but adjacent landowners objected. In 1996, the county lost its case

---

### *Directions* →

**Take Interstate 76 west from Philadelphia. After 16.8 miles, take Exit 328A, merge onto US 202–US 422, and travel west. After 0.5 miles, take Exit 328A to merge onto US 422 going west, toward Pottstown. After 9.2 miles, take the PA 29 exit and turn right at the end of the ramp toward Collegeville/Phoenixville. After 2.4 miles, turn right at East Main Street and left at the next intersection to stay on PA 29. Follow PA 29 for 4 more miles, then turn right onto Plank Road. The park entrance is on the right; the trail begins at the ranger station next to the parking lot. *1 Plank Road, Schwenksville, PA 19473.***

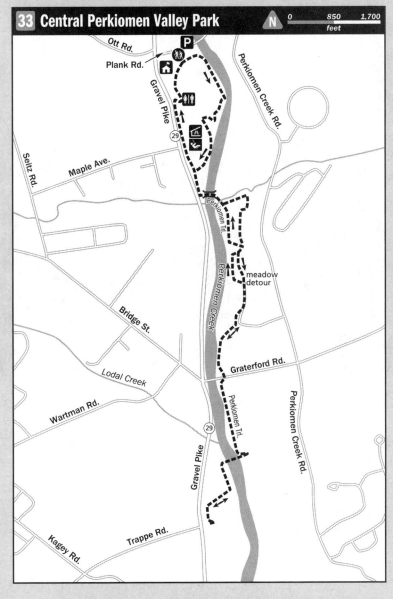

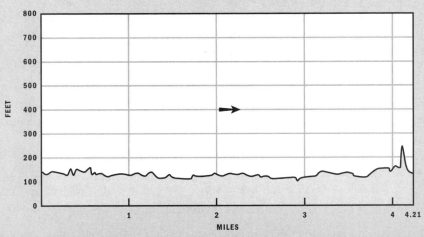

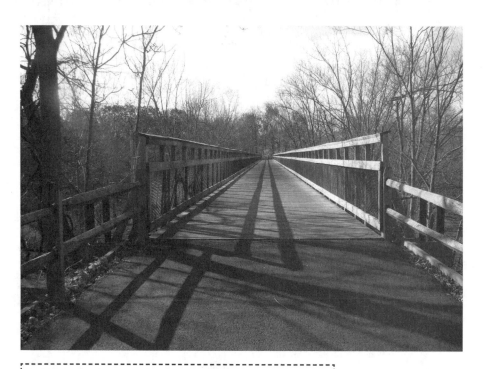

A railroad bridge converted to a footbridge along the Perkiomen Trail

against land claimants, and it was forced to reassemble the corridor through purchases and easements totaling 215 parcels from 157 landowners. The Natural Lands Trust and the Montgomery County Lands Trust spent more than $7 million to help establish an easement to ensure that this trail remains open space.

Today the multiuse trail runs 19 miles along Perkiomen Creek, passing through ten Montgomery County municipalities and connecting three county parks: Lower Perkiomen Valley Park, Green Lane Park, and Central Perkiomen Valley Park, the start of this hike. You begin at the park ranger station in the parking lot off Plank Road. Maps of the park and the Perkiomen Trail are inside the kiosk in front of the ranger station.

Across Plank Road are the entrance and parking lot for the Old Mill House, built in the early 1900s as a summer retreat for Dr. and Mrs. Hiram Rittenhouse-Loux. It is now part of the park, rented out for private parties.

You can see the Old Mill House from the ranger-station parking lot. At the other end of the parking lot from the ranger station, a sign marks the nature trail. A gravel path hugs the Perkiomen Creek, where ospreys swoop, mallards swim, and herons wade among the marsh grass. The creek also harbors turtles, frogs, salamanders, and water snakes.

Follow this path, which starts eastward, then turns south. Enjoy the water view for about 0.25 miles until you see a cabin on your right. This section of the park parallels a small catch basin, so in heavy rain you may need to hop from rock to rock to avoid wet feet and to reach the path behind the cabin. This path winds through woodlands along the creek, then turns right and meets the Perkiomen Trail. Turn left and follow the Perkiomen Trail south.

In about 0.2 miles, cross a pedestrian bridge where anglers fish for brook trout and Canada geese nap midcreek. It's easy to follow the trail's yellow floral signs as the trail turns right and heads southwest. Woodlands border meadows, which border the creek, providing prime bird-watching. Stay on the paved trails here when you see the dirt paths. The red-bellied woodpecker, American robin, northern cardinal, and northern flicker can be easily spotted near nesting boxes and tree stumps.

After you cross Graterford Road, the maximum-security Graterford Prison looms on your left. In 1993, on an outcrop of Lockatong Formation rocks along a tributary of the Perkiomen Creek, an inmate discovered dinosaur footprints. Hundreds of other fossilized footprints from at least four dinosaur species were also found in the area. Several specimens were removed and placed in the William Penn Museum in Harrisburg for conservation and study. Despite the possibility of more such finds, the Department of Corrections stresses that you stay on the trail.

Just before a railroad bridge that has been converted to a footbridge, the Skippack Township Trail intersects on your right (for more information on this trail, see **www.skippacktownship.org/TrailInfo.htm**). It connects with Palmer Park, Skippack Village, and Evansburg State Park (see Hike 34, page 175). This is an alternative route for another day, however, so continue to follow the signs for the Perkiomen Trail and walk west over the bridge.

Less than a half mile past the bridge you will reach Berthie's Café, where you can stop for refreshment any time of day or night. Just past Berthie's, a shady gazebo provides the perfect spot for a rest before you retrace your steps north, back over the bridge and toward Central Perkiomen Valley Park. This time, follow the two dirt-path detours to change the scenery slightly and have a look at the birds and, in spring and summer, the butterflies and wildflowers. After the second detour, the dirt meets a gravel path, turn left where you will continue until you reach the paved Perkiomen Trail again in about 0.1 mile. Turn right onto the Perkiomen Trail and walk across the bridge. Stay on the Perkiomen Trail until you reach Central Perkiomen Valley Park. There are restrooms on the right and a pavilion and playground straight ahead. Beyond the playground lies the parking lot from which you started.

The Reading Railroad no longer hauls its "clean" coal along the Perkiomen Trail, and the term "clean coal" has developed a whole new meaning, even though the world is still many years away from a zero-emissions coal solution (not to mention solutions for the safety and environmental hazards of strip mining). But no matter what the nation settles upon for its energy resources, the good news is that this branch of the Reading Railroad that once carried cars full of anthracite to heat homes, buildings, and schools is now a trail for all to enjoy.

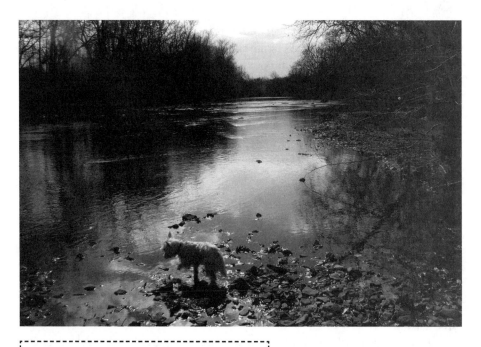

Crystal Kear near the clear waters of Perkiomen Creek

*For more information on other access points along the Perkiomen Trail, see* **trails.montcopa.org.**

## NEARBY ACTIVITIES

SKIPPACK VILLAGE
*(Antiques, craft, and specialty shops,
art galleries, and restaurants)*
On Route 73 (Skippack Pike)
between Routes 113 & 363,
Skippack
**www.bestofskippack.com**

WILLOW CREEK ORCHARDS
*(Organic fruits and vegetables;
pick-your-own and farmers' market)*
3215 Stump Hall Road, Collegeville
(610) 584-8202
**www.willowcreekorchards.com**

# EVANSBURG STATE PARK  **34**

## IN BRIEF

Take the Farm Trail to Skippack Creek, where at one time more than seven mills lined the creek's banks. Hike to a unique four-story mill, which still stands on land most likely once owned by a man who belonged to an obscure religious sect that broke from the Mennonites to speak in favor of American independence.

## DESCRIPTION

There once was a religious sect in the United States that many people don't know about: the Funkites. No, they didn't worship James Brown or Bootsy Collins; to the contrary, their faith was pretty mainstream and their principles patriotic—they believed in freedom of religion and the rights put forth in the U.S. Constitution.

In the late 1700s, Mennonite Bishop Christian Funk spoke in favor of supporting the colonies' separation from British rule. Many people who lived in eastern Pennsylvania at the time had fled Europe because of

---

### *Directions* ———————————→

Take Interstate 76 west from Philadelphia. After 12.7 miles, take Exit 331B to merge onto US 476 north. After 14.8 miles, take Exit 31 toward Lansdale. After 0.6 miles, turn left at PA 63–Sumneytown Pike. After a few blocks, turn right at Bustard Road. After 2.8 miles, take a right on PA 73; soon after, take a left onto Cedar Road. After 0.5 miles, stay left on Stump Hall Road. Go right onto Kratz Road, then veer left onto Lesher Road. Now take a right onto Thompson Road and look for May Hall Road on the left. Soon after is the park entrance—drive to the nature center at the dead-end. The trail starts in the nature-center garden and goes behind to the bridge in back. *851 May Hall Road, Collegeville, PA 19426.*

---

**KEY AT-A-GLANCE INFORMATION**

**LENGTH: 5.6 miles**

**CONFIGURATION: Balloon**

**DIFFICULTY: Moderate**

**SCENERY: Historic farmland, creek, forests, meadows, historic mill, bridge, and cemetery**

**EXPOSURE: Full shade–full sun**

**TRAIL TRAFFIC: Light**

**TRAIL SURFACE: Dirt, gravel, asphalt, grass**

**HIKING TIME: 2 hours**

**DRIVING DISTANCE FROM CENTER CITY: 34 miles**

**ACCESS: Daily, dawn–dusk, year-round; free admission**

**MAPS: USGS Collegeville; maps available at ranger station**

**WHEELCHAIR TRAVERSABLE: No**

**FACILITIES: Restrooms in main park area off May Hall Road**

**SPECIAL COMMENTS: Park workers are creating new trails and preparing a new park map, which should be available in 2010. More information: (610) 409-1150; dcnr.state.pa.us/stateparks/parks/evansburg.aspx.**

---

GPS Trailhead
Coordinates
UTM Zone (WGS84)  18T
Easting   0465881
Northing   4450057
Latitude   N 40° 12' 0.8"
Longitude   W 75° 24' 3.3"

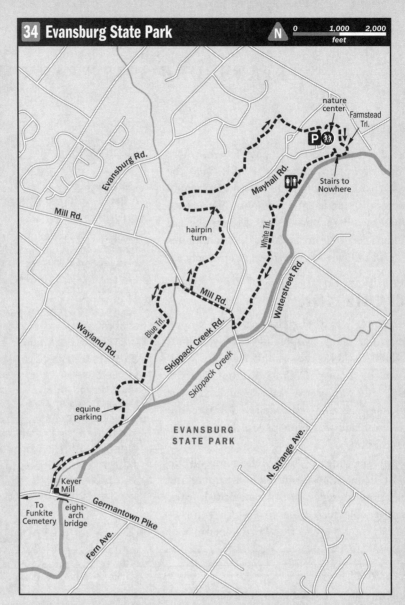

nature center

Farmstead Trl.

Evansburg Rd.

P

Mayhall Rd.

Stairs to Nowhere

hairpin turn

White Trl.

Mill Rd.

Waterstreet Rd.

Blue Trl.

Wayland Rd.

Skippack Creek Rd.

Skippack Creek

EVANSBURG
STATE PARK

N. Strange Ave.

equine parking

Keyer Mill

To Funkite Cemetery

eight-arch bridge

Germantown Pike

Fern Ave.

N    0    1,000    2,000
feet

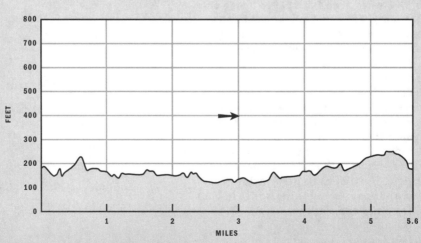

800
700
600
500
400
300
200
100
0

FEET

1          2          3          4          5.6

MILES

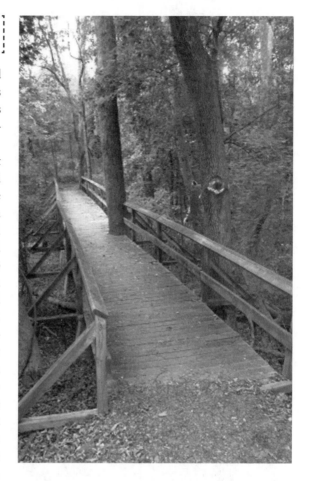

One of the many wooden footbridges within Evansburg State Park

religious persecution, and they enjoyed the freedoms created by William Penn's "holy experiment" to worship as they pleased.

Funk preached that Mennonites should stand up against European rule and support the American Revolution, lest they lose all the religious rights they had gained. This ran contrary to the Mennonites' beliefs in nonviolence, pacifism, and not swearing allegiances. Funk also believed in supporting a Revolutionary War tax, but this also ran contrary to standard Mennonite doctrine. Because of his beliefs, Bishop Funk was ordered to step down from the order and was excommunicated in 1778. He and about 50 of his followers broke from the main congregation and formed the Funkites. After Funk's death, the congregation continued to worship in Lower Providence Township and Evansburg.

This hike weaves through former farm country now converted to Evansburg State Park, visits an old mill and eight-arch bridge, and searches for the Funkite Cemetery, which serves as a memorial to Christian Funk.

Your quest begins left of the nature center, where the Farmstead Trail leads you over one wooden bridge and then another, heading east, following orange markers. German Mennonite Paul Friedt bought the land surrounding the present-day nature center in 1725; his descendants farmed this area for nearly two centuries. The wood lot near the creek provided them with timber and water, necessary for farming and survival.

The maples were used for firewood, barrels, and woodenware. The oak was bendable and suitable for box covers, barrel staves, and handles. The shrubs, weeds, root, and bark were gathered for medicines and teas. An 18th-century colonist might have used grapevine sap to try to grow hair on his bald head;

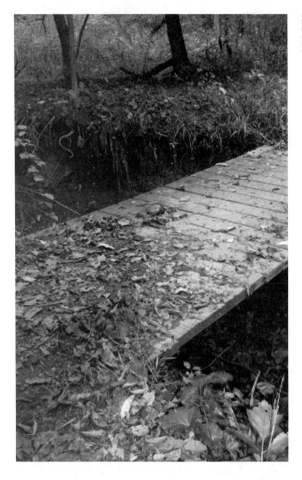

This wooden bridge crosses over a deep gully.

goldenrod tea would have been used as a diuretic to flush out urinary-tract infections. Wild deer, rabbits, and squirrels supplied the main food staples.

Soon the trail, well maintained with wooden footbridges, leads to the Skippack Creek, where you turn right, heading west, following white trail markers that lead onto the White Trail. The Lenape Indians frequented this area and called the creek *Skippauhacki,* which means "wetland." The reddish-brown sandstone rock formations along the creek were used for brownstone homes and buildings, popular in the late 19th and early 20th centuries.

Continue to hug Skippack Creek while you enjoy the trees' reflection in the clear water and the hawks flying overhead. Pass through the picnic area, and continue as the trail ascends. The trail heads downhill, and then the White Trail joins the Blue Trail, weaving west and then south, crossing near the edge of an aromatic pine forest. At about the 1-mile point, bear left to stay on the White Trail.

Soon you come to a stone-and-steel bridge, where you turn right and head southwest until you reach Skippack Creek Road. Cross the road and stay to the right of a meadow, heading west-northwest on an equine trail. After the meadow, hop over a small stream. Stay on the trail because hunting is permitted in this part of the park, but the trails are considered safety zones.

When you reach Wayland Road, cross it, turn right, and regain the trail, which is to your left. Continue straight at a large whitewashed barn. Pass an overgrown, closed trail and continue to the equestrian parking lot. Here turn right on Skippack Creek Road, heading southwest on the shoulder of the road until you reach the Keyser Mill. The creek provided the primary energy source during Colonial times for more than seven mills: five gristmills, a combination sawmill-gristmill, and a fulling mill (for weaving cloth).

The Keyser Mill operated as a flour- and gristmill for 95 years, until 1930. This unique structure stands four stories, making it larger than the typical two-story 18th-century mill, and is the last of the water-powered mills still standing in the area. The land on which the mill was built originally belonged to one Abraham Funk, who more than likely was a Funkite.

The hustle of Germantown Pike looms loudly close by, but beside the mill, an eight-arch stone bridge casts its peaceful shadow across the creek.

Once you've enjoyed the view of the bridge's reflection, return on Skippack Creek Road (northeast) to the equestrian parking lot. From here, retrace your route to the meadow you crossed after seeing the stone-and-steel bridge.

From the meadow's edge, cross the street and head north on the equine trail, on your left. Continue to a **T**-junction, where you turn left (west) and follow the trail back to a ranger station, the nature center, and the parking lot.

Before you leave the small town of Evansburg, take the time to stop at another cemetery, less than a mile from the park. In the middle of the Saint James Cemetery, at the corner of Evansburg Road and Germantown Pike, stands the tomb of unknown soldiers who died in the Revolutionary War. During the Battle of Germantown in 1777, the St. James Chapel was used as a hospital. Some 150 soldiers are buried in this cemetery.

By 1783, when the Treaty of Paris was signed, the 13 colonies were recognized as free, sovereign, and independent states. Thanks to the young men and women who fought to establish this country, and to people like the Funkites, who weren't afraid to stand up for their rights and for what they believed in, the Bill of Rights was adopted in 1791, and freedom of religion and the press were incorporated into the First Amendment.

## NEARBY ACTIVITIES

SKIPPACK VILLAGE
*(Antiques, craft, and specialty shops, art galleries, and restaurants)*
On Route 73 (Skippack Pike) between Routes 113 & 363, Skippack
**www.bestofskippack.com**

WORCESTER HISTORICAL SOCIETY
*(Museum of local history, especially of industry and farming)*
2011 Valley Forge Road, Village of Center Point
**www.worcesterhistorical.org**

# 35 FORT WASHINGTON STATE PARK

## KEY AT-A-GLANCE INFORMATION

**LENGTH: 5.5 miles**

**CONFIGURATION: Out-and-back, with a nature-trail-and-picnic detour**

**DIFFICULTY: Moderate**

**SCENERY: Bridges, trees, creek, and seasonal raptor migration**

**EXPOSURE: Full sun–full shade**

**TRAIL TRAFFIC: Light–medium**

**TRAIL SURFACE: Paved, gravel, dirt**

**HIKING TIME: 2 hours**

**DRIVING DISTANCE FROM CENTER CITY: 25 miles**

**ACCESS: Daily, year-round, dawn–dusk; free admission**

**MAPS: USGS Germantown**

**WHEELCHAIR TRAVERSABLE: Parts**

**FACILITIES: Restrooms near Militia Hill day-use and Flourtown day-use areas; see map at www.dcnr.state. pa.us/stateparks/parks/fortwash ington/fortwashington_mini.pdf**

**SPECIAL COMMENTS: Bring binoculars, especially in fall for the hawk migration. You may want to pack a picnic lunch to enjoy toward the middle of this hike at the Flourtown day-use area. More information: (215) 591-5250; dcnr.state.pa.us/ stateparks/parks/fortwashington .aspx.**

## GPS Trailhead Coordinates

UTM Zone (WGS84) 18T

Easting 0480982

Northing 4441211

Latitude N 40° 7' 15.5"

Longitude W 75° 13' 23.5"

## IN BRIEF

This hike offers lots of greenery and shade in the summer, paved trails all year round, and flowering plants and shrubs in springtime. In the fall it comes alive with color, in time for the migration of hawks, vultures, ospreys, and even eagles.

## DESCRIPTION

Fort Washington State Park takes it name from the temporary fort used by George Washington's troops in the fall of 1777, before they marched to Valley Forge. In recent years, the park has gained popularity as a place to view migrating birds and butterflies—190 bird species and 60 butterfly species have been reported. In addition, the park's 493 acres are home to 30 species of mammals, 16 species of fish, 300 species of wildflowers, and 37 species of trees and shrubs.

Although the park offers ample shade in the summertime, flowering trees and shrubs in springtime, and paved trails for mild-winter walking, most folks visit for the fall raptor migration. Then, broad-winged hawks

## *Directions*

**From Philadelphia, take Interstate 76 west via the ramp to Valley Forge. After 12.7 miles, take Exit 331B to merge onto I-476 heading north. Take Exit 20 for the Pennsylvania Turnpike/ Plymouth Road/I-276/Germantown Pike. Keep left at the fork and follow the signs for Plymouth Road. Turn right onto Plymouth Road, then left at Butler Pike. Take a slight right at Militia Hill Road, then turn left at Stenton Avenue. Go slightly right at Militia Hill Road. Parking is on the right. *500 Bethlehem Pike, Fort Washington, PA 19034.***

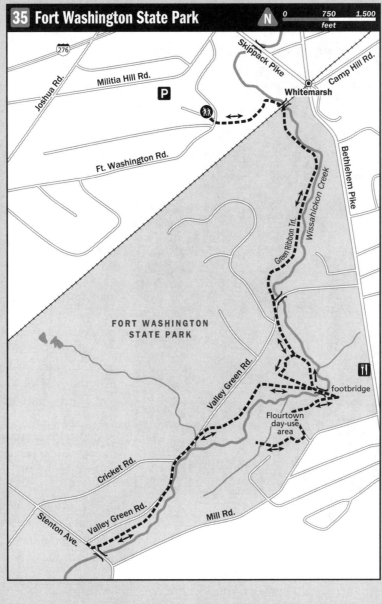

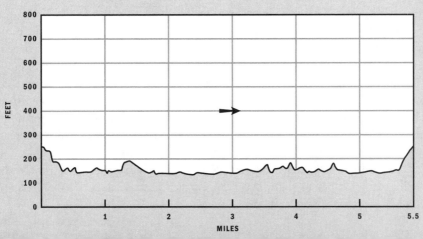

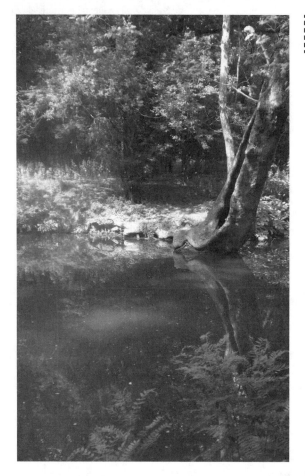

A quiet spot along the
Wissahickon Creek

are abundant, sharing the sky with red-shouldered hawks, northern harriers, ospreys, Cooper's hawks, and sharp-shinned hawks. One hawk species, the red-tailed hawk, often nests in the park.

Other raptors to look for include northern goshawks, peregrine, merlins, and American kestrels, all of which are falcons; turkey vultures and black vultures may also be soaring overhead. If you're lucky, you may spot the all-American bird of prey, the bald eagle, which has made a comeback in eastern Pennsylvania thanks to the Endangered Species Act of 1973, which helped to restore the birds by importing them from states where they were more numerous, establishing safe habitats, and imposing penalties for shooting or poisoning eagles. The 1973 banning in the United States of the pesticide DDT, which contaminates the food source of many birds, also aided the recovery of eagles and other raptors.

This hike begins in the parking lot on Militia Hill, where a tall deck provides visitors with a prime hawk-viewing area. By the steps of this watchtower, signs help visitors identify vultures, hawks, and eagles. When looking for an eagle, bird watchers should note how the bird soars and glides—eagles glide with their heads far in front of their level wings (which can span 90 inches), and when swooping for fish will get only their feet wet. Ospreys hold their wings in an M-shape and flap their wings more than soar; they will plunge completely into the water when catching their fish. A turkey vulture will rock from side to side as it flies, forming more of a V-shape with its wingspan. When perched, the turkey vulture looks slumped as it scavenges for scraps. The bald eagle, on the other hand, holds its head high and has a shorter beak. The osprey looks humble and innocent with its feathered head, but in flight it can appear just as majestic as the bald eagle, with a wingspan of between 52 and 72 inches.

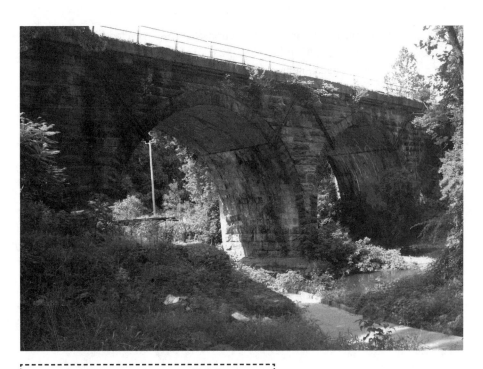

Stone-arched bridge inside Fort Washington State Park

Once you've caught your fill of high-flying friends, walk to the front of the watchtower, where a butterfly garden and bird feeder give you the lowdown on *Lepidoptera* (butterflies and moths). According to a brochure, compiled between 1980 and 1997 by Richard W. Boscoe, in the park there are 3 species of swallowtails, 4 of whites and sulfurs, 18 of brush-footed butterflies, 12 of *Lycaenidae* (hairstreaks, coppers, blues, and harvesters), and 23 of skippers. Pick up the brochure in the wooden compartment near the tower, and see how many species you can spot both in the garden and on your walk.

Now go downhill and left to pick up the Green Ribbon Trail, which partially hugs Wissahickon Creek. Although, this hike covers only about 6 miles, the Green Ribbon Trail is almost 20 miles long. It starts in Philadelphia, where the Wissahickon Creek meets the Schuylkill River and continues all the way to Upper Gwynedd in Montgomery County; much of the trail contains well-maintained walking paths, and updates and improvements to the trail continue.

Continue to yield left by the railroad tracks, marching downhill and under the pines, until you reach the paved trail, where you turn right. In midsummer, wild raspberries speckle the brush with sweetness, but beware of poison ivy, which often twists about the berry's thorny branches. You soon go under a stone underpass, where the creek waters flow beside you, washing away the stress of the day. The cool shade accompanies you through the first leg of this trail and continues until you reach a road straight ahead, where the route turns right and becomes a gravel path.

Soon you are faced with an option of choosing a less-traveled trail or continuing along the gravel path. This hike takes the trail less traveled and makes a left to align with the creek. Search nearby for small woodland animals such as squirrels and chipmunks. Eventually the nature trail wends its way back to the main path. The trail continues to weave close to the creek, offering smatterings of black-eyed Susans in summertime and a plethora of color provided by the changing foliage in fall. The far end of this out-and-back ends at Stenton Avenue and West Valley Green Road, where you turn and retrace your route, this time taking the gravel path, rather than the nature trail, so that you can see what you missed.

At this point along the hike, you may be growing tired, so instead of continuing directly back to Militia Hill, look for a sign where the path splits, leading you to the right and to the Flourtown day-use area, which has restrooms, a shady picnic pavilion, and a fountain to refill your water bottle. Before reaching the turnoff to the recreation area, cross a long footbridge. Stop in the middle to see if you can catch a glimpse of one of the park's massive great blue herons, and then move on to relax and eat lunch at one of the many picnic tables.

After resting your feet, return to the split in the trail, and continue back toward Militia Hill and a last glimpse at the many majestic migratory birds that make this park a special stop on your trek through eastern Pennsylvania.

## NEARBY ACTIVITIES

BOYD ANTIQUES
509 Bethlehem Pike
Fort Washington
(215) 646-5126
www.boydsantiques.com

THE CLIFTON HOUSE
(Library and museum of
local importance)
473 Bethlehem Pike
Fort Washington
(215) 646-6065
www.amblerhistory.com

HOPE LODGE
553 South Bethlehem Pike
Fort Washington
(215) 646-1595
www.ushistory.org/hope/index.html

ZAKES CAFE
444 South Bethlehem Pike
Fort Washington
(215) 654-7600
www.zakescafe.com

# GREEN LANE PARK

## IN BRIEF

This 6.5-mile hike can easily be shortened or stepped up to 16 miles. It winds around a glistening reservoir with scenery reminiscent of the Adirondacks, but without the seven-hour drive. This vast park of more than 3,400 acres lies only 40 miles from Philadelphia.

## DESCRIPTION

From the Hill Road Park Office, you can catch a glimpse of the 800-acre Green Lane Reservoir. With your back to the boat launch, you will see the Whitetail Nature Trail trailhead to the right of the parking lot. Take the trail into the woods, where it hugs the reservoir for the most part, providing views of the pine-lined water. The park is aptly named—many of the reservoir's inlets glisten in shades of hunter and Kelly green due to algae and the trees' reflection.

The park becomes even greener during the popular Scottish-Irish Festival and Highland Games in late August or early September. The free festival features top-line Celtic music, comedy, pipe bands, dancers, falconry, sword fighting, arts and crafts, food, and much more.

### Directions ——————→

**Take Interstate 76 west from Philadelphia. After 12.6 miles, take Exit 331B and merge onto I-476. After almost 15 miles, take Exit 31 and turn right at the end of the ramp onto PA 63. After 9.5 miles. turn right onto Gravel Pike; then, after 0.2 miles, take the first left onto Park Road, which splits into Hill Road. About 1 mile down Hill Road, look for the park entrance (boat-rental entrance) on your right. In the front of the parking lot is the Hill Road Office; the Whitetail Nature Trail trailhead is toward the back of the parking lot. *2144 Snyder Road, Green Lane, PA 18054*.**

### i  KEY AT-A-GLANCE INFORMATION

**LENGTH:** 6.5 miles

**CONFIGURATION:** Out-and-back

**DIFFICULTY:** Hard

**SCENERY:** Pine-lined reservoir, shady woodlands

**EXPOSURE:** Mostly shaded

**TRAIL TRAFFIC:** Light

**TRAIL SURFACE:** Grass, dirt, rocky at times

**HIKING TIME:** 2.25 hours

**DRIVING DISTANCE FROM CENTER CITY:** 40 miles

**ACCESS:** Daily, dawn–dusk, year-round; free admission

**MAPS:** USGS Perkiomenville and Sassamansville; maps at ranger station

**WHEELCHAIR TRAVERSABLE:** No, but the park does have paved trails.

**FACILITIES:** Restrooms near boat launch

**SPECIAL COMMENTS:** No bikes on the Blue Trail. More information: (215) 234-4528; parks.montcopa .org (click the link for this park in the list on the left).

### GPS Trailhead Coordinates

UTM Zone (WGS84)  18T

Easting  0458289

Northing  4466591

Latitude  N 40° 20' 55.77"

Longitude  W 75° 29' 28.1"

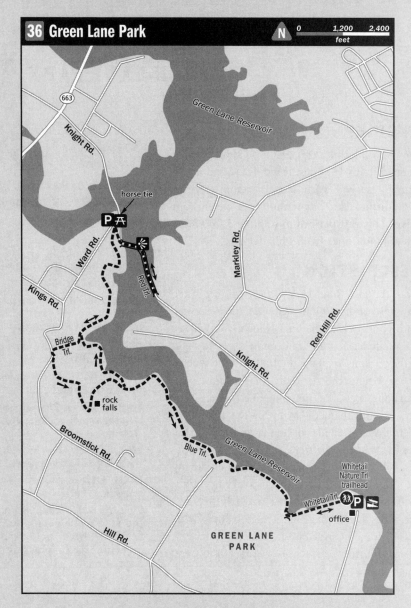

N

0          1,200      2,400
              feet

Green Lane Reservoir

663

Knight Rd.

Ward Rd.

Kings Rd.

horse tie

P

Red Trl.

Markley Rd.

Red Hill Rd.

Bridge
Trl.

rock
falls

Knight Rd.

Broomstick Rd.

Blue Trl.

Green Lane Reservoir

Whitetail
Nature Trl.
trailhead

Whitetail Trl.

P

Hill Rd.

office

GREEN LANE
PARK

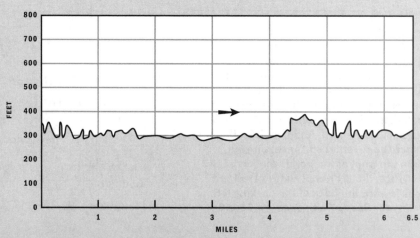

| FEET | | | | | | | |
|---|---|---|---|---|---|---|---|
| 800 | | | | | | | |
| 700 | | | | | | | |
| 600 | | | | | | | |
| 500 | | | | | | | |
| 400 | | | | | | | |
| 300 | | | | | | | |
| 200 | | | | | | | |
| 100 | | | | | | | |
| 0 | 1 | 2 | 3 | 4 | 5 | 6 | 6.5 |

MILES

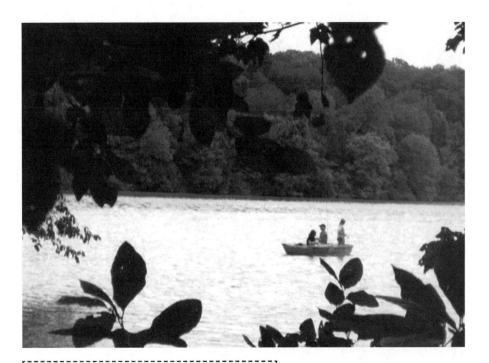

A young family out for a day of fishing on the reservoir

Continue southwest on the Whitetail Nature Trail until you see blue paint markers indicating that the trail joins with the Blue Trail. Continue west on the combined trails until you cross a small bridge with split-rail fencing. The clearings that open to the reservoir make excellent spots to look for ospreys or bald eagles, which have returned to the area in recent years. Other birds to watch for include red-throated and common loons, grebes, cormorants, and diving ducks.

Turn right approximately 100 feet after the bridge to stay on the Blue Trail as it splits off from the Whitetail Nature Trail, continues to hug the reservoir, and heads northwest. The trail continues over a small stream. Do not follow the equestrian trails that venture uphill into the woods.

About a mile into the hike, the trail turns left and crosses large boulders, heading farther into the woods and then uphill, but still not straying far from the glistening waters and the anglers trying for crappie, carp, and catfish. Trout, northern pike, and muskie also inhabit the Green Lane Reservoir. This part of the Blue Trail includes loose rocks and narrow crossings appropriate for the experienced hiker. Bikers are not permitted on this trail, but it is shared with equestrians, so watch out for horse manure.

Continue on the Blue Trail as it dips into a steep ravine and back uphill. You soon reach a sign that says TURN AROUND. To cut the 6-mile hike in half, take this left. Otherwise, continue down the steep hill. At the bottom of the hill, turn left to stay on the Blue Trail.

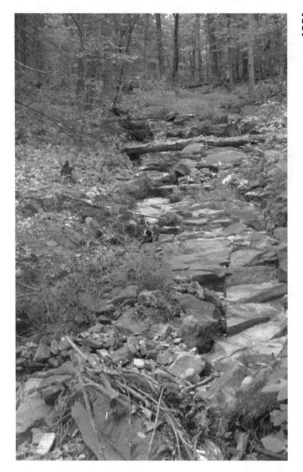

A rocky inlet along the Blue Trail

Once you've hiked a total of approximately 2 miles, the blue markers become fewer and farther between. A sign points toward the Bridge Trail, which bends to the right. This begins an out-and-back section to a scenic overlook above the northwest side of the reservoir. The trail widens at the 2.5-mile mark as you near the bridge. Soon you walk into a parking lot. At the bottom of the lot, a walkway turns right and brings you over the scenic bridge.

If you want an ambitious walk, you can continue across the bridge and pick up the 10-mile Red Trail, which loops around the trails on the eastern side of the reservoir. If you find a 6-mile jaunt sufficient, then turn around and continue back through the parking lot the way you came. Stop at the picnic bench next to the lot for a snack and water break. The bench marks the hike's halfway point.

Head back to the Blue Trail (where you started the out-and-back), but instead of going left on the Blue Trail, turn right and head south into the woods on an unmarked trail. Follow it to Broomstick Road and turn left onto the road, picking up the trail again in approximately 50 yards, on the left. There are no markers on this trail, but it is well maintained and easy to follow.

This part of the trail can be steep and slippery. The unnamed trail again meets the Blue Trail, where you turn right and head uphill until you reach a sign for Rock Falls. The falls can dry up during late summer. Wild ferns grow abundantly in this part of the hike.

Continue on the Blue Trail as you see the reservoir once again. The trail turns right and heads east. Continue east when you see the TURN AROUND sign, and follow the Blue Trail back to the Whitetail Trail, which leads you back to the parking lot and the Hill Road office. There, you can rent a boat and see

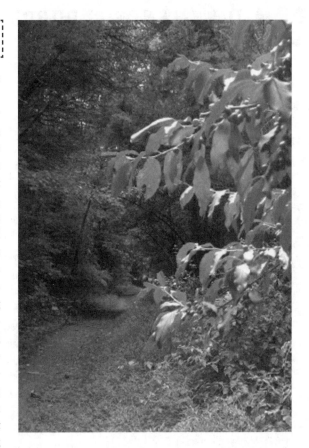

A quiet path before the scenic bridge

the reservoir from a whole new perspective.

Thanks to community workers, county staff, park staff, and volunteers, these 3,400 acres of open space offer a perspective not often obtained these days, especially less than 40 miles from a major commercial mecca. This park offers fishing; boating; picnicking; horseback-riding, hiking, and mountain-biking trails; family and equestrian camping; tennis; sand volleyball courts; playgrounds; cross-country skiing; ice skating; ice fishing; and a nature center with environmental classes. But most importantly, the park provides preserved lakes, forestland, and wetlands so imperative to the survival of the ecosystem and to the planet in general.

## NEARBY ACTIVITIES

BARBARA ANN'S VICTORIAN TEA ROOM
(Breakfast, lunch, private parties)
120 Main Street, Green Lane
(215) 234-9292

THE BARN ATTIC
*(Store with new, preowned, collectible, vintage, and antique items)*
324 Harleysville Pike, Harleysville
(215) 256-9305
**www.barnattic.net**

WYNN'S CREEKSIDE INN
*(Restaurant, pub, and bed-and-breakfast)*
1840 Perkiomenville Road,
Perkiomenville
(215) 234-2292

# 37 JOHN JAMES AUDUBON CENTER AT MILL GROVE

 **KEY AT-A-GLANCE INFORMATION**

**LENGTH:** 2.7 miles

**CONFIGURATION:** Balloon

**DIFFICULTY:** Hard

**SCENERY:** Museum, stone barn, nearby farm, meadows, ruins of springhouse and smoke stack, and lots of birds

**EXPOSURE:** Full sun–full shade

**TRAIL TRAFFIC:** Light

**TRAIL SURFACE:** Paved, dirt

**HIKING TIME:** 2 hours

**DRIVING DISTANCE FROM CENTER CITY:** 25 miles

**ACCESS:** Museum open Tuesday–Saturday, 10 a.m.–4 p.m.; Sunday, 1–4 p.m. Grounds open Tuesday–Sunday, 7 a.m.–dusk. Trails and parking are free; museum admission is $4 adults, $3 seniors age 60+, and $2 children ages 4–17.

**MAPS:** USGS Valley Forge and Collegeville

**WHEELCHAIR TRAVERSABLE:** Partially

**FACILITIES:** Restrooms in visitor center

**SPECIAL COMMENTS:** No dogs allowed. More information: (610) 666-5593; pa.audubon.org/centers_mill_grove.html.

## GPS Trailhead Coordinates

UTM Zone (WGS84)  18T

Easting    0462162

Northing   4441508

Latitude   N 40° 7' 22.89"

Longitude  W 75° 26' 38.82"

## IN BRIEF

Ideal for art and ornithology enthusiasts, this hike traverses the original American homestead of John James Audubon. A visit to the museum sets the stage for a natural connection with the man who would inspire generations of artists and conservationists.

## DESCRIPTION

Flocks of passenger pigeons create a massive gray wave a mile wide overhead, seeming to last for days; droves of great auks waddle ashore for their yearly incubation; the Carolina parakeet nestles in a tree hollow as its kin perch nearby, painting the river with reflective color in motion. These are the sights you won't see during your 60 hikes within 60 miles of Philadelphia, or anywhere else for that matter: all three of these birds are extinct. You can, however, view the birds as they were drawn by the artist and ornithologist John James Audubon in his famous print collection, *Birds of America*—his personal magnum opus, which contains a detailed visual record of more than 400 bird species.

Although John James Audubon shot the birds he wanted to draw—this was standard

---

### Directions

Take Interstate 76 west from Philadelphia. After 17 miles, take Exit 328B-A to merge onto US 422 toward Swedesford Road/Pottstown. After 4 miles, take the PA 363 exit north toward Trooper/Audubon. Soon after, take a slight right at PA 363–South Trooper Road. Turn left at Audubon Road; continue for about 1 mile, then turn left at Pawlings Road. Look for parking for the Audubon Center. The hiking trail starts at the museum. *1201 Pawlings Road, Audubon, PA 19403.*

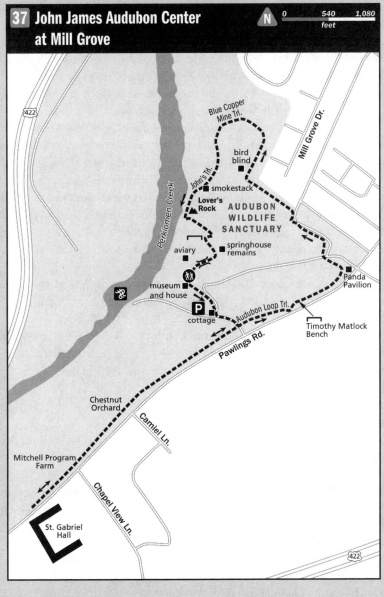

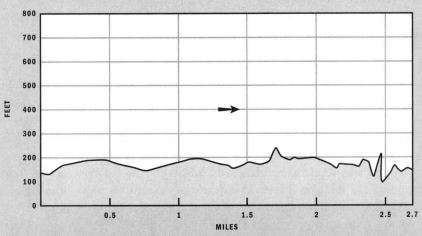

practice in the days before lightweight binoculars—his artistic work inspired and educated countless people about the importance of birds and nature. Fifty-four years after Audubon's death, the conservationist group, the National Audubon Society was created in his name.

If not for a small twist of fate, however, the National Audubon Society might not exist. Audubon's father encouraged his son to become a mariner, but chronic seasickness discouraged that dream, and the young Audubon became more of a landlubber, observing and drawing the natural surroundings of his adopted American countryside. Audubon had left his native France, fleeing service in Napoleon's army, to live in peaceful Penn country at his father's estate in Mill Grove. During his three years there, Audubon fell in love with wildlife, honed his artistic talents, and conducted the first bird-banding studies to trace migratory behavior.

The estate, which in 2004 became a museum dedicated to John James Audubon, houses a collection of prints, portraits, and memorabilia related to Audubon, the Audubon Society, and Mill Grove itself. A long driveway leads to the house and grounds—park at the first lot on the left, in front of the park pavilion. Signs point you to a paved path, which leads to the museum.

The museum's gift shop has tour tickets and trail maps. The self-guided house tour includes a short film on John James Audubon, which describes the 13-year process he perfected to draw, paint, and print his work before modern printing techniques or photography.

An early printing of *Birds of America* sits under glass, with a modern version of the book nearby for viewing. Several other prints adorn the walls, along with one original painting and a painting of the artist, as well as a bust of him and his wife. Upstairs, Audubon's room has been restored to how it looked in the early 19th century. The walls and windowsills contain garlands of blown eggs; stuffed specimens of frogs, squirrels, opossums, and raccoons line the mantle and shelves. A table with candle, plume, and paper depicts the presence of a prodigious and dedicated artist. Another room has models of a hawk and an owl—along with large sheets of paper, stools, and tables—so that young Audubons can try their hand at drawing birds.

In the next room is a painting depicting the great egret. This species, almost hunted out of existence in the late 19th century to provide plumes for ladies' hats, was saved through conservation measures by the Audubon Model Law, passed in 1901. (The great egret later became the symbol for the Audubon Society.) Other treasures include prints from the octavo edition of *The Viviparous Quadrupeds of North America,* which was completed by Audubon's son John Woodhouse Audubon, also a talented artist. There is also an array of Native American artifacts collected at Mill Grove, as well as a mineral collection taken from mines that operated on the property during the 18th and 19th centuries.

The museum holds an abundance of artifacts and information, but the trails surrounding the museum also hold nature's copious treasures, so once you've

The Pennsylvania chapter of the American Chestnut Foundation has reintroduced the tree to the greater Philadelphia area.

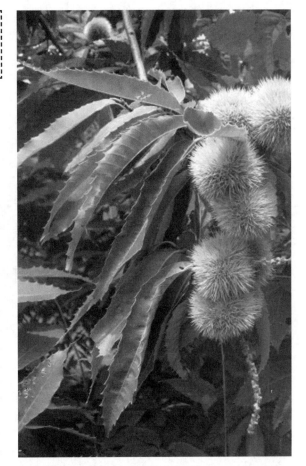

browsed sufficiently, grab your trail map and exit the front door for a hike of the grounds. Before you start this hike, visit the small raptor aviary, which is behind a small white shed, nestled in the hillside to your left as you descend toward the creek. A red-tailed hawk, eastern screech owl, great-horned owl, and American kestrel reside inside, but you may need to search the far corners of their cages to find them. The park takes the birds out in public during its Harvest Market Fair and also on its Raptor Day, which occur annually.

Turn right from the aviary and follow the paved path down a slope until you come to a green-and-white cottage on your right. Turn left and continue to a **T**-junction. Here turn right and head southwest on the Audubon Loop Trail (look for yellow markers). This portion of the trail hugs the outer meadows of the park. In the eastern United States, many grasslands have been vanishing due to overdevelopment. This means that many grassland-dependent birds, such as the eastern bluebird and tree swallow, have lost their habitats and are declining in numbers.

In fact, according to a report by the U.S. Department of Agriculture Economic Research Service, during the period between 1982 and 1992, nearly 16 million acres of land was newly developed in the United States, consisting mostly of forestland, pasture, and cropland. The Sierra Club estimates that in the span of three human generations, 3 percent of the America's bird population has become extinct. The National Audubon Society has made efforts to restore grasslands and add nesting boxes to help stabilize these bird populations.

The park's outer meadows contain butterflies galore, and rabbits race across the fields to hide in the brush. Dragonflies buzz by the rich green chestnut trees,

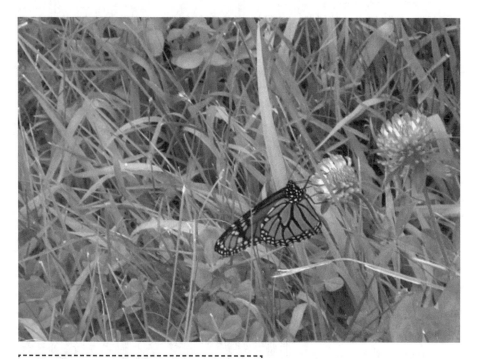

A butterfly weaves through the restored grasslands.

which are part of the Pennsylvania Chapter of American Chestnut Foundation's attempts to reintroduce the tree to this area. America's chestnut trees were all but destroyed by a blight in the first half of the 20th century. Recent attempts to restore the tree, through hybridization with a Chinese variety, have been promising. With success, these trees should be bred into blight resistance within the next decade or so.

Continue on the Audubon Loop Trail until you come to a farm with llamas and donkeys, on the right. This farm is part of the Mitchell Program, an intensive 120-day residential treatment program for delinquent male youth. Now turn around and head back the way you came, going northeast on the Audubon Loop Trail to see more meadows and birds.

A historical marker is just ahead on the trail. Timothy Matlock, a statesman and Revolutionary War patriot, helped found the "Fighting Quakers," a society of Free Quakers who believed in the importance of fighting for American independence. A bench near this marker provides a place from which to count the species of birds that circle the nearby meadows: mourning doves, northern cardinals, blue jays, American robins, sparrows, and goldfinches. More than 175 species of birds have been seen at Mill Grove.

Continue along the Audubon Loop Trail until you arrive at the main entrance of the park. Here turn left, cross the entrance road, and then continue on the Audubon Loop Trail, heading northwest. With a meadow on your left, stop at the bird blind for an even closer look at resident fauna. Pick up the Blue Copper Mine Trail, and look at a smokestack from the engine house of a copper mine that operated in the mid–19th century. Take a left after the Blue Copper Mine Trail and stay southwest on the outer portion of the trail to pick up John's Trail, with its bright-green markers. This part of the route is not paved or wheelchair accessible.

The trail now descends a set of wooden steps and provides a scenic view of Perkiomen Creek. Lover's Rock, at the bottom of the steps, is a popular stopping spot. Stay on John's Trail, hugging the creek, until you come to a junction near a bench and a marker. Here turn left and descend more steps, heading east. The stone remains of an old springhouse sit beside trail. Cross a stone-pillar bridge for a closer view of the structure that once provided water and food storage for the estate and mill.

You are now on the last leg of this hike through history, heading south toward an open meadow from which the parking lot and the museum can accessed. Audubon kept detailed journals in which he warned of the dangers of overhunting and loss of habitat. Although it may be too late to witness waves of carrier pigeons, droves of great auks, and flocks of Carolina parakeets, with the efforts of the National Audubon Society and other conservation groups, there may still be time to spy the enormous wingspan of the California condor; hear once again the song of Bachman's warbler, which has not been spotted since 1988; or glimpse an ivory-billed woodpecker, whose extinction status is yet to be determined. Without preservation and conservation efforts, these birds and many others may become just illustrations like those in Audubon's *Birds of America*.

## NEARBY ACTIVITIES

LOWER PERKIOMEN VALLEY PARK
101 New Mill Road, Oaks
(610) 666-5371
**parks.montcopa.org**

VALLEY FORGE NATIONAL
HISTORICAL PARK
*(See Hike 40, page 206)*
1400 North Outer Line Drive,
King of Prussia
(610) 783-1099
**www.nps.gov/vafo**

# 38 LORIMER PARK:
## Council Rock and Dairy Farm Trail

**KEY AT-A-GLANCE
INFORMATION**

**LENGTH:** 2.5 miles

**CONFIGURATION:** Double loop

**DIFFICULTY:** Easy

**SCENERY:** Council Rock, Pennypack Creek, woodlands, dairy farm

**EXPOSURE:** Mostly shaded

**TRAIL TRAFFIC:** Light

**TRAIL SURFACE:** Gravel

**HIKING TIME:** 1–2 hours

**DRIVING DISTANCE FROM CENTER CITY:** 17 miles

**ACCESS:** Daily, dawn–dusk; free admission

**MAPS:** USGS Frankford; maps available at ranger station

**WHEELCHAIR TRAVERSABLE:** Mostly; park near the ranger station.

**FACILITIES:** Restrooms in welcome area near ranger station

**SPECIAL COMMENTS:** Trails are unsigned; obtain map at the ranger station. No dogs or alcoholic beverages permitted in park. Old McVeagh Mansion is a private residence, despite being listed on park map. More information: (215) 947-3477; parks.montcopa.org (click the link for this park in the list on the left).

GPS Trailhead
Coordinates

UTM Zone (WGS84)  18T

Easting    0493672

Northing   4438501

Latitude   N 40° 5' 48.42"

Longitude  W 75° 4' 27.24"

## IN BRIEF

This park's unsigned trails wind through shady woodlands, hug a babbling creek and trickling stream, and then ascend to a pastoral scene worthy of a Norman Rockwell painting.

## DESCRIPTION

*You've got to get up every morning with determination if you're going to go to bed with satisfaction.*

—George Horace Lorimer

An editor who worked with the likes of Willa Cather, F. Scott Fitzgerald, Rudyard Kipling, Sinclair Lewis, H. G. Wells, John Galsworthy, and Stephen Crane, George Horace Lorimer helmed the *Saturday Evening Post* from 1899 to 1937. He was the first of the magazine's editors to commission covers from Norman Rockwell, starting a business relationship with this all-American art icon that would last 45 years. While Lorimer was in charge of the *Post*, subscriptions grew to 3 million copies per week.

*Directions* ⟶

Take Interstate 95 north from Philadelphia. After 8 miles, take Exit 30 for Cottman Avenue/ Rhawn Street/PA 73, and merge onto Cottman Avenue. After 4 miles, turn right at Oxford Avenue. After 1.2 miles, continue on Huntingdon Pike. Stay on Huntingdon Pike for almost 1 mile, then turn right at Rockledge Avenue. In less than 0.25 miles, turn left at Old Ford Road. After 1 mile, turn right at Moredon Road. Park across the street from the Lorimer Park sign, on the left. Walk down the steps, cross the street, and follow the park entrance to the ranger station. The trailhead is at the bridge. *183 Moredon Road, Huntingdon Valley, PA 19006.*

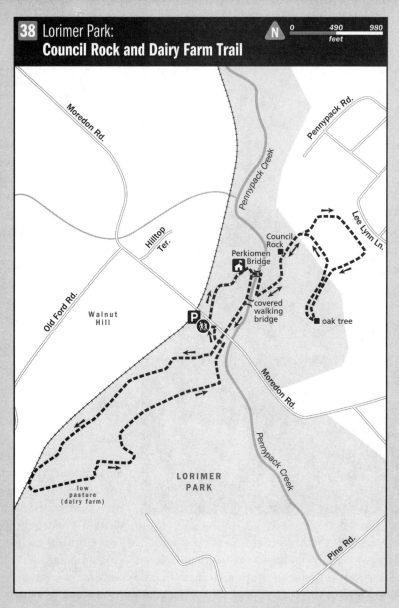

N

0     490     980
feet

Moredon Rd.

Pennypack Rd.

Pennypack Creek

Lee Lynn Ln.

Hilltop Ter.

Council Rock

Perkiomen Bridge

covered walking bridge

Old Ford Rd.

Walnut Hill

oak tree

Moredon Rd.

LORIMER PARK

low pasture (dairy farm)

Pennypack Creek

Pine Rd.

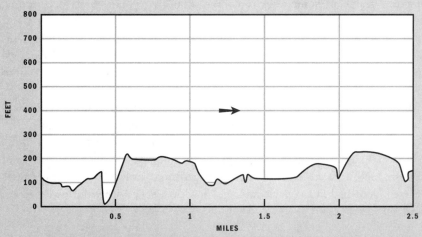

FEET

800
700
600
500
400
300
200
100
0

0.5     1     1.5     2     2.5

MILES

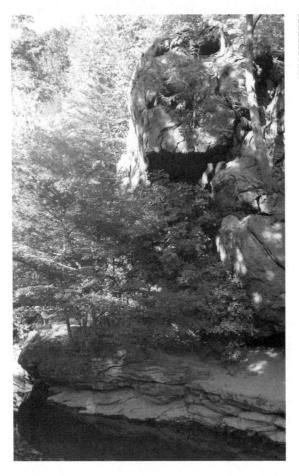

Council Rock, an outcrop of Wissahickon schist, may have once been used as a meeting spot for Native Americans.

Like many successful people, Lorimer invested in land. He chose the rich countryside of Montgomery County for his home and other investment property. His estate in Wyncote, Pennsylvania, eventually became a private Catholic grammar school, but he donated 230 acres in eastern Abington Township—land that would become Lorimer Park—to the county in memory of his mother and daughter, "for the enjoyment of its natural beauty."

That natural beauty bursts through the moment you enter. Babbling Pennypack Creek passes underneath a wooden footbridge to the right of the ranger station. As you walk across the bridge, the sun may reflect the water's ripples on the majestic Council Rock, an outgrowth of Wissahickon schist. Residents of the area claim that this massive rock was once used as a meeting spot by Native Americans. Couples now meet atop the rock to share a romantic moment, sometimes returning months or years later for wedding photographs.

Once across the bridge, look for another small bridge, on the right. This covered footbridge, which spans a small stream, was constructed in 1997 by Eagle Scout Timothy Egger and Troop 72. Cross this bridge and take the gravel trail to your left, which passes beside Council Rock and heads east, then northeast. The first of today's double loop is well shaded and well populated by deer, which have lost much of their forage land to development in this part of Pennsylvania.

Some of the abundant trees growing within the park include red, white, and black oaks and blackgum, maple, pine, and tulip. The understory consists of spicebush, mountain laurel, and witch hazel. All told, at least 70 species of trees have been identified in the park, and the meadows glow with wildflowers in the spring and summer.

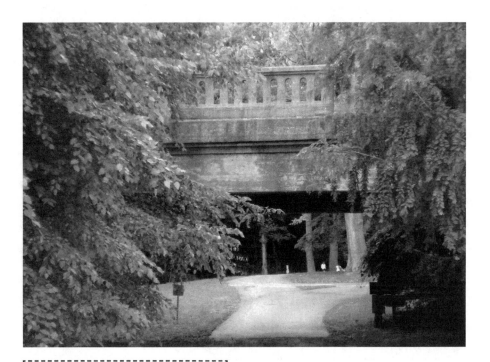

Moredon Road bridge over Lorimer Park trail

Climb the gravel trail, heading north, to a fork, where you stay right, heading east and then southeast. Pass a residential area on the left. The trail curves right, hugging a meadow and then returning to shady woodlands. Continue on an outer loop until you come to a **T**-junction near a giant oak tree. Here turn right, heading back toward the creek. Soon you rejoin the original trail, heading west toward Council Rock and the wooden footbridges.

When you return to the first bridge, the trail hugs Pennypack Creek for about 0.25 miles. An underpass takes you beneath Moredon Road. The mature trees, the creek, and the stone underpass lend a remote and quiet feel to this part of the park. Continue to hug Pennypack Creek until you come to another bridge; here the creek turns left. You may see an occasional angler here, biding for the trout that are stocked here seasonally by the Pennsylvania Fish and Boat Commission. After crossing the bridge, take a right and walk along a trail that hugs a stream called Harper's Run. Trail traffic is light most of the time, and birds are abundant even in the wintertime. Bring your binoculars to see migrating raptors, warblers, and a slew of resident birds.

Continue to follow the trail as it climbs upward. Your strenuous efforts on this leg are amply rewarded at the top of the hill by a pastoral scene of dairy cows grazing amid rolling hills. On a sunny day, they look like black silhouette cutouts moving slowly through the fields. Stop here to meditate before continuing to a junction. Here you can opt for a shorter route by turning left and following the trail as it returns to forest, or you can continue straight, beside a fenced

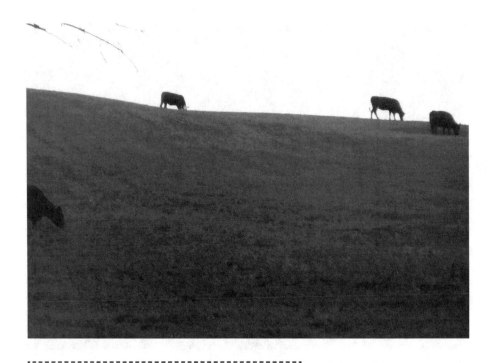

The cows look like black silhouettes as they graze the fields.

pasture. Either way, you will be heading back toward the creek and the bridge you crossed just before coming to Harper's Run. After the bridge, look for a concrete pathway with white arrows, pointing you back toward the parking lot.

The hike you've just completed scratches the surface of this natural haven, which lies 35 minutes from Philadelphia's Center City. The park's trails turn off in many different directions but are not marked. You never know what awaits around each corner, and you can only imagine George Horace Lorimer losing himself after a long day of editing—probably not realizing that someday the authors he published in the *Post* would become literary legends, nor how much future generations would enjoy losing themselves in the nature that he preserved.

## NEARBY ACTIVITIES

BRYN ATHYN CATHEDRAL
*(Gothic-Norman church built in 1919; its stained glass was created with a medieval process.)*
Open daily, 1 to 4 p.m.
900 Cathedral Road, Bryn Athyn
(215) 947-6225
www.brynathyncathedral.org

BRYN ATHYN COLLEGE
*(Picturesque college campus)*
2965 College Drive, Bryn Athyn
(267) 502-2511
www.brynathyn.edu

JOSEPH'S PIZZA
7947 Oxford Avenue, Philadelphia
(215) 722-7000
www.josephsfoxchase.com

# PENNYPACK ECOLOGICAL RESTORATION TRUST

## IN BRIEF

Enjoy the diverse restored and preserved landscapes and naturally restored wildlife of the central Pennypack Creek valley. Walk along the creek, through forests, and past historic homes and buildings, then finish in a divine meadow.

## DESCRIPTION

The role of organizations such as the Pennypack Ecological Restoration Trust, which seek to protect, restore, and preserve land, has become ever more important. The trust protects natural areas in central Pennypack Creek valley through land acquisitions, restoring meadows and woods through stewardship, and maintaining trails, meadows, and forests through endowments.

Parking is available on the shoulder of Creek Road. Start this hike on Creek Road Trail, heading north. Immediately, you are transported from the buzz and business of city and suburbia to a world of flowing waters and a restored stream habitat with plenty of turtles and toads. Beside the creek, butterflies flutter among snapdragons, goldenrods, and other wildflowers.

------------------------------------------------

## *Directions* ———————————➤

Take PA 611 north from Center City, Philadelphia. After 10 miles, bear right on Washington Lane and continue 1.3 miles. Turn left at PA 2017/Susquehanna Road. Within a block, turn right on Valley Road. After about 0.5 miles, bear left at Washington Lane and continue 2 miles. Turn right at Terwood Road, drive 0.25 miles, then look for Creek Road on your left. Creek Road ends within several hundred feet. Find off-street parking.
*2955 Edge Hill Road (Headquarters), Huntingdon Valley, PA 19006*

### KEY AT-A-GLANCE INFORMATION

**LENGTH:** 6.17 miles
**CONFIGURATION:** Balloon
**DIFFICULTY:** Moderate
**SCENERY:** Creek, historic homes and building, grasslands, forests
**EXPOSURE:** Full sun–full shade
**TRAIL TRAFFIC:** Light–moderate
**TRAIL SURFACE:** Pavement, gravel, dirt, grass
**HIKING TIME:** 2 hours
**DRIVING DISTANCE FROM CENTER CITY:** 15 miles
**ACCESS:** Year-round, daily, 8 a.m.–dusk; free admission
**MAPS:** USGS Hatboro; access at www.pennypacktrust.org/trails .htm#maps
**WHEELCHAIR TRAVERSABLE:** Much of the creek path is accessible.
**FACILITIES:** No public restrooms
**SPECIAL COMMENTS:** No pets are permitted on Raytharn Trail. The Pennypack Ecological Restoration Trust is part of the larger Pennypack Greenway Preservation plan to protect land along the entire Pennypack Creek, which is endangered by development and water pollution. For more information about the Pennypack Greenway, visit www.pennypackgreenway.org or call (215) 657-0830.

------------------------------------------------

## GPS Trailhead Coordinates

UTM Zone (WGS84)  18T
Easting   0493794
Northing   4442480
Latitude   N 40° 7' 57.4"
Longitude   W 74° 4' 22.3"

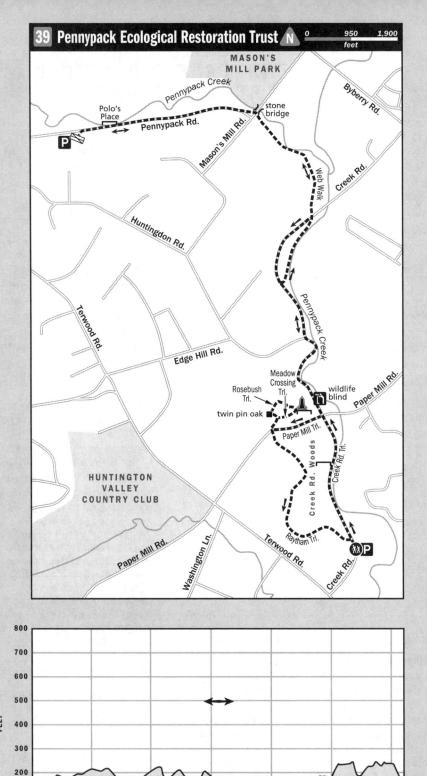

0    950    1,900
feet

MASON'S
MILL PARK

Pennypack Creek

Byberry Rd.

Polo's
Place

stone
bridge

Pennypack Rd.

P

Mason's Mill Rd.

Web Walk

Creek Rd.

Huntingdon Rd.

Pennypack Creek

Terwood Rd.

Edge Hill Rd.

Meadow
Crossing
Trl.

wildlife
blind

Paper Mill Rd.

Rosebush
Trl.

twin pin oak

Paper Mill Trl.

Creek Rd. Woods

Creek Rd. Trl.

HUNTINGTON
VALLEY
COUNTRY CLUB

Raytham Trl.

P

Paper Mill Rd.

Washington Ln.

Terwood Rd.

Creek Rd.

FEET

800
700
600
500
400
300
200
100
0

1    2    3    4    5    6.17

MILES

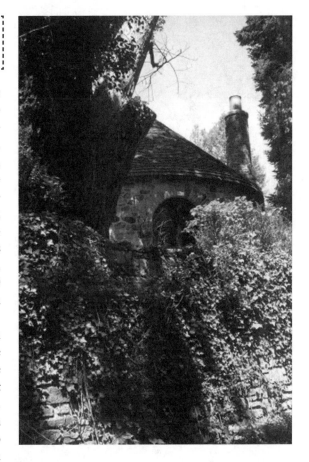

A stone building on the grounds of the Lord's New Church, which borders the Creek Trail.

The creek and the nearby forest provide excellent bird-watching opportunities; phoebes, bluebirds, kestrels, red-tailed hawks, red-winged blackbirds, sparrows, white-breasted nuthatches, warblers, swallows, cardinals, mockingbirds, woodpeckers, robins, and wrens may be spotted. In fact, sightings of more than 150 species of birds have been recorded here.

As you continue north along the creek, watch the mallards napping and notice the large boulders that dot the stream to your right. Healthy saplings sprout in the Creek Road Woods to your left. Shortly after you cross Paper Mill Road, you come upon a wildlife blind that provides a chance for up-close birding and observation of a wetland.

Soon the gravel trail turns to pavement, continuing about 50 yards beside a quiet road before narrowing again. The nearby cream-colored colonial homes recall a slower time in the history of southeastern Pennsylvania. Creek Road Trail continues past an open gate to where tall pines scent the air with the smell of Christmas.

Stone buildings with walls of cascading ivy and a picturesque chapel belonging to the Lord's New Church are farther north along the trail. The New Church is a Christian religious movement that closely follows the writings of Emanuel Swedenborg. These picturesque grounds are closed at dusk. If you have time, walk around if you wish; if not, continue north on Creek Road Trail.

Just before a stone bridge in the distance, pick up the dirt path on your left that hugs the western side of the creek. Soon, the open trail, which is warm in the summer, gives way to lots of trees, ensuring shade and cooler temperatures.

This trail crosses Mason's Mill Road, another popular parking spot for visitors to the Trust's property. This road can be busy with traffic at times, but serenity

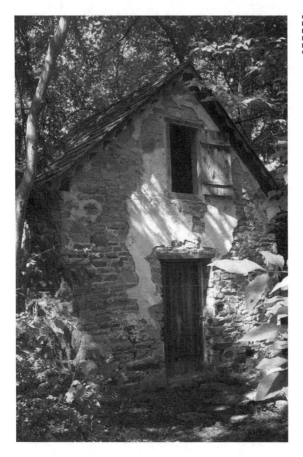

Old stone shed along the Web Walk

resumes on the other side. A bench by the creek bears a plaque reading POLO'S PLACE and signifies that you are coming close to the western end of the trail at the Parkway Gate.

At this point, turn around and head back to the junction near the stone bridge. Here, instead of turning right, keep straight on the Web Walk, heading southwest, for a closer look at the creek. The narrow trail weaves close to the creek, over wooden walkways, and past an old stone shed. Web Walk leads you back to Creek Road Trail, where you turn left, heading south.

Past the wildlife blind, find the Paper Mill Trail on your right. This last leg of the hike uses Paper Mill Trail and part of Rosebush Trail, then follows Raytharn Trail south to the parking area. Pets are not allowed on Raytharn Trail, so if Rover is in tow, you may need to save your exploration of these trails that circle the meadow restoration and head straight back to the parking lot. If Rover stayed home, however, you can head west, past the wetland and uphill on the Paper Mill Trail.

At the top of Paper Mill Trail, turn sharply right and then right again. You now reach a lookout with a bench and a memorial stone to a woman named Kathryn Adelberg Greenhouse (1944–1987), who likely saw the trust take the first steps in its master plan, adopted in 1975, to preserve undeveloped and environmentally sensitive land in the central watershed of Pennypack Creek.

The trust's association began to assemble the preserve in 1976, through land donations, purchases, and conservation easements. What started in 1970 with the efforts of a small environmental group fighting to improve the water quality of Pennypack Creek has grown into 720 acres of protected land only 35 minutes from Center City, Philadelphia.

After the trail loops, turn left and head southwest for a short stroll on Rosebush Trail to reach Meadow Crossing Trail, where an enormous twin pin oak stands to your right. The wooden trail markers are well labeled and in plain view, so pick up Raytharn Trail heading southeast at a meadow clearing.

These restored meadows constitute a collaborative restoration-research program with the U.S. Department of Agriculture, the Natural Resources Conservation Service, the Natural Lands Trust, and the Pennypack Trust. The meadow plots, with 21 different planting dates and pre-planting treatment combinations, will eventually guide other land-management organizations to the best measures for establishing native-grass meadows, which create habitats for diverse animals and plants.

At two neighboring benches, Raytharn Trail turns right, heading southwest and into a wooded area. You soon return to meadowlands and a scenic view of a farm in the outlying valley. The trail turns left, and you are rewarded with a view of the towers and spires of the Bryn Athyn Cathedral in the distance. As you walk downhill toward the parking area, you are reminded of nature's divine qualities, and see that restored ecosystems promise a gradual renewal of life where you can not only connect with nature, but also fall in love with it again and again.

## NEARBY ACTIVITIES

ALLWAYS CAFÉ
*(Salads, sandwiches, pastas)*
634 Welsh Road,
Huntington Valley
(215) 914-2151
(215) 914-2165 (fax)
**www.allwayscafe.com**

GLENCAIRN MUSEUM
*(Art on the history of religion)*
1001 Cathedral Road,
Huntingdon Valley
(215) 938-2600
**www.glencairnmuseum.org**

*See also Hike 38, Lorimer Park, page 196.*

# 40    VALLEY FORGE NATIONAL HISTORICAL PARK

## KEY AT-A-GLANCE INFORMATION

**LENGTH: 7.1 miles**

**CONFIGURATION: Balloon**

**DIFFICULTY: Hard because of length, not terrain**

**SCENERY: Revolutionary War head-quarters, historic mud huts**

**EXPOSURE: Sun and some shade**

**TRAIL TRAFFIC: Moderate**

**TRAIL SURFACE: Mostly paved; Historic Trace Road is grass and dirt**

**HIKING TIME: 3 hours**

**DRIVING DISTANCE FROM CENTER CITY: 25 miles**

**ACCESS: Year-round, daily, 6 a.m.– 10 p.m.; Welcome Center, 9 a.m.– 5 p.m.**

**MAPS: USGS Valley Forge. Maps available at www.nps.gov/vafo/ planyourvisit/upload/vafo_trails_ 2007.pdf**

**WHEELCHAIR TRAVERSABLE: Yes, by staying on the bike path instead of Historic Trace Road**

**FACILITIES: Restrooms in Welcome Center**

**SPECIAL COMMENTS: Carry water and sunscreen, especially in the summer; see www.nps.gov/vafo or call (610) 783-1099 for additional park information.**

## GPS Trailhead Coordinates

UTM Zone (WGS84)  18T

Easting   0464000

Northing   4439090

Latitude   N 40° 6' 5.1"

Longitude   W 75° 25' 20.3"

## IN BRIEF

This hike is a step back in time to a preserved historic encampment that turned a hungry, ragtag bunch of young enlisted men into a mature militia that would march forth from this valley to ultimately win independence for the American colonies.

## DESCRIPTION

Just a year ago, in 1776, you were on top of the world. General Washington had led your division, torn and tattered, across the Delaware River to a surprise attack and victory against the British-hired Hessian troops in Trenton. After this, you defeated a British brigade in Princeton. The tide of the war was changing; freedom and independence seemed within reach.

But today, you are plagued with insecurity. Although news traveled south regarding General John Burgoyne's surrender to Major General Horatio Gates at Saratoga, you have since fought two failed battles and have lost friends and hopes. Your ancestors fled their homeland to find freedom, and England has come across the ocean to take it all away.

You have been relocated to a camp northwest of the besieged Philadelphia, in

## Directions

From Philadelphia, take US 76 west. After 16 miles, take Exit 328B-A to merge onto County Line Expressway/US 422 west toward Swedes-ford Road/Pottstown. After 3 miles, exit onto PA 23 West/West Valley Forge Road toward Valley Forge. Continue to follow West Valley Forge Road. After 0.25 miles, turn right on Outer Line Drive, where you will see the Welcome Center just 100 feet ahead. *1400 North Outer Line Drive, King of Prussia, PA 19406.*

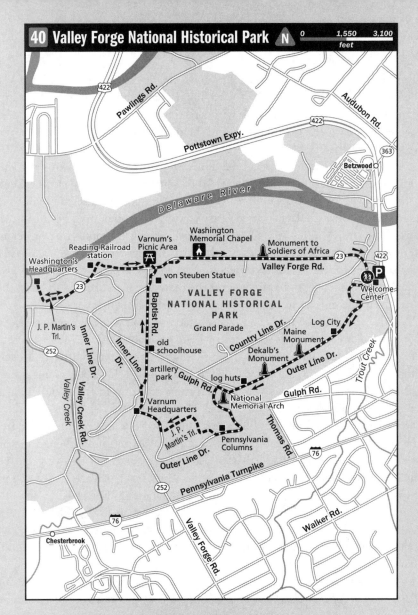

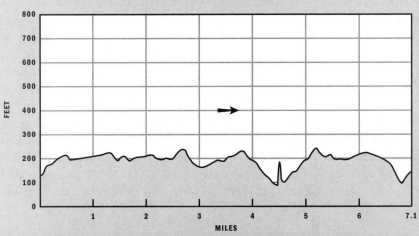

rural Valley Forge. Your log hut offers some shelter, but there hasn't been a surplus delivery in almost a week. You're hungry, cold, and you miss your family. Many of your comrades are sick with pneumonia and dysentery. Some of the new recruits have already deserted, and the rest of them don't look like they will hold up in battle.

Nonetheless there is work to be done. So grab your backpack to start military exercises about the encampment. To the northeast, at the Welcome Center, comrades await with maps and information. Once you have secured your map, leave the building, and make two lefts: you are now marching uphill, directly toward General Muhlenberg's Brigade, which anchor the outer line of defense. Here you will see the beginnings of a log city. Orders from the general have set specifications for these huts at 16 feet long by 14 feet wide by 6.5 feet high, with a door near the street and a fireplace at the rear. The men ordered to build these were given one dull ax to cut the wood and perform their labor.

After you pass the fields and inspect the huts, you will eventually arrive at a monumental arch honoring your service—you have now entered the 21st century, and you learn that the Continental Army was victorious, years after that wicked winter. In February 1778 a French alliance was formed. Inspector General Baron Friedrich Wilhelm Augustus von Steuben came to camp to train soldiers in the essentials of military drill and discipline. The sad soldiers you left back at the log city were transformed into a well-trained militia worthy of the "land of the free." The stay at Valley Forge matured the Continental Army, and although it would be another five years of battles—some successful, some less so—you and your remaining comrades eventually saw victory. The Treaty of Paris ended the war, released all war prisoners, and proclaimed the colonies as free states.

Look proudly upon this majestic arch, dedicated in 1917, which exalts "the incomparable patience and fidelity of the soldiery." A centennial in 1877, with reenactments and fanfare, featured a speech by the lawyer and renowned orator Henry Armitt Brown:

*"And here in this place of sacrifice, in this vale of humiliation, in this valley of the shadow of that dead out of which the life of America rose regenerate and free, let us believe with an abiding faith that to them union will seem as dear and liberty as sweet and progress as glorious as they were to our fathers and are to you and me and that the institutions which have made us happy preserved by the virtue of our children shall bless the remotest generation of the time to come."*

Before marching out of this fort in June of 1778, you watched 2,000 soldiers die—not from the winter's bitter cold or starvation, for the supply flow had improved with the appointment of Nathanael Greene as quartermaster general—but from disease that plagued the camp during the spring thaw. Influenza, typhus, typhoid, and dysentery took many men, but you were spared because of capable nurses and surgeons, as well as a smallpox inoculation program and camp-sanitation regulations. The huts were aired out daily, kitchen waste and bedding straw were burned, and drinking water was disinfected with whiskey

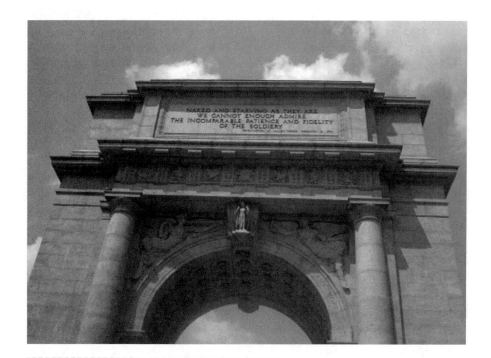

NAKED AND STARVING AS THEY ARE
WE CANNOT ENOUGH ADMIRE
THE INCOMPARABLE PATIENCE AND FIDELITY
OF THE SOLDIERY

A monumental arch honors Revolutionary War heroes.

and vinegar. A captain was appointed daily to visit the sick within his brigade to see that they had proper care.

Fill your canteen with water at the fountain before the arch and continue your march, turning left in front of the arch and picking up a paved walkway at the south section of Outer Line Drive. If the spirits of fallen soldiers have returned to the park, surely they ride on the backs of the countless deer that dominate the fields. These deer stare boldly at visitors, enjoying the protection of the National Park Service, while they meander from meadow to mud hut. The abundance of deer has led some locals to lobby for controlled hunting, but this has not yet been approved.

Ascend the trail until you see the towering Pennsylvania Columns on your left, with winged Eagles silhouetted against the sky. Continue the path along J. P. Martin's Trail. After serving in the war, Joseph Plumb Martin wrote a book called *Private Yankee Doodle,* which details "Some of the Adventures, Dangers, and Sufferings of a Revolutionary Soldier." Ahead are a parking lot and rest-room—sanitary facilities and transportation have come a long way since the 18th century. Picnic benches to your right provide a fine lunch spot.

Snake fencing lines the trail until you reach a roadway; stay right where the fence angles left. The pastoral meadow and rolling hills look untouched and undeveloped, like a memory preserved in time. Follow the trail to a sign for Varnum's Headquarters, right. Brigadier General James Mitchell Varnum served in the Continental Army from 1777 until 1779. Varnum campaigned to allow

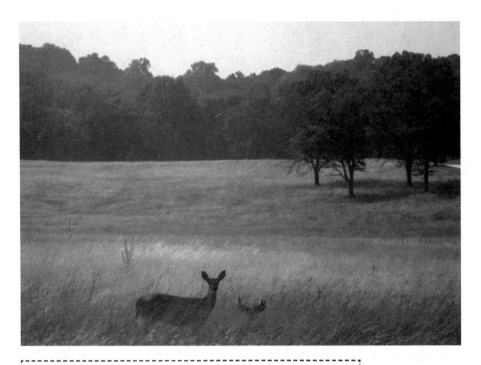

Spirits of fallen soldiers ride on the backs of the abundant deer population.

African Americans to enlist in the Continental Army, which resulted in the formation of the 1st Rhode Island Regiment as an all-black unit.

Before reaching Varnum's headquarters and a picnic area, look for the Knox Artillery Park on the right; cross the grassy patch to see the cannons standing at attention. Under orders from Brigadier General Henry Knox, the artillery was stored and repaired here, and gun crews trained and drilled, so that in the event of attack, the cannons could be dispatched from this central location to wherever they were most needed.

Once you have inspected the artillery, march due north on a grassy path called Historic Trace Road. The only unpaved portion of this hike, it offers open views of rolling meadows and a historic one-room stone schoolhouse. This structure, built approximately 35 years after the encampment, resulted from the industrial expansion of the Valley Forge area. Later, a newer schoolhouse would be erected across Gulph Road, and this building would fall into disrepair, serving as a storage shed and stable for local farmers.

Continue straight, admiring the fortifications within the valley. Your grassy path intersects the paved bike path at the top of the hill. Here, bear right; admire the von Steuben Statue, and picture the awe and respect of the Continental soldiers as this seasoned Prussian military professional taught them the proper use of the bayonet.

Cross the park road and bear left along J. P. Martin's Trail for an out-and-back to Washington's Headquarters, following the trail until it starts to dip and signs point you to a humble stone home. Here the most famous man in U.S. history took shelter with his wife and family during the encampment. Inside, a small dining area has been recreated; you can imagine the dinner conversations during this crucial period in America's history.

Upstairs is a room with a canopy bed; George Washington slept here—really. Tour the other rooms; a knowledgeable park ranger can answer your questions regarding the history of this house. Washington's guard huts sit in front of the house, a testimony to the threat of British attack. Return to the trail, and notice a Reading Railroad stationhouse, under renovation as of this writing, that sits to the left. The Reading once brought Philadelphians up to visit this site that eventually became Pennsylvania's first national historic park.

The trail arrives at a parking lot; cross it and return to Varnum's Headquarters and picnic area. Nearby is the Grand Parade, where military exercises occurred.

You are now on the last leg of your long march. You may want to stop at the Washington Memorial Chapel, built to commemorate George Washington's service to our country. Every Sunday afternoon from June to September, glorious carillon music echoes through the fields from this towering Gothic Revival building.

Continue on the trail to the next monument, which pays tribute to patriots of African descent, who, enticed by freedom, joined the fight. Some sources document that at least 500 African Americans served in the Continental Army at Valley Forge. You are now less than a mile from the end of this historic march.

On the half hour, a theater beside the park's Welcome Center shows an 18-minute film describing life at the Valley Forge encampment. Seasonal trolley tours and bike rentals offer alternative vehicles to view the park. A store in the Welcome Center sells historical literature and cold drinks.

You leave this park with a sense that you are a small part of something special—that the events that occurred here, preserved so well, live in the hearts and minds of all Americans, and that the concept of freedom, for which these soldiers fought with bravery and fierce determination, is an ideal to be cherished and appreciated by all who are fortunate to live within its protected embrace.

## NEARBY ACTIVITIES

JOHN JAMES AUDUBON CENTER AT
MILL GROVE *(see page 180)*
1201 Pawlings Road, Audubon
(610) 666-5593
**pa.audubon.org/centers_mill_grove.html**

LOWER PERKIOMEN VALLEY PARK
101 New Mill Road, Oaks
(610) 666-5371

VALLEY FORGE CONVENTION CENTER
1160 First Avenue, King of Prussia
(610) 337-4000
**www.vfconventioncenter.com**
*(See Web site for calendar.)*

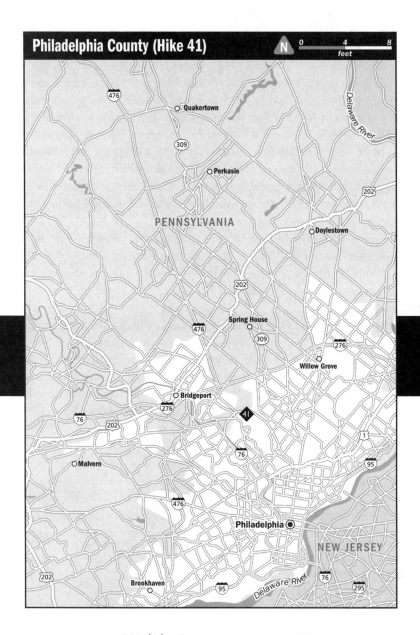

N

0    4    8
feet

Quakertown

476

309

Perkasie

PENNSYLVANIA

202

Doylestown

202

Spring House

476

309

276

Willow Grove

Bridgeport

276

76

202

41

76

Malvern

1

95

476

Philadelphia

NEW JERSEY

202

Brookhaven

95

Delaware River

76

295

Delaware River

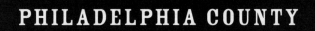

PHILADELPHIA COUNTY

# 41  WISSAHICKON GORGE

### KEY AT-A-GLANCE INFORMATION

**LENGTH:** 5.55 miles

**CONFIGURATION:** Loop

**DIFFICULTY:** Moderate

**SCENERY:** Gorge, creek, bridges

**EXPOSURE:** Mostly shaded

**TRAIL TRAFFIC:** Medium

**TRAIL SURFACE:** Dirt, gravel, rocky at times

**HIKING TIME:** 2.25 hours

**DRIVING DISTANCE FROM CENTER CITY:** 12 miles

**ACCESS:** Year-round, daily, dawn–dusk; free

**MAPS:** USGS Germantown; detailed map at Environmental Center

**WHEELCHAIR TRAVERSABLE:** No

**FACILITIES:** Private restrooms at Valley Green Inn

**SPECIAL COMMENTS:** See www.fow.org for more details.

## GPS Trailhead Coordinates

UTM Zone (WGS84)  18T

Easting    0480120

Northing   4436920

Latitude   N 40° 4' 56.1"

Longitude  W 75° 13' 59.3"

## IN BRIEF

Inside the western city limits of Philadelphia is a natural retreat hidden in a rugged gorge, with a covered bridge, an old inn, and a statue that commemorates the last Native American chief in the Wissahickon Valley.

## DESCRIPTION

The sides of the Wissahickon Gorge rise about 200 to 300 feet on both sides in many spots along the creek. This gives the hike a feeling of being far away from the very city within which it lies. The Forbidden Drive hike in Wissahickon Valley offers both scenic beauty and intriguing history. The name Forbidden Drive comes from the fact that no traffic is allowed on the trail, even though, in places, it is wide enough to accommodate cars.

To enter Forbidden Drive, walk back down the dirt road from the Environmental

## *Directions* ————————→

**From Philadelphia, follow Interstate 76 west 4.7 miles. Take Exit 340A, merge onto City Avenue, then take the right fork just across the bridge, and merge onto Ridge Avenue. Proceed 1.3 miles, turn right onto Walnut Lane and then, at the second intersection, turn left onto Henry Avenue. After 3.2 miles, Henry becomes Ridge Avenue; continue 0.7 more miles, then turn right onto Northwestern Avenue. Go about 1 mile, to the intersection of Northwestern Avenue, Andorra Road, and Thomas Road. At this intersection, take a hard right onto a dirt road, which leads to the Environmental Center after just a few hundred feet. Park here and walk back down the dirt road to the park entrance on the right, across from where all the roads intersect. *The Environmental Center is located at 300 Northwestern Avenue, Philadelphia, PA 19118.***

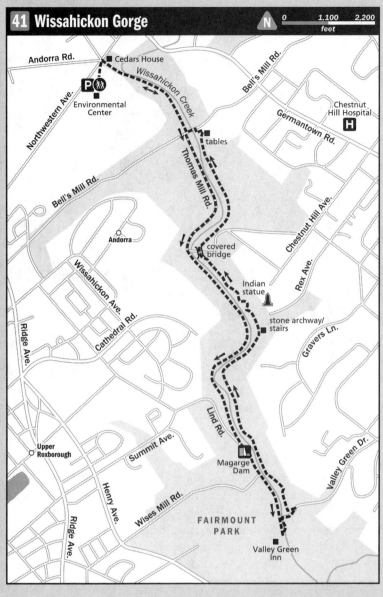

N

0    1,100    2,200
feet

Andorra Rd.

Cedars House

Wissahickon Creek

Bell's Mill Rd.

Northwestern Ave.

Environmental
Center

Chestnut
Hill Hospital   H

Germantown Rd.

tables

Bell's Mill Rd.

Thomas Mill Rd.

Chestnut Hill Ave.

Andorra

Wissahickon Ave.

Cathedral Rd.

covered
bridge

Rex Ave.

Indian
statue

stone archway/
stairs

Gravers Ln.

Ridge Ave.

Summit Ave.

Lind Rd.

Upper
Roxborough

Magarge
Dam

Valley Green Dr.

Henry Ave.

Wises Mill Rd.

FAIRMOUNT
PARK

Ridge Ave.

Valley Green
Inn

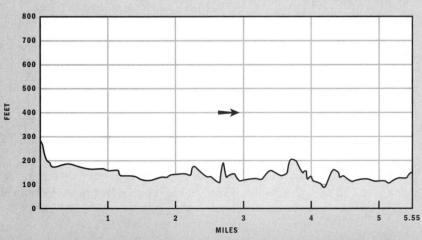

FEET

800
700
600
500
400
300
200
100
0

1    2    3    4    5    5.55

MILES

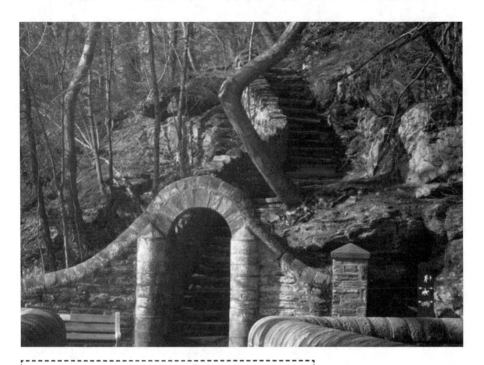

A stone bridge crosses Rex Avenue to an archway and staircase.

Center parking area and look for the Cedars House on the right. The drive is covered with mainly dirt and is as wide as a country road. In fact, it was a road-way in the horse-and-carriage days. Along the path, you may notice old water wells and even a natural-spring drinking fountain (closed because of pollution since the 1950s).

Within the first 0.5 miles, you cross Bell's Mill Road. Along the creek, remnants of several dams commemorate what was once the area's thriving mill industry. The most significant, Margaree Dam, impounded water for the last active mill in the valley, which closed in 1883. Signs throughout the park explain this and other historical points.

Just past the 1-mile mark, a covered bridge, built in 1737 and renovated in the 1990s, spans the creek. In the 1800s it was the only covered bridge of the five bridges over the creek. Now it is the only covered bridge within a major U.S. city's limits.

At about the 1.5-mile mark, on the other side of the creek, stands the Tedy-uscung statue, which has been overlooking the Wissahickon Valley since 1902 and commemorates the last Native American chief in the valley. The statue may be blocked by trees, but a plaque on Forbidden Drive describes its location and history.

On the right at the 2.5-mile mark is Valley Green Inn, the only inn in the valley that is still in operation. Built in 1850, it catered to travelers on Forbidden

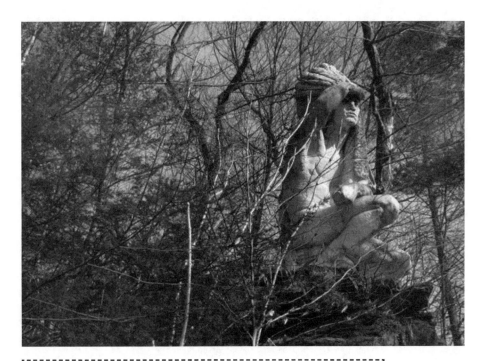

A statue commemorating the last Native American chief looks out upon the trail.

Drive. The two-story inn looks just as it did in century-old photographs, complete with a horse stable. This is the hike's turnaround point and a good place to stop to eat. While here, check out the inn's interesting collection of local artifacts.

After lunch, simply turn around at Valley Green Inn, head north a few hundred feet, and turn right onto the stone arch bridge. There are other stone arch bridges in Wissahickon Valley, but the one here at Valley Green is distinctive for its closed spandrel arch. After crossing the bridge, turn left onto a narrow wooden bridge leading into the woods, and bear left to climb to an outlook post that provides a different view of the bridge and inn. The trail starts just to the right of the lookout. This trail (simply referred to as one of the "upper trails") is a lot more challenging than Forbidden Drive.

Stay on the upper path. The secondary trail closer to the creek is extremely narrow and can be quite treacherous, especially after rain or snow. This side of the creek affords a different view of the valley. After a half mile, you can see the foundations of the old mills, which now resemble nothing more than shattered collections of rocks. Near the 3.5-mile mark (or 1 mile after turning around), a stone bridge crosses Rex Avenue to a stone archway and stone staircase directly north. Take the staircase up the hill to continue on the trail. The masonry work here looks like something from an old castle. Just a few hundred feet beyond the staircase's end, you can see the Tedyuscung statue directly overhead. Avoid the short climb up to the statue; it's steep and slippery.

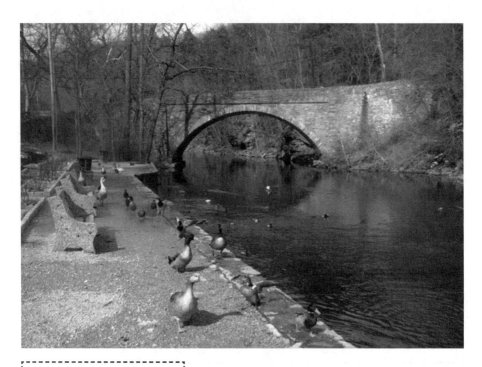

Stone bridge at Valley Green Inn

Near the end of the trail, you return to West Bells Mill Road, at the edge of which is a picnic area, a few feet to the right of the creek. Cross West Bells Mill Road, turn left to cross the bridge, then turn right onto Forbidden Drive. Within a half mile, you'll see the Cedars House on the left, and you'll be back where you started.

## NEARBY ATTRACTIONS

PHILADELPHIA ZOO
*(America's first zoo)*
34th Street and Girard Avenue
Fairmount Park, Philadelphia
(215) 243-5235
**www.philadelphiazoo.org**

VALLEY GREEN INN
*(Restaurant)*
Wissahickon Gorge,
Philadelphia
(215) 243-5235
**www.valleygreeninn.com**

MORRIS ARBORETUM
100 East Northwestern Avenue,
Philadelphia
(215) 247-5777
**business-services.upenn.edu/arboretum**

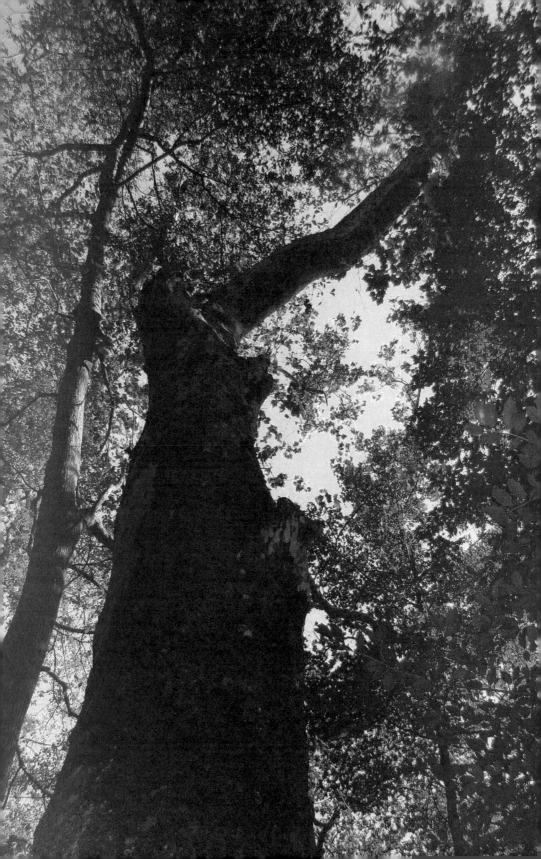

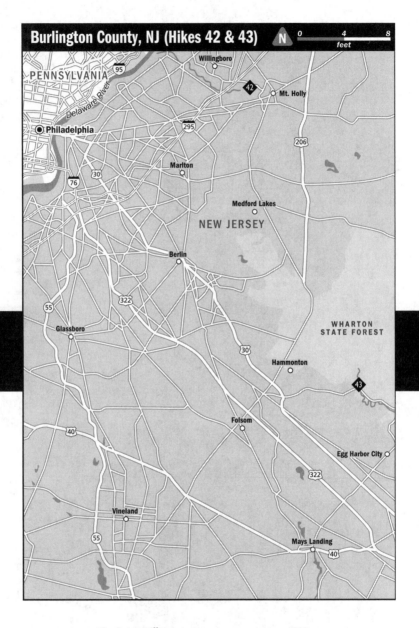

**Burlington County, NJ (Hikes 42 & 43)**

N

0        4        8

feet

Willingboro

PENNSYLVANIA

95

Delaware River

42

Mt. Holly

Philadelphia

295

206

Marlton

30

76

Medford Lakes

NEW JERSEY

Berlin

322

55

WHARTON
STATE FOREST

Glassboro

30

Hammonton

43

Folsom

40

Egg Harbor City

322

Vineland

55

Mays Landing

40

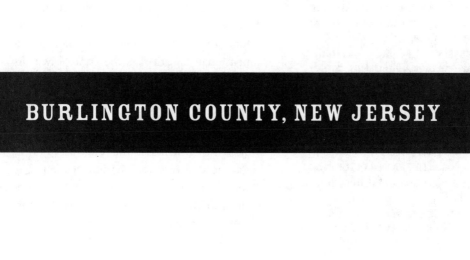

BURLINGTON COUNTY, NEW JERSEY

# 42  BATSTO VILLAGE

## KEY AT-A-GLANCE INFORMATION

**LENGTH:** 4.18 miles

**CONFIGURATION:** Loop

**DIFFICULTY:** Moderate

**SCENERY:** Pinewoods, lake, old restored village

**EXPOSURE:** Mostly shaded

**TRAIL TRAFFIC:** Medium

**TRAIL SURFACE:** Pine-needle-covered

**HIKING TIME:** 1 hour, 15 minutes

**DRIVING DISTANCE FROM CENTER CITY:** 44 miles

**ACCESS:** Visitor center, museum, museum shop, and nature center open 9 a.m.–4 p.m. daily; sawmill demonstration (starting May 25) Saturdays, Sundays, and holidays at 1:30, 2, and 2:30 p.m.

**MAPS:** USGS Atsion; maps at kiosk by visitor center

**WHEELCHAIR TRAVERSABLE:** No

**FACILITIES:** Restrooms in visitor center

**SPECIAL COMMENTS:** For more information, call (609) 561-0024 or visit www.batstovillage.org.

## GPS Trailhead Coordinates

UTM Zone 18S (WGS84)

Easting 0530257

Northing 4388259

Latitude N 39° 38' 37.1"

Longitude W 74° 38' 50.5"

## IN BRIEF

A pinewoods hike and preserved village are among the highlights of the huge Wharton State Forest, in New Jersey's Pine Barrens.

## DESCRIPTION

The Batsto Trail is next to Batsto Village, which was an industrial center from 1766 to 1867 and is now a well-maintained tourist attraction. From the parking lot (in front of the visitor center), the most visible landmark is the mansion in the middle of the town square. Behind the visitor center, a detailed three-dimensional map depicts the entire town. As you head north past the mansion and village, the Batsto Trail is directly in front of you and runs to the right of Batsto Lake.

The Batsto Trail links to several other trails, all of which give the hiker an interesting glimpse of the area's natural habitat. The Batona Trail extends 50 miles and provides an idea of the vast size of the Pine Barrens. The Wharton State Forest, which includes the Batsto Trail, covers more than 115,000 acres

## Directions

Take Interstate 76 east 5.7 miles from Philadelphia, entering New Jersey. Continue on NJ 42, which after 8 miles becomes the Atlantic City Expressway. From this point, continue 15.9 miles and take Exit 28. At the end of the ramp, turn left onto NJ 54. After 2.1 miles, make an angled right turn onto NJ 542–Central Avenue. Stay on 542 for 7.5 miles, including a jog to the right at US 30; the Batsto Village entrance is on the left. The Batsto Trail hike starts at the lake's east side, next to the village dam crossover.
*31 Batsto Road, Hammonton, NJ 08037.*

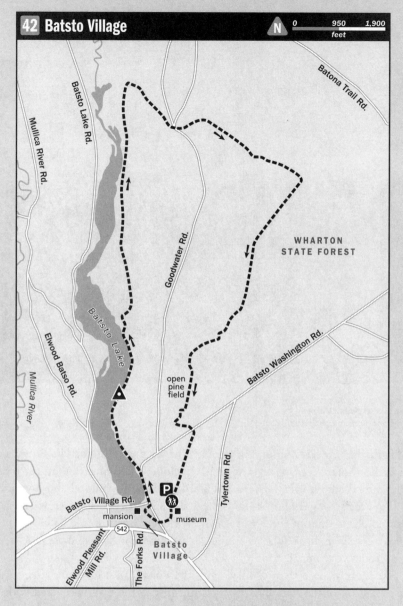

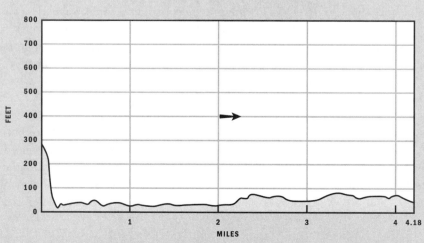

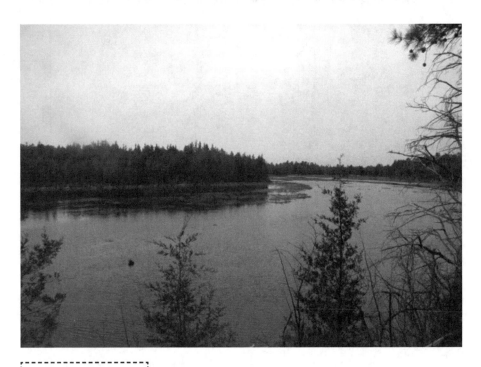

The lake at Batsto Village

and is the largest tract of land in the New Jersey park system. The Pine Barrens represent a quarter of New Jersey's undeveloped land and the largest tract of undeveloped land on the Eastern Seaboard between Richmond and Boston.

An area so vast and mysterious inevitably gives rise to some strange legends. Most notable is that of the Jersey Devil, a winged creature said to have haunted the Barrens since the 1700s. As you look through a forest of endless pine trees, it is easy to let your imagination run wild.

At slightly more than 4 miles long, the Batsto Trail gives the hiker a good representation of the Pine Barrens terrain. Most of the trail is covered with pine needles, and a pine aroma. Early European settlers found the sandy soil useless for agriculture, but the area has since become a major cranberry producer (cranberry fields can be seen from many area roads). The nutrient-poor soil also supports orchids and carnivorous plants. Plaques convey information about local wildlife. The trail is relatively flat, like most of the Pine Barrens. Follow the white markers.

From an overlook just past the 1-mile mark, you get a good view of a Batsto Lake peninsula. The lake and river played a vital role in the development of Batsto Village. The gristmill (1828) and circular saw–equipped sawmill (1882) used water from the lake for power. Batsto Village also had an elaborate hydraulic pump that delivered water to the mansion and piggery. The local rivers were a source of bog ore, which was processed at the village iron furnace. When the

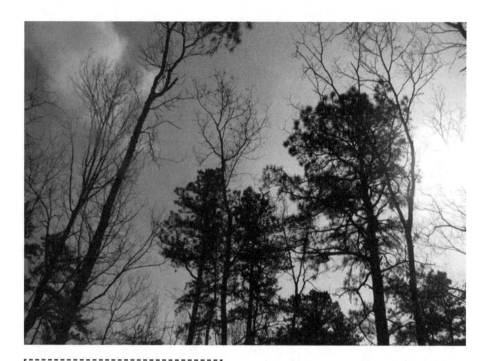

It's not called the Pinelands for nothing.

dam created the lake, boats could move bog ore from rivers and streams to the now-vanished furnace.

Past the overlook, the trail suddenly turns right (east) and crosses an access road. At the 3.75-mile mark. The trail reaches a clearing with a bench on the right. Dry soil conditions and frequent fires have created a forest populated by pitch pines no taller than 6 feet. As you walk through this scattered forest, the hike ends at a picnic area in front of the visitor center.

While you're here, tour the restored buildings of Batsto Village, which will transport you to New Jersey's industrial past of more than a century ago. The iron- and glassmaking facilities have long since disappeared, but the sawmill still actively cuts wood.

The village centerpiece is the mansion, the one-time home of the village iron-master. A wealthy Philadelphia industrialist, Joseph Wharton, redesigned it in an Italianate style. The general store, corn crib, gristmill, and several other buildings survive, including workers' houses across the dam. Several other old villages, now ghost towns, can be seen along Pine Barrens highways. They, and Batsto Village, memorialize the area's lost industry.

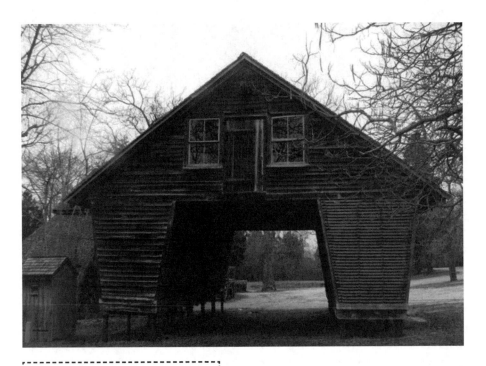

Old corn-storage building

## NEARBY ACTIVITIES

ATSION VILLAGE & RECREATION CENTER
*(19th-century colonial ironworks and
community with recreation facilities)*
Route 206, Shamog
**www.batstovillage.org/atsion.htm**

BELHAVEN LAKE RESORT
*(Resort and campground with swim-
ming, boating, golf, and fishing)*
1213 Route 542, Egg Harbor City
**www.beachcomber.com/NJ/Camping/
Shore/belhav.html**

TOMASELLO WINERY
*(Third-generation winery; 30 varieties
of grapes)*
225 White Horse Pike, Hammonton
**www.tomasellowinery.com**

# RANCOCAS NATURE CENTER AND POWHATAN INDIAN RESERVATION  43

## IN BRIEF

This hike in Rancocas State Park visits the Rancocas Nature Center (New Jersey Audubon Society) and the Powhatan Renape Indian Reservation.

## DESCRIPTION

The Rancocas Nature Center, run by the New Jersey Audubon Society, maintains trails that lead directly into the Powhatan Renape Indian Reservation, which is part of the Powhatan Renape Indian Nation. Both organizations share a deep passion for the earth, and their properties border each other within Rancocas State Park.

In these parts of the park, young trees and shrubs stand near older forestland that reaches for the sky. This demonstrates the process of forest succession, in which one community of plants, trees, or shrubs gradually supplants another, usually because of differences in shade tolerance. Fields of wildflowers border conifer plantations rich with white pine, Austrian pine, Norway spruce, and European larch.

------------------------------------------

## *Directions* ⟶

From Philadelphia, take US 676/US 30 east over the Benjamin Franklin Bridge into New Jersey. After 1.7 miles, bear left at US 30 east and continue 2.2 miles. Bear left at Kaighns Avenue/NJ 38 and continue for miles on NJ 38. Look for NJ 73 south and bear left. After a mile, merge onto US 295 north to Trenton. Drive 8.2 miles on US 295, and take Exit 45A. Then, merge onto Rancocas Road and look for the nature center's entrance about 1 mile ahead on the right, just past the Indian reservation entrance. *794 Rancocas Road (Nature Center), Westampton, NJ 08060.*

### KEY AT-A-GLANCE INFORMATION

**LENGTH: 2.47 miles**

**CONFIGURATION: Balloon**

**DIFFICULTY: Moderate**

**SCENERY: Wildflower meadow, creek, conifer forest, hardwood forest, Indian reservation**

**EXPOSURE: Full sun–full shade**

**TRAIL TRAFFIC: Light**

**TRAIL SURFACE: Grass, dirt**

**HIKING TIME: 1 hour**

**DRIVING DISTANCE FROM CENTER CITY: 21 miles**

**ACCESS: Nature Center is open Tuesday–Saturday, 9 a.m.–5 p.m.; Sunday, noon–5 p.m.; closed Monday**

**MAPS: USGS Bristol and Mount Holly; maps at nature center**

**WHEELCHAIR TRAVERSABLE: No**

**FACILITIES: Restrooms in Audubon Center**

**SPECIAL COMMENTS: Dogs, bicycles, and motorized vehicles are not allowed on the trails. Kids are welcome. For more information, call (609) 261-2495 or visit www.njaudubon.org/centers/rancocas and www.powhatan.org.**

------------------------------

### GPS Trailhead Coordinates

UTM Zone (WGS84)  18T

Easting   0515302

Northing   4428150

Latitude   N 40° 0' 12.2"

Longitude   W 74° 49' 14.7"

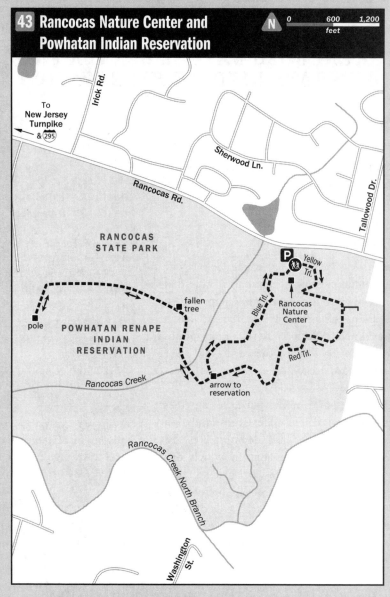

N
0   600   1,200
feet

RANCOCAS
STATE PARK

To
New Jersey
Turnpike
& 295

Irick Rd.

Sherwood Ln.

Rancocas Rd.

Tallowood Dr.

Yellow Trl.

Rancocas
Nature
Center

Blue Trl.

Red Trl.

fallen
tree

pole

POWHATAN RENAPE
INDIAN
RESERVATION

Rancocas Creek

arrow to
reservation

Rancocas Creek North Branch

Washington St.

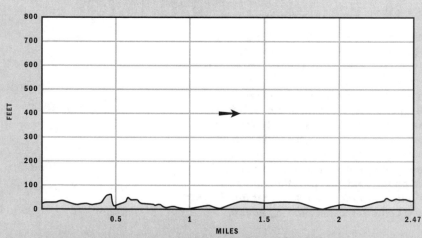

FEET

800
700
600
500
400
300
200
100
0

0.5   1   1.5   2   2.47

MILES

Several habitats come together near the freshwater tidal marsh by Rancocas Creek, offering both food and cover for birds and varied habitats for plants and other animals. In fact, 150 species of birds and 200 species of plants have been documented here.

The hike starts at the Rancocas Nature Center, located in a small farmhouse, where the staff cares for turtles, reptiles, and bunnies. The center offers a touch table, a natural-history exhibit, and a wildlife-viewing area. The grounds—meadows, flower gardens, and trails—are well groomed. A small store with nature guides, other books, and T-shirts helps support this organization, which offers children's programs, garden walks, nature-photo exhibits, bird walks, scouting programs, and more.

From the nature center, follow the Yellow Trail, which begins off the back porch. Soon you are lost in the cricket's song, sunshine illuminating your face and mind. When you come to a T-junction, turn left and follow the Red Trail. In a little more than 0.1 mile, you come upon a bench. Slow down to watch the cardinals, brown thrashers, robins, cedar waxwings, and gray catbirds, or to spot a red-tailed hawk or bald eagle hovering overhead.

Continue along the trail until you come to a conifer forest. Here the grass trail turns to a dirt path and the temperature drops at least 10 degrees. When you reach a sign with blue arrows, turn left. There is a bench to your right, in case you want a cool spot to stop and listen to the sounds of birds chirping in the distance.

Go straight when you see the markers for the Orange Trail on your left, and continue on the Blue Trail until you see a large yellow arrow. Turn left and cross the bridge. Beyond the bridge, turn right and hug the stream on your left, heading northwest. You have now officially entered the reservation of the Powhatan Renape Indians, where the trails are unmarked.

At the time of the first European settlement, the Powhatan Indians resided in what is now called eastern Virginia. Like many Native American tribes, they were eventually driven from their lands, and a number of them gradually migrated to Pennsauken Township in Camden County in the late 19th century, later settling in Medford in Burlington County.

The tribe has become most famous in modern pop culture for the myth of Pocahontas, perpetuated by Walt Disney. The truth is that "Pocahontas," whose true birth name was Matoaka, was kidnapped by the British and assimilated into their culture. She agreed to marry the widower John Rolfe, but there is great uncertainty regarding whether she truly loved him or was trying to promote peace between the settlers and the Powhatans. The Powhatans were attacked soon after Captain John Smith, who established the first permanent English settlement in North America, returned from Jamestown to England. In fact, the widely accepted idea that John Smith was saved by Pocahontas from bludgeoning is also unfounded. There is no evidence that the Powhatans practiced this means of killing.

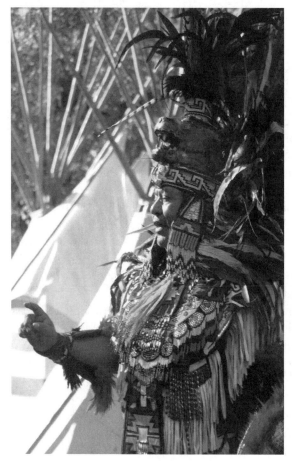

A Powhatan chief, in traditional garb, speaks at the Renape Nation's biannual arts festival.

The Powhatans, like so many Native American tribes, suffered at the hands of the European settlers, who believed them to be savages. The settlers came rumbling in, burned the Powhatans' homes to the ground, and confiscated or destroyed the resources the tribe needed for survival, leaving them hungry and homeless.

In 1982, with the help of Chief Roy Crazy Horse, a writer, educator, and advocate for Native Americans, the Powhatan Renape Nation, which now runs a museum, gallery, and gift shop to promote education about the Native American people, was able to secure a lease from the state for a portion of Rancocas State Park in Westampton Township. The Powhatan Renape Nation also provides social services to the New Jersey Native American community and education about Native American customs, beliefs, traditions, and culture.

Twice a year, the Powhatan Renape Nation hosts a colorful arts festival with traditional dances, demonstrations, performances, crafts, food, and more. This hike brings you into the area where the festival is held biannually and where a replica of a precolonial Native American village has been reconstructed.

Continue northeast until you come to a large fallen tree in the middle of the path, which you will need to maneuver under or climb over. Dead and fallen trees provide food and shelter for hundreds of animals. Cavity-nesting birds, such as owls and woodpeckers, in addition to insects, squirrels, salamanders, mice, and chipmunks are just a few of the animals that benefit from dead and fallen trees. Fungi and mushrooms also develop around fallen trees, assisting the process of biodegradation that allows nutrients to return to the earth.

Stay on this trail to head directly into a large field, the center of the Powhatan Renape Indian Reservation. Here you will find a museum that displays Native American tools, weapons, clothing, crafts, and instruments, and also dioramas. The museum is open only September to June, on the first and third Saturday of each month, from 10 a.m. to 3 p.m. and on Tuesday and Thursday by appointment. A full-size re-creation of a Powhatan village can also be found on the grounds, along with a few resident buffalo.

To end the hike, retrace your route across the bridge to the yellow arrow. Here, turn left and follow the Blue Trail as it loops back to the Rancocas Nature Center. Leave no litter, and take with you only these thoughts from Chief Roy Crazy Horse, who died in 2004 at age 79:

*Ours is the arrogant generation, which has taken upon ourselves to use an eternity's resources for our own benefit.*

*. . . We do not consider the birds and animals, the plants and forests, when we seek "progress and "development." We do not honor our Mother Earth and her gifts. We do not respect other peoples in other places. We act as if the Creation exists solely for our own benefit. Corporate profit triumphs. Exploitation becomes virtue.*

*. . . We still hold the keys to the future: our Original Instructions as human beings. It is not too late for all those who came here from elsewhere to adopt a new way of life, which is the oldest way of life on this land. It is not too late to seek balance, to sustain a future, to establish in our time a new economic order, which puts people, not profits, first."*

From "A Message To Our Doubly-Arrogant Generation," **www.powhatan .org/ageneration.html.**

## NEARBY ACTIVITIES

CENTER STAGE ANTIQUES
Open Saturday and Sunday, 10 a.m. to 5 p.m., or by appointment
King Street and Rancocas Road, Mount Holly
(609) 261-0602
**www.centerstageantiques.com**

MILL RACE VILLAGE
*(Unique shopping village)*
2 Washington Street, Historic Mount Holly
**www.millraceshops.com**

ROBINS NEST RESTAURANT
*(Restaurant and bakery)*
2 Washington Street, Historic Mount Holly
(609) 261-6149
**www.robinsnestmountholly.com**

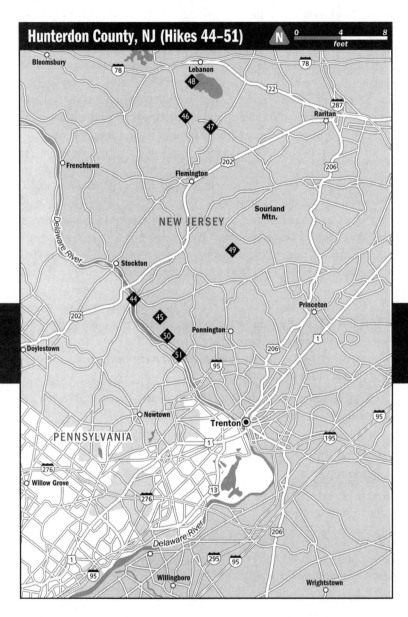

## Hunterdon County, NJ (Hikes 44–51)

N

0    4    8
feet

Bloomsbury
78
Lebanon
48
78
22
287
Raritan
46
47
Frenchtown
202
206
Flemington
NEW JERSEY
Sourland Mtn.
Delaware River
49
Stockton
44
Princeton
202
45
50
Pennington
Doylestown
51
206
1
95
Newtown
Trenton
95
PENNSYLVANIA
1
195
276
Willow Grove
276
13
Delaware River
206
1
295  95
95
Willingboro
Wrightstown

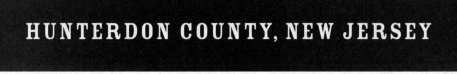

HUNTERDON COUNTY, NEW JERSEY

# 44   DELAWARE CANAL: New Jersey Side

### KEY AT-A-GLANCE INFORMATION

**LENGTH: 7.2 miles**

**CONFIGURATION: Out-and-back**

**DIFFICULTY: Moderate**

**SCENERY: Canal, river, farms, and old homes**

**EXPOSURE: Full sun–full shade**

**TRAIL TRAFFIC: Moderate**

**TRAIL SURFACE: Pavement and gravel**

**HIKING TIME: 2 hours**

**DRIVING DISTANCE FROM CENTER CITY: 41 miles**

**ACCESS: Daily, sunrise–sunset; free admission**

**MAPS: USGS Lambertville; www.dandrcanal.com/maps.html**

**WHEELCHAIR TRAVERSABLE: Partially; some bridges may be too narrow.**

**FACILITIES: Restrooms in Lambert-ville at nearby restaurants or at the Hometown Deli in Stockton**

**SPECIAL COMMENTS: This is the ulti-mate hike for viewing the Delaware River. More information: (609) 924-5705; www.dandrcanal.com.**

## IN BRIEF

This out-and-back hike offers 19th-century architecture in a natural setting, sandwiched between two historic river towns. There are farmhouses, riparian wildlife, butterflies, and birds to enjoy, and you may also meander the shops and boutiques of Lambertville at the hike's end.

## DESCRIPTION

There are a few ways one may hike along the Delaware Canal. You can walk out and back from Lambertville to Stockton, or you can drop off your bike in Stockton and bike back to Lambertville. Many parts of the canal path can be easily accessed from adjacent road-ways. What makes this slice of river unique is that once you have completed your hike, you can explore Lambertville Borough, with its boutiques, antique shops, galleries, and restaurants.

To hike along this portion of the canal, park your car at the South Union Street park-ing lot, next to Caballo Park, and take the towpath at the end of the lot, heading north.

## Directions

Take Interstate 95 north from Philadelphia. After approximately 31 miles, take the first exit in New Jersey, Exit 1, for NJ 29/Lambertville. After 0.5 miles, merge onto NJ 29. Continue north on NJ 29 for 9.2 miles, and turn left onto NJ 179–Bridge Street in Lambertville. Within a few blocks, look for South Union Street on the left. Turn left on South Union Street and con-tinue about 0.75 miles until the road ends. The parking lot for Caballo Park will be on the right. You can also park in town and simply start the hike near the Lambertville Inn.
*South Union Street, Lambertville, NJ 08530.*

## GPS Trailhead Coordinates

UTM Zone (WGS84)  18T

Easting   0504708

Northing   4467992

Latitude   N 40° 21' 44.8"

Longitude   W 74° 56' 40.3"

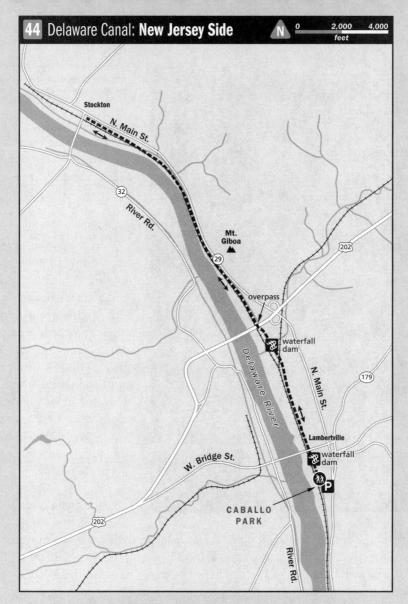

Stockton

N. Main St.

32

River Rd.

Mt.
Giboa

29

202

overpass

waterfall
dam

N. Main St.

179

Lambertville

waterfall
dam

P

CABALLO
PARK

W. Bridge St.

202

River Rd.

Delaware River

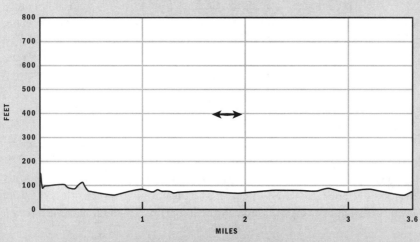

| FEET | | | | |
|---|---|---|---|---|
| 800 | | | | |
| 700 | | | | |
| 600 | | | | |
| 500 | | | | |
| 400 | | | | |
| 300 | | | | |
| 200 | | | | |
| 100 | | | | |
| 0 | 1 | 2 | 3 | 3.6 |

MILES

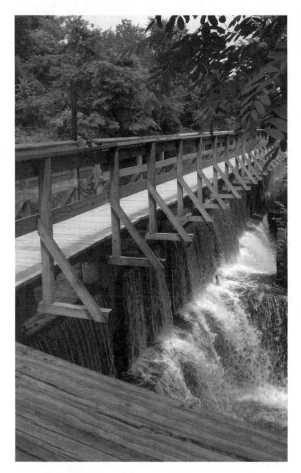

A short jog along the path and past a small waterfall, you reach Lambertville's Main Street. Cross the street and continue on the canal path all the way to Stockton.

Victorian residences and other 19th-century dwellings, such as bridge-tender homes, line the canal path. Each home displays a different facade, with potted plants and cast-iron fences, window boxes and garnished patios. Even the stone and brick storefronts take you back to a simpler time, when all houses were not built from the same architectural plan.

If those houses could talk, they would tell a few tales about the winners and losers of the Industrial Revolution. Canals helped provide the link to transport raw materials and manufactured goods from Eastern ports to points throughout New Jersey and the rest of the country. The state chartered the Delaware and Raritan Canal in 1830.

Over the next few years, Irish immigrants toiled under deplorable conditions, for as little as 75 cents per a day, to create the canal and its neighboring path. Most of these immigrants came from extremely poor families and had been persecuted in Ireland because of their religion. They used picks, shovels, and their bare hands as tools. Workers who were too poor to afford shoes, tied rags around their calloused feet. When Asiatic cholera swept the area in 1832, some of the workers collapsed from illness and were buried along the canal, with no subsequent record of their identity.

The canal was completed in 1834. Its mule-drawn boats would later be used to transport troops and supplies during the Civil War. Toward the end of the 19th century, steam trains and steamboats became the preferred methods for transporting both goods and people. During Prohibition, bootleggers used barges on the canal to transfer liquor. In the long run, the canal became a haven

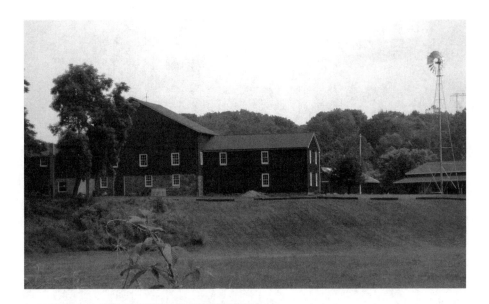

A farmhouse stands in view along the canal walk.

for boaters, bikers, and hikers. Restored thanks to citizen activists, the canal and its adjacent path became the Delaware & Raritan Canal State Park in 1974.

The villages from Lambertville to Stockton have maintained their small-town feel. You pass Neice Lumber and Finkles Hardware as you stroll along, watching mallards and Canada geese as they swim the canal. From spring to summer, the nearby bushes and trees echo with a chorus of different birds, including mourning doves, sparrows, robins, and thrushes. Snapping turtles are occasionally seen; do not approach them too closely—you could lose a fingertip.

Soon you pass another waterfall gushing under a walking bridge, and the houses become fewer and farther between. You may notice a scenic farmhouse on your right; a nearby bench provides the best break for your water bottle and trail snack. Once you've rested both body and mind, continue straight toward Route 202, where the trail turns left and bridges over to the opposite side of the canal. This part of the path, until it narrows, is shared by bicyclists and an occasional maintenance vehicle, so be alert.

If you hear a chugging sound in the distance, it is not a train but the mechanical workings of a nearby quarry. Don't let the noise distract you from the hawks flying over the oaks and white birches, or the reflection in the river of Queen Anne's lace. Butterflies are abundant and dragonflies speed past.

You may hear the sound of mourning doves as you get closer and closer to Stockton and its residential neighborhood. The Stockton Food Store will be the halfway point on your out-and-back adventure, so feel free to grab a sandwich and eat on the picnic benches behind the store. Restrooms can be found at the gas station or in any of the nearby restaurants in Stockton, such as the Stockton Inn, Meil's, and Via Ponte. Art enthusiasts can peruse the pottery, sculpture,

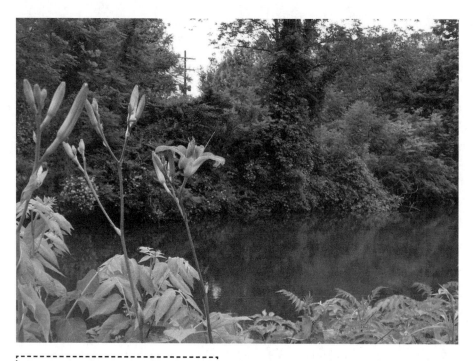

Wild lily and fern sprout beside the canal.

and paintings at Riverbank Arts, across the street from the food store. Many pieces were inspired by the local scenery.

Once you've rested and explored this quaint river town, retrace your route to the parking lot—hopefully with camera in hand—to capture your favorite memories of this unique hike of preserved canal history.

## NEARBY ACTIVITIES

HAMILTON'S GRILL ROOM
*(Restaurant)*
8 Coryell Street
Lambertville
(609) 397-4343
**www.hamiltonsgrillroom.com**

LAMBERTVILLE HOUSE
*(Lodgings and wine bar)*
32 Bridge Street
Lambertville
(888) 867-8859
**www.lambertvillehouse.com**

LILY'S ON THE CANAL
*(Restaurant)*
2 Canal Street
Lambertville
(609) 397-6242

# HOWELL LIVING HISTORY FARM  45

## IN BRIEF

This slow-paced view of what a working farm was like during the 19th and early 20th centuries includes rolling pastures, orchards, crop fields, barn animals, waterfowl, and much more.

## DESCRIPTION

*March 10, 1974*

*I am offering the farm as a gift to Mercer County in memory of Charley. To be used as a Living History Farm, where the way of living in its early days could not only be seen but actually tried by the public, especially children— milking a cow, gathering eggs in a homemade basket—helping to shear sheep, carding wool, spinning, and weaving . . .*

*Older people could teach the young how to sew a fine seam, or find hickory nuts to crack with a stone on the hearth, or find wild herbs for curing the miseries, or just go off fishing with a hickory stick pole . . .*

*Sleigh bells and up before dawn, fragrance of mint as you herd the cows up from the meadow, with the sun slanting across the Delaware. And church. And spring again . . .*

*Sincerely,*

*Inez Howe Howell*

### KEY AT-A-GLANCE INFORMATION

**LENGTH: 0.8 miles**

**CONFIGURATION: Loop**

**DIFFICULTY: Easy**

**SCENERY: Pastoral 19th-century farm**

**EXPOSURE: Full sun–full shade**

**TRAIL TRAFFIC: Light–moderate**

**TRAIL SURFACE: Gravel, dirt, grass**

**HIKING TIME: 1 hour or less**

**DRIVING DISTANCE FROM CENTER CITY: 40 miles**

**ACCESS: Tuesday–Saturday, 10 a.m.–4 p.m., February–November; Sunday, noon–4 p.m., April– November (self-guided tours only); closed Monday and holidays. Free admission and parking; fee for children's crafts and corn maze**

**MAPS: USGS Lambertville**

**WHEELCHAIR TRAVERSABLE: Partially**

**FACILITIES: Restrooms in visitor center**

**SPECIAL COMMENTS: No dogs allowed. More information: (609) 737-3299; www.howellfarm.org. For a longer outing, this hike can be combined with the Ted Stiles Preserve hike (see page 261).**

## *Directions*

**Take Interstate 95 north from Philadelphia. After approximately 31 miles, take the first exit in New Jersey, Exit 1, for NJ 29/ Lambertville. Travel north on NJ 29 for 7.5 miles to Valley Road. Turn right and travel 1.5 miles to Woodens Lane. Turn left; the Howell Farm entrance lane is 0.25 miles on the right. Park in the lot and pass through the visitor center to access the trail. *70 Woodens Lane, Titusville, NJ 08560.***

### GPS Trailhead Coordinates

UTM Zone (WGS84)  18T

Easting  0508248

Northing  4465580

Latitude  N 40° 20' 26.63"

Longitude  W 74° 54' 10.45"

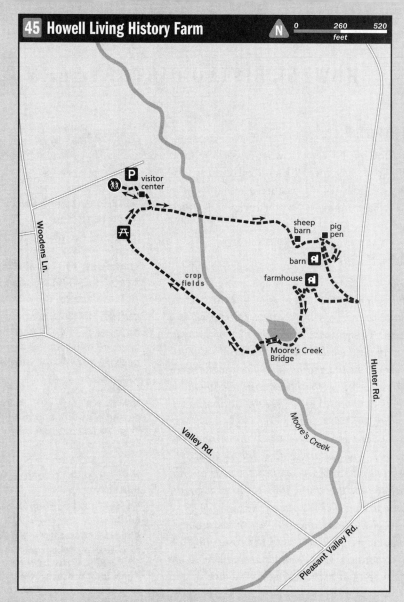

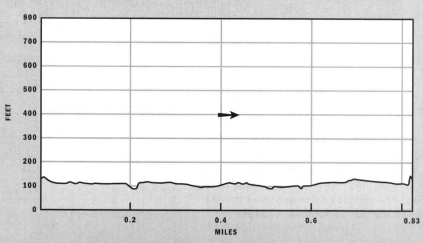

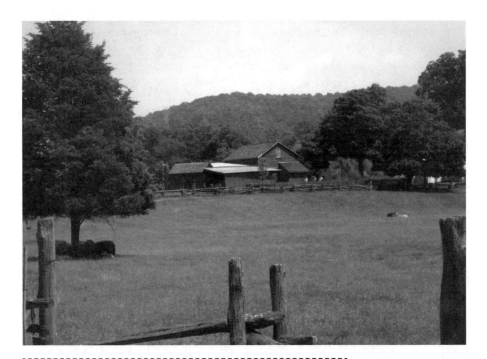

A 19th-century barn lies beyond the pasture at the Howell Living Farm.

If you stumbled across the Howell Living History Farm without knowing its origins, you might think you stepped into some mysterious time machine and traveled back to when children skipped through the fields and balanced upon creek rocks in their overalls; when baseball was still played with a fallen branch as a bat; and when, after the game, you could lie down on your quilt and imagine different shapes among the clouds. Life is slower on the farm, and that may well be what Inez Howell had in mind when she donated her farm to Mercer County, New Jersey.

In 1974, after the passing of her husband, Charley, Inez gave the farm to the county in his memory. Today, the property and its country surroundings depict farming the way it was performed in New Jersey in the 19th and early 20th centuries. This 130-acre park was a working farm for more than 240 years before being donated to the county. The Mercer County Park Commission has restored and now continually maintains the farm with help from donations and volunteers. On almost any given day, a walk here can slow the pulse within your body.

Old-time breeds of horses, cows, sheep, chickens, and other farm animals are kept as they were a century ago. Volunteers and visitors are often put to work milking, mixing feeds, and collecting eggs. Eighty acres of pastures, meadows, and woodlands nestle against neighboring Ted Stiles Preserve (see Hike 50, page 261) and stream corridors. Forty-five acres of period crops and gardens grow near the farm's buildings. These structures, which are listed in both state and federal registers of historic places, include an 18th-century farmhouse, a

19th-century barn, a wagon house, a corncrib, and an icehouse. Two miles of lanes can be accessed by foot or by horse-drawn wagon.

This hike circles the perimeter of the main farm and pasture. The visitor center on the edge of the parking lot is your gateway to bygone days. Pass through and collect literature regarding the farm and its many year-round activities. Exit the door toward the farm, and bear left to mosey along a dirt path that crosses a wood bridge and hugs a split-log fence. Behind the fence, sheep huddle under a tree for shade. The oxen often brave the sun and let it scorch their rugged hides or stand in seeming praise to the rain while it trickles down their snouts.

Continue along the path toward the sheep barn, which is usually empty during the day while the sheep graze. This century-old wagon house was moved to this location in 1981 from another farm to replace an earlier one. Straight ahead are other animals, including pigs that wallow in their muddy pens—years ago these pigs would likely have been fattened and then hauled to Philadelphia to be sold for pork. Circle the Phillips Barn and wink at the horses of tan, black, gray, and bronze, lined in their stables like large toys.

Once you've had your fill of the farm animals, trek down the hill and take a look at the apple orchard, which was restored in its original location in 1987, using a photograph of the farm from the 1930s. Angle right by the Moore's Creek Bridge, to admire a large willow tree—its branches measuring the wind. Moore's Creek, which once provided waterpower for local gristmills, captures the streams from nearby mountain slopes and meanders until it reaches the mighty Delaware River. Hunter Road, which runs across the bridge, was the original entry to the Howell Farm and is sometimes open as an alternate walking route.

The route now takes you back up the hill, toward the well-preserved farm-house. Like many farmhouses in the area, this one was built in stages, based on the changing needs of the family throughout the years. The last addition was made in 1900 and included a "modern" kitchen. Stay right, beside the pasture fence, for a view of the kitchen garden, which features vegetables, herbs, and wildflowers, some exploding into bloom in spring and summer. Next to the garden stands a two-seat outhouse—no need for waiting. The corncrib, another outbuilding, was designed to keep a year's worth of feed corn fresh by allowing fresh air to pass through and dry the grain. The wagon house, built in the mid-1800s, reflects the need for wagons and other equipment that came with the growth of the farm.

Walk to the back of the farmhouse to find the icehouse. From 1989 to 1991, the Friends of Howell Farm restored this building so it could once again store ice cut from the pond. It can hold 25 tons of ice and keep it frozen year-round. The pond provides a convenient nesting area for local waterfowl and feeds a creek that flows beneath another wooden bridge.

This small creek contains crayfish and pollywogs. Children like to explore its cattail-lined banks for dragonflies. Just past the bridge is an open meadow dotted with shade trees, where a blanket and a backpack snack could lead to an afternoon snooze, lulled by an orchestra of crickets.

The trail continues around a bend to where more farming took place. Here, a truck garden contained vegetables for canning, cooking, and sale. (Tomatoes, for example, were a popular cash crop in this geographical area at the end of the 19th century.) Just past the truck garden, the south crop fields rotated corn, oats, wheat, and hay. To your right is a scenic view of the farm through a thicket that provides a refuge for wild rabbits and a natural sanctuary for birds.

Continue straight and return to the visitor center, where you can end your hike, sit a while at the picnic area, or go behind the pines at the back of the building to see the beehives. Each of these hives can produce 30 to 50 pounds of honey annually. Honey was not only an important sweetener but also could be used for medicinal purposes, from relieving cold symptoms to treating small burns.

You've now concluded your walk through living history, and hopefully you've felt inspired by this slower-paced lifestyle and shared in the vision of Inez Howe Howell, who preserved this slice of time, knowing how quickly the world was a-changin'.

## NEARBY ACTIVITIES

BOWMAN'S HILL TOWER AND
WILDFLOWER PRESERVE
*(See Hike 1, page 16)*
1635 River Road
New Hope
(215) 862-2924
www.bhwp.org

GOLDEN NUGGET ANTIQUE MARKET
1850 River Road (NJ 29)
Lambertville
(609) 397-0811
www.gnmarket.com

HISTORIC LAMBERTVILLE, NEW JERSEY
www.lambertville.org

WASHINGTON CROSSING HISTORIC PARK
*(See Hike 51, page 266)*
1112 River Road
Washington Crossing
(215) 493-4076
www.ushistory.org/washingtoncrossing

# 46 HUNTERDON ARBORETUM

## KEY AT-A-GLANCE INFORMATION

**LENGTH:** 1.31 miles

**CONFIGURATION:** Loop

**DIFFICULTY:** Easy

**SCENERY:** Gardens, shady woodlands

**EXPOSURE:** Mostly shaded

**TRAIL TRAFFIC:** Light

**TRAIL SURFACE:** Grass, wooden boardwalk

**HIKING TIME:** 30 minutes

**DRIVING DISTANCE FROM CENTER CITY:** 58 miles

**ACCESS:** Daily, dawn–dusk, year-round; free admission

**MAPS:** USGS Flemington; maps available at arboretum office and online at www.njtrails.org/trailmap.php?TrailID=84

**WHEELCHAIR TRAVERSABLE:** No

**FACILITIES:** Restrooms near parking lot

**SPECIAL COMMENTS:** For more information, call (908) 782-1158 or visit co.hunterdon.nj.us/depts/parks/guides/Arbortum.htm.

## GPS Trailhead Coordinates

UTM Zone (WGS84) 18T

Easting 0511790

Northing 4491965

Latitude N 40° 34' 42.4"

Longitude W 74° 51' 38.5"

## IN BRIEF

This short hike offers botanical richness and scenic ponds and gazebos that make for an enjoyable stop, especially in spring, summer, and fall.

## DESCRIPTION

In only 73 acres, the Hunterdon County Arboretum in Clinton Township, New Jersey, contains an impressive variety of exotic plants and trees in a diverse habitat. Few areas in the Atlantic states can match its botanical richness. The Outer Loop trail is only 1.3 miles long, but because of the variety in the natural surroundings, it seems longer.

The walk starts at the entrance gate, which is directly off the parking lot. It leads to a 20,000-square-foot, wire-fence-enclosed nursery harboring dogwoods, weeping cherries, flowering crab apples, rhododendrons, azaleas, and other shrubs and trees. In the middle of the garden is the two-story Deats Gazebo, constructed in 1892 and relocated here from nearby Flemington. The gazebo and the colorful surrounding garden have become popular for weddings. To the right, just past the gazebo, a gated exit leads to several trails

## Directions

Take Interstate 95 north from Philadelphia, entering New Jersey. After 33.7 miles, take Exit 4, then turn left at the end of the ramp onto NJ 31. Stay on NJ 31 for 23 miles, through a traffic circle, a merger with US 202, and another traffic circle. The Arboretum is on the right, 5.8 miles after the second traffic circle. The parking lot is next to the road, and the trail starts just beyond the parking area. *1020 State Route 31, Lebanon, NJ 08833.*

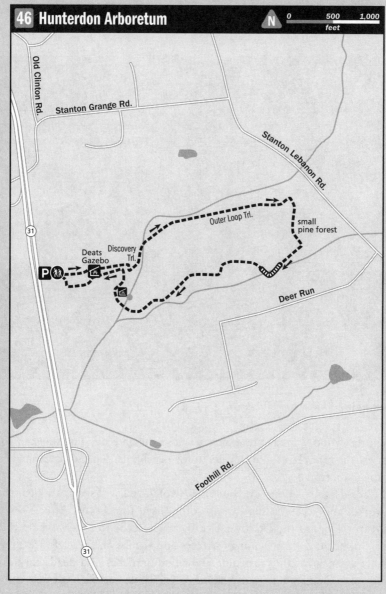

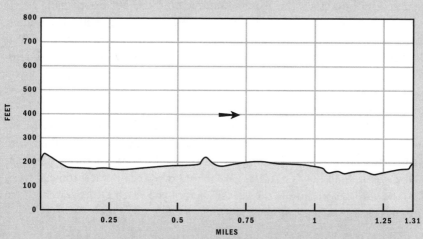

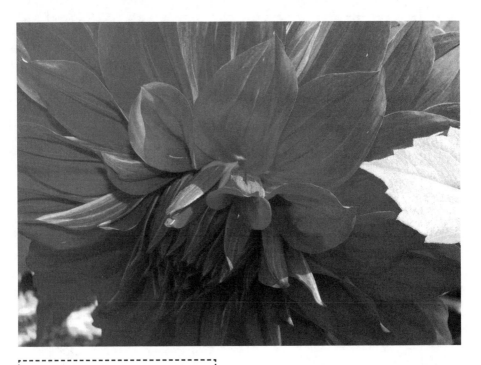

Flowers are in full bloom by mid-summer.

through the wooded area. Make sure to close the gate on your way out so deer do not eat the rare plants and flowers in the gazebo garden. Across a small gravel road, the main trail begins.

Head east past a pond on your right (which you will see again near the end of the hike) and across a small bridge often used for photos. After a few more yards, turn left onto the Discovery Trail, which leads to a field where the trail turns right, heading east. Among the trees and shrubs on your left are a few oak trees that are nearly 200 years old. The white branches of a dead, barkless tree contrast with the green growth behind it. Continue east into a forest until you reach a sign indicating a right turn to continue on the Outer Loop Trail.

Make the turn and travel south through a pine forest carpeted with needles. The path turns abruptly right, heading west to a wooden boardwalk above wetlands that shrink during dry weather. After approximately 50 feet, the boardwalk splits; bear left until the boardwalk ends. (If you turned right instead, you would end up at the same spot.) This is the wetland study area, which showcases skunk cabbages, cattails, and ferns.

After the boardwalk, the trail continues up a small incline and then yields right, heading north, until you approach a quaint, shaded pond abundant with life. You may hear an occasional frog. Overlooking the pond, on the right side, is a small gazebo. Walk north past the gazebo and take the next left to head west, back to the garden gate. Inside the garden, before you reach Deats Gazebo, turn left to see a little pool with stone sculptures.

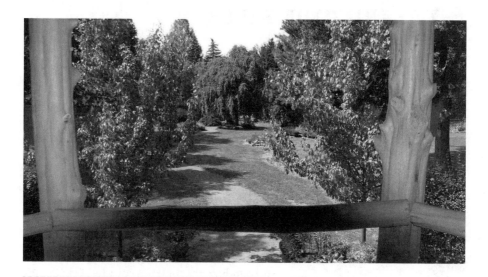

Walk up the steps of Deats Gazebo for a wider scope of the arboretum below.

Just south of the little pool is the Wizard Garden. There, turn right and travel down a tree-shaded pathway heading west. On your left are a small children's castle and some game-themed kiosks. At the end of the path, turn right and cross a small wooden bridge. You are back to where you started.

A brochure available at the Hunterdon County Parks Department Headquarters office in front of the hiking area explains the 27 markers you see on the hike. In fact, the first thing you see from NJ 31 is the headquarters. The Edmund Laport Greenhouse is at the south wing of the headquarters.

George Bloomer first cultivated the property that is now the arboretum in 1953, when he created a commercial nursery. The site included his office and residence, a horse barn, a greenhouse, and several other structures. His wife, Esther, an avid animal-rights activist, founded the Hunterdon County Society for the Prevention of Cruelty to Animals in 1965. In 1974, the state bought the nursery from the Bloomers. The arboretum offers tours in the spring and fall.

## NEARBY ACTIVITIES

HISTORIC CLINTON, NEW JERSEY
*(Quaint shopping, dining, museum, gallery)*
**www.clintonguild.com**

HUNTERDON COUNTY HISTORIC COURTHOUSE
*(Site of famous Lindbergh trial)*
75 Main Street, Flemington
(908) 782-2610

SPRUCE RUN RESERVOIR
*(State park)*
68 Van Syckels Road, Clinton
(908) 638-8572
**state.nj.us/dep/parksandforests/parks/spruce.html**

# 47 READINGTON RIVER BUFFALO FARM

## KEY AT-A-GLANCE INFORMATION

**LENGTH:** 2.57 miles

**CONFIGURATION:** Balloon

**DIFFICULTY:** Moderate

**SCENERY:** Buffalo, horses, pigs, rolling hills, valley, forest

**EXPOSURE:** Full sun–full shade

**TRAIL TRAFFIC:** Light

**TRAIL SURFACE:** Asphalt, gravel, grass, dirt

**HIKING TIME:** 1 hour

**DRIVING DISTANCE FROM CENTER CITY:** 58 miles

**ACCESS:** Daily, dawn–dusk; free admission. The store is open 9 a.m.–4 p.m. on weekends, or by appointment (see contact information below)

**MAPS:** USGS Flemington; maps at store and buffalo-farm trailhead

**WHEELCHAIR TRAVERSABLE:** No

**FACILITIES:** No public restrooms

**SPECIAL COMMENTS:** Examine yourself for ticks after hiking; *do not touch the electric fencing.* More information: (908) 806-0030; www .njbison.com or www.readington twp.org/Round-Mountain.html.

## GPS Trailhead Coordinates

UTM Zone (WGS84)  18T

Easting  0515236

Northing  4490614

Latitude  N 40° 33' 58.2"

Longitude  W 74° 49' 12.1"

## IN BRIEF

Green, rolling hills and swooping valleys spotted with grazing buffalo await you on this hike through a working bison farm, meadows, and hardwood forests.

## DESCRIPTION

The 230-acre Readington River Buffalo Farm raises bison for retail and wholesale products; the owners kindly permit hikers on the fields surrounding the buffalo pastures. This stunning parcel of land adjoins an open-space trail called the Woodschurch Farm Loop.

This hike may make you feel as though you've stepped into another time. Seeing the herds graze brings you back to precolonial times when buffalo roamed many parts of North America. In fact, at one time the buffalo population of 60 million to 120 million may have been larger than that of any other large mammal on earth.

Native Americans relied heavily on the buffalo for their everyday needs. They not only

## *Directions*

Take Interstate 95 north from Philadelphia, entering New Jersey. After 33.7 miles, take Exit 4 for NJ 31 north toward Pennington. At the end of the ramp, turn left onto NJ 31–Pennington Road. After 1.3 miles, take the third exit from the traffic circle to stay on NJ 31. After 10.1 miles, turn right onto the ramp for NJ 31–US 202. After 5.7 miles, take the second exit from another traffic circle to stay on NJ 31. After 2.5 miles, turn right onto County Road 523– Bartles Corner Road. After 4.6 miles, look for the READINGTON RIVER FARM sign on the left. Drive approximately 0.75 miles to the buffalo store and park. The hike starts next to the store, going up the paved hill to the buffalo fields. *937 County Road 523, Flemington, NJ 08822.*

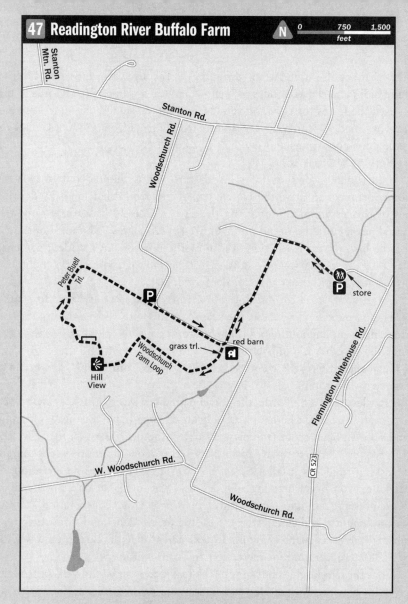

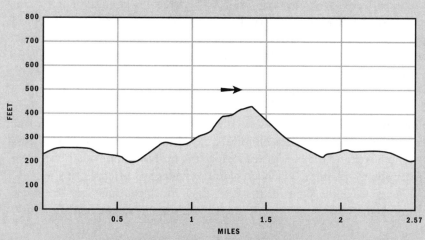

ate the meat but also used buffalo droppings to fuel fires. They used the brains for tanning hides and the gallstones for yellow paint. They boiled the hooves to make glue, used the horns for cups and spoons, and carved small bones into knives and tools. They made clothing, tepees, shoes, and blankets from the hides. They used the sinew for bowstrings and sewing thread, and even used the tails for shooing flies. Nothing was wasted.

Unfortunately, in the 1800s bison were almost hunted out of existence, in some instances to drive the Native Americans from their lands by depriving tribes of this essential resource. By the turn of the 20th century, only a few hundred bison could be found in the entire United States. A handful of ranchers saved the bison from extinction, and now these herds have made a comeback. Today they are raised for meat and other specialized products throughout the United States and in other parts of the world.

This hike starts at the parking lot in front of the store and next to a buffalo pen. There you can view these massive animals, with their dark-brown coats, as they snack on hay and nap. From the store, continue along the asphalt drive toward the silo, barn, and back fields. Follow the asphalt-and-gravel road west and then south. Enjoy the views of grazing buffalo, rolling hills, and green valleys strewn with round bales of hay.

After less than a half mile, the gravel path gives way to grass. Then look for a red barn on your left, where a kiosk indicates the trailhead for the Woodschurch Farm Loop, an open-space trail owned by Readington Township. In 1978, Readington became the first township in New Jersey to hold an open-space referendum, asking residents to allot $1 million toward open-space preservation. The referendum won overwhelming support, and the township developed a master plan to preserve land for agriculture, recreation, and conservation. Through township, county, and state efforts, Readington residents and visitors now reap the benefits of this plan, enjoying 16,000 acres of undeveloped land—with at least 2,700 acres allotted for recreation and conservation.

From the Woodschurch trailhead the trail bends right and walks through an open field, heading west-southwest. Follow the yellow hiker icons, which then lead you northwest over a wooden bridge. The stream below can be dry during the summer. Horses also use the trail, so watch where you step. The trail bends left, heading south, then twists once again to the right, heading north. The path around the grassy field is mowed, and the markers are easy to follow.

Soon you walk into woods, where you ascend. A chestnut horse with a white blaze may peer from a private wooden barn on your right. About a mile in total from the buffalo pen, you reach another field. Here you can see the town of Flemington in the valley below, especially on a clear day. Head west on the trail, following the electric transmission towers; now bear right, heading northeast at the second tower and then northwest, where the trail leads into a hardwood forest. After about 0.5 miles, a wooden bench provides an optional rest stop.

When you see the signs for the Peter Buell Trail, continue straight (northwest) rather than left onto the bridle trail. Follow the yellow markers on this

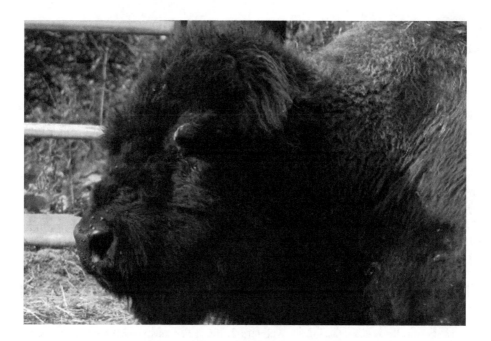

This buffalo happily naps in the afternoon sunshine.

trail as it descends and turns eastward. Watch for a right turn onto a parallel trail that brings you back into the meadow from which you entered the woods. This trail heads southeast and leads to a gravel parking area. Turn left onto dirt-surfaced Woodschurch Road. A red barn indicates that you've returned to the back entrance of the buffalo farm, where you'll turn left to retrace your steps to the farm and your car.

If you enjoy steak, stop at the farm store and buy some bison meat, which is claimed to be lower in fat and cholesterol than beef. (If the store is closed, one of the farmers may open it for you.) If you don't like meat, simply take home the memory of the mighty buffalo and the land you just hiked—both saved through rigorous conservation efforts.

## NEARBY ACTIVITIES

HISTORIC CLINTON
*(Village with shopping, dining, museum, and stone mill, 10 to 15 miles northwest of the buffalo farm)*
www.clintonguild.com

HUNTERDON COUNTY ARBORETUM
*(Trees, flowers, and trails)*
1020 Route 31, Lebanon
(908) 782-1158

SCHAEFER FARMS
*(Family-owned farm; seasonal produce and events)*
1051 Flemington/Whitehouse Road, Flemington
(908) 782-2705
www.schaeferfarms.com

# 48　ROUND VALLEY RESERVOIR

## KEY AT-A-GLANCE INFORMATION

**LENGTH:** 10.12 miles

**CONFIGURATION:** Out-and-back

**DIFFICULTY:** Very hard

**SCENERY:** Hills along reservoir, shady woodlands

**EXPOSURE:** Mostly shaded

**TRAIL TRAFFIC:** Light

**TRAIL SURFACE:** Grass, dirt, rocky at times

**HIKING TIME:** 4 hours

**DRIVING DISTANCE FROM CENTER CITY:** 60.5 miles

**ACCESS:** Memorial Day–Labor Day fee is $5 per vehicle weekdays, $10 weekends; otherwise free. Year-round, daily, 8 a.m.–dusk

**MAPS:** At Ranger Station; USGS Flemington

**WHEELCHAIR TRAVERSABLE:** No

**FACILITIES:** Restrooms near parking lot

**SPECIAL COMMENTS:** For additional information, visit state.nj.us/dep/parksandforests/parks/round.html or call (908) 236-6355.

## GPS Trailhead Coordinates

UTM Zone (WGS84)　18T

Easting　0512720

Northing　4496480

Latitude　N 40° 37' 8.8"

Longitude　W 74° 50' 58.3"

## IN BRIEF

This tough trail, which curves around a large reservoir, is worth the challenge for adventurous hikers who aren't afraid of hills.

## DESCRIPTION

Round Valley Reservoir in Hunterdon County, New Jersey, is known for its scenic walks and unusually clear blue water. Mountain ridges surround the reservoir, forming a 160-million-year-old caldera—a collapsed volcanic crater. In 1960 the New Jersey Water Authority built two dams to flood the valley. The reservoir covers 2,000 acres and is 180 feet deep, making it the deepest lake in New Jersey. The park offers fishing, hiking, boating, biking, and swimming. The 55-billion-gallon reservoir is stocked with trout, and contains other fish, such as bass, pickerel, and catfish. Facilities include a swimming area, two playgrounds, and numerous cookout spots.

Round Valley's most notable landmark is Cushetunk Mountain, which references the Lenape phrase meaning "place of hogs." Early

## Directions

From Philadelphia, follow Interstate 95 north 33.7 miles, entering New Jersey. Take Exit 4 and turn left at the end of the ramp onto NJ 31. Continue 25.2 miles, through a traffic circle, a merger with US 202, and another traffic circle, and then turn right onto Allerton Road. After 1.3 miles, bear right onto Valley Crest Road. After 0.3 miles, turn left at the T-intersection onto Stanton Lebanon Road. The Round Valley entrance is on the right. Once through the entrance, take the first right to reach the south parking lot and boat launch. Cushetunk Trail starts at the lot's message board. *1220 Stanton Lebanon Road, Lebanon, NJ 08833-3115.*

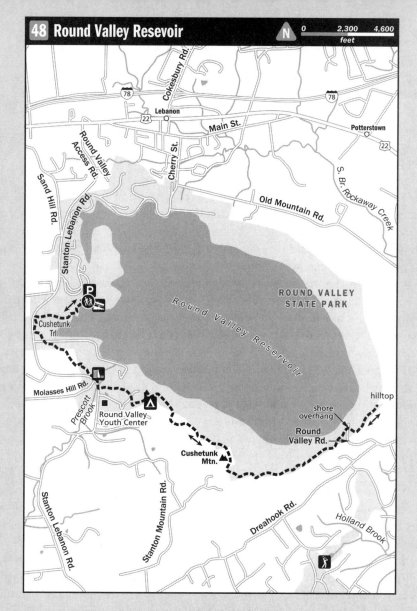

N

0        2,300        4,600
feet

Cokesbury Rd.

78

Lebanon

Main St.

Pottterstown

22

Round Valley Access Rd.

Cherry St.

S. Br. Rockaway Creek

Sand Hill Rd.

Stanton Lebanon Rd.

Old Mountain Rd.

P

ROUND VALLEY STATE PARK

Cushetunk Trl.

*Round Valley Resevoir*

hilltop

Molasses Hill Rd.

Prescott Brook

Round Valley Youth Center

shore overhang

Round Valley Rd.

Cushetunk Mtn.

Stanton Lebanon Rd.

Stanton Mountain Rd.

Dreahook Rd.

Holland Brook

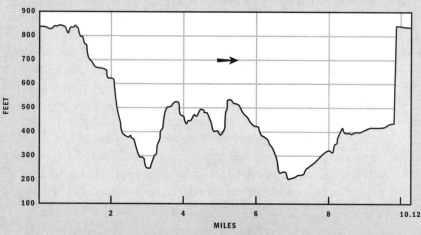

FEET

900
800
700
600
500
400
300
200
100

2        4        6        8        10.12

MILES

white settlers, who found the rocky landscape unsuitable for farming but appropriate for timber production, just called it "Hog Mountain."

During the Revolutionary War, patriots hid from the British in this valley, which having only one entrance, could be effectively defended. Among those who took refuge were members of the Stevens family; after the war they relocated to Hoboken, where they later founded the Stevens Institute of Technology.

Round Valley's main trail is Cushetunk Trail, which starts at the south parking lot's message board. From there, walk west down a small dirt hill and past a rocky shoreline, and then continue up a mountain, where the landscape changes to forest in 1.25 miles. The trail is a roller-coaster experience, continually taking you up and down mountain slopes. Red markers indicate the trail, but even without them, the trail is pretty clear.

The most challenging part of the hike is the mountainside descent that follows the south dam. Climbing this incline on the way back takes some effort. The south dam, a favorite place for deer to graze, is just more than 1 mile into the hike, on your left, and looks more like a mountainside than a dam. Past the dam and over Prescott Brook, the trail passes Round Valley Youth Center, heading east. This is about the 1.5-mile mark. The left fork, which leads to the youth center, is off-limits. Continue to bear right on Cushetunk Trail. From here, you get the impression you are in the middle of nowhere instead of in central New Jersey.

Farther into the hardwood forest, several signs warn that you are in bear territory. You may see deer, foxes, and, yes, perhaps even a bear running away in the distance. You may also notice hawks, opossums, turkey vultures, and bald eagles. Along the trail at the 3-, 3.5-, and 5-mile marks, log benches provide a place to sit while you enjoy the impressive views of the reservoir's north shore.

As you climb the mountain slopes, the path becomes narrower and rockier. In the fall, leaves obscure the rocks, so watch your step. Sturdy hiking shoes help. Below the main trail on the eastern side of the park, at about the 3-mile mark, are campsites that are accessible only by those boating or hiking in. You will pass an access road just before the 5-mile mark. If you turn left onto this road, you can see a picnic pavilion, telephone, and water fountain. Continue straight on the path another 0.25 miles until you reach the highest peak of Cushetunk Mountain. From here there is an impressive view of Hunterdon County: Looking east, you'll see housing developments in the distance, and roads crisscrossing the landscape. To the west, you can see the reservoir and the surrounding valley. This vista gives the illusion that you have traveled farther than you actually have. After taking in the view, retrace your steps to return west, to the south parking lot. If you want to complete the entire hike, continue on this same trail until you hit the north dam at the 9-mile mark, then head back. Remember, if you want to do the whole hike, it is an 18-mile all-day event.

Cushetunk Trail is one of the better-maintained and -marked trails in central New Jersey, so it is easy to retrace your steps, even if you venture off the trail to explore the various campgrounds facing the reservoir. Because of the mountainous nature of this trail, you should allow at least 4 hours to complete this 10-mile hike. The Cushetunk Trail hike is not a casual walk, but an intensive day out for the serious hiker. The entire trail runs 18 miles from the south parking lot to the dam at the north side of the reservoir and back. It is 9 miles to the north dam and another 9 miles to retrace your steps to the south parking lot, so it is not possible to circumnavigate the reservoir.

Occasionally, the park service gives guided tours of Round Valley's trails, including Cushetunk Trail. Usually, a sign at the park entrance announces these tours. There are many shorter trails at Round Valley as well, which the whole family can enjoy. Several are less than 1 mile long and are perfect for children and recreational bird-watchers.

## NEARBY ACTIVITIES

HISTORIC CLINTON, NEW JERSEY
*(Quaint shopping, dining, museum, gallery)*
**www.clintonguild.com**

HUNTERDON COUNTY HISTORIC COURTHOUSE
*(Site of famous Lindbergh trial)*
75 Main Street, Flemington
(908) 782-2610

SPRUCE RUN RESERVOIR
*(State park)*
68 Van Syckels Road, Clinton
(908) 638-8572
**state.nj.us/dep/parksandforests/parks/spruce.html**

# 49 SOURLAND MOUNTAIN PRESERVE

## KEY AT-A-GLANCE INFORMATION

**LENGTH:** 3 miles

**CONFIGURATION:** Loop with out-and-back

**DIFFICULTY:** Moderate

**SCENERY:** Woods, boulder field

**EXPOSURE:** Sun and some shade

**TRAIL TRAFFIC:** Moderate

**TRAIL SURFACE:** Dirt

**HIKING TIME:** About 1 hour

**DRIVING DISTANCE FROM CENTER CITY:** 45 miles

**ACCESS:** Year-round, daily, dawn–dusk; free admission

**MAPS:** USGS Hopewell; co.hunter don.nj.us/depts/parks/guides/Sourland.htm#trails

**WHEELCHAIR TRAVERSABLE:** No

**FACILITIES:** No public restrooms

**SPECIAL COMMENTS:** The Sourland Mountains are supposedly haunted! For more information, visit www.somersetcounty parks.org/activities/parks/sourland_mt.htm.

## GPS Trailhead Coordinates

UTM Zone (WGS84)  18T

Easting  0517942

Northing  4474545

Latitude  N 40° 25' 16.4"

Longitude  W 75° 47' 18.8"

## IN BRIEF

This moderate hike guides you through supposedly haunted woods and boulder fields in New Jersey's Sourland Mountain range.

## DESCRIPTION

East Amwell Valley, in Hunterdon County, features rolling hills and pastoral meadows. The vastness of the Delaware Valley becomes apparent from the open views along its many country drives. Although farther from Philadelphia than other hikes in this book, its scenic drives and local vineyards make it worth the trip.

Arriving at the Rileyville Road entrance, you won't feel like you're in the mountains—it's such a gradual drive up the 500 feet, and the forest is heavily wooded. So pay attention to signs. At the parking lot, you can't miss the trailhead, with its wooden gate on the northeast side.

After about 0.25 miles on the Service Road Trail, turn right on South Loop Trail, just past a small stream crossing. The trail is marked by small diamonds on almost every third tree. South Loop Trail quickly morphs

## Directions

**Follow US 95 north 34 miles from Philadelphia to Exit 4 (NJ 31 north). Turn left at Pennington Road/NJ 31 north. Drive 1.3 miles from the traffic circle, then take the third exit, onto NJ 31 north. Continue 3.6 miles, then bear right at Pennington Hopewell Road. After 2.5 miles, continue on West Broad Street about 1 mile. Turn left at North Greenwood Avenue, which becomes Hopewell Wertsville Road before becoming Rileyville Road after a couple of miles. Look for the park entrance, on the right.** *Rileyville Road, Hopewell, NJ 08525.*

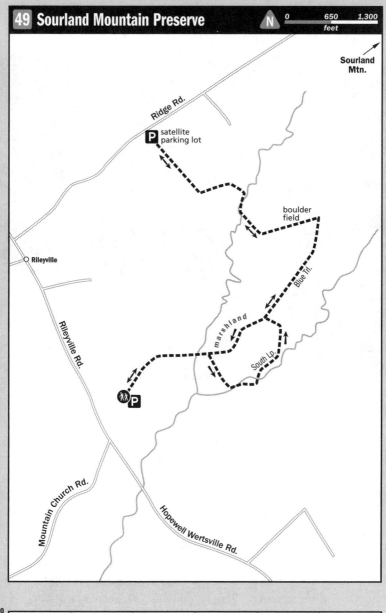

Sourland
Mtn.

Ridge Rd.

P satellite
parking lot

boulder
field

Blue Trl.

Rileyville

*marshland*

South Lp.

Rileyville Rd.

Mountain Church Rd.

Hopewell Wertsville Rd.

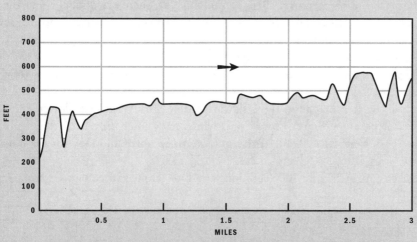

800

700

600

500

400

300

200

100

0

FEET

0.5        1        1.5        2        2.5        3

MILES

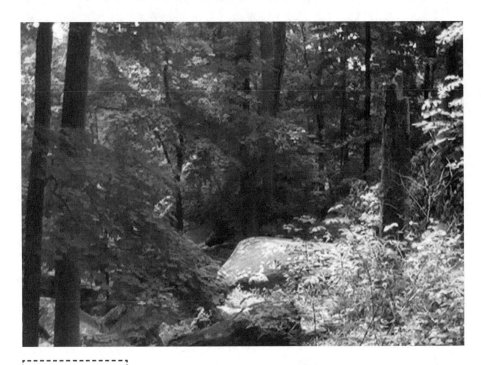

Top of boulder field

into a path that winds between little boulders and meanders around drainage brooks. In general, stay to the left while on the short South loop.

Whether you are moving east or otherwise, you may have to rely on your sense of direction: legend has it that compasses do not work in these hills, which locals claim to be haunted. One of the signers of the Declaration of Independence, John Hart, fled into these hills ahead of the British, hiding out for almost a year; some claim to have since seen his ghostly figure. But by far the most haunting event that occurred in these hills was the tragic kidnapping and murder of 20-month-old Charles Lindbergh Jr., which resulted, in 1937, in the sensational "trial of the century." Because, to this day, there are doubts about the guilt of the convicted and subsequently executed Bruno Richard Hauptmann, the case remains an enigma and further adds to a somewhat creepy atmosphere within these woods.

Despite the chilling past of these mountains, these woods provide a great hike for tree lovers, who can wander through a deciduous forest that showcases almost all the trees native to the Delaware Valley area. Great wildflowers blossom in spring along South Loop Trail, which ends after only 0.25 miles and rejoins the Service Road Trail. Turn right, continue north and look for the Blue Trail on your left.

After approximately 100 feet along the Blue Trail, you come to a boulder

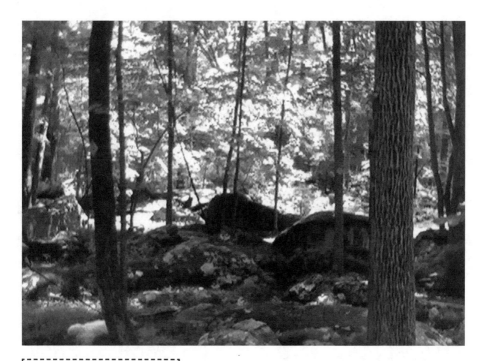

Winding path through the rocks

field. These diabase, or "trap rock," boulders were once used for railroad bal-last—the foundation for railroad tracks. Fissures in the boulders testify to long-ago quarrying activity. Continue along the Blue Trail and cross the same stream you crossed near the start of the Service Road Trail. The stream has no bridge here, so you may have to jump over to the other side.

At this point, you traverse a small easement belonging to the Delaware and Raritan Greenway Land Trust, so the signs may change a bit. Some of the signs that mark trails diverging from the main Blue Trail read, THIS IS *NOT* A TRAIL (thank you, D&R). A small clearing marks the Ridge Road parking lot; here you may want to rest and have a snack before retracing your route on the Blue and Service Road trails.

On your way back, look for the marshland on your right, which you don't see on the way in, when taking the South Loop Trail. Like most wetlands in New Jersey, it is protected because it is crucial to the surrounding ecosystem. Also, without these wetlands, nearby roads would likely flood. Look for some rare birds, such as the grasshopper sparrow and scarlet tanager; the Sourland Preserve is a stopover for migratory birds traveling from South America to the Arctic.

After crossing the stream again, you are back at the parking lot. Reward yourself with a trip to Unionville Vineyards.

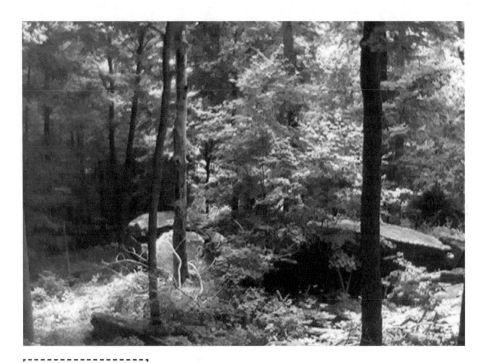

Bottom of boulder field

## NEARBY ACTIVITIES

HUNTERDON COUNTY HISTORIC
COURTHOUSE
*(Site of famous Lindbergh trial)*
75 Main Street, Flemington
(908) 782-2610

UNIONVILLE VINEYARDS
9 Rocktown Road, Ringoes
(908) 788-0400
**www.unionvillevineyards.com**
(Directions from park: Turn right from
park exit, onto Rileyville Road. Go
left onto Wertsville Road. Look for
Rocktown Road on your left. Follow
signs to winery.)

# TED STILES PRESERVE  50

## IN BRIEF

This hike offers rocky terrain, rolling meadows, and historic farmland with 19th-century ruins, plus an old apple orchard where migrating birds stop to enjoy the berries.

## DESCRIPTION

Edmund "Ted" Warner Stiles, a respected ornithologist, taught at Rutgers University for 35 years, and staunchly fought for environmental issues, inspiring many of his students to continue his mission.

Stiles was instrumental in preserving the land surrounding the Hutcheson Memorial Forest in Somerset County, New Jersey, and helped preserve tens of thousands of acres in and near Hopewell Valley, New Jersey. He served on dozens of nonprofit boards, volunteering countless hours for environmental causes. He has been called one of New Jersey's most accomplished and tireless activists for protection of natural lands. One of Stile's greatest contributions involved a ten-year campaign that led to the preservation in 1998 of Baldpate Mountain, the highest point in Mercer County, New Jersey. These are just some of the reasons that, after Ted's passing in March 2007, the 1,800-acre park was renamed the Ted Stiles Preserve. So, as

### KEY AT-A-GLANCE INFORMATION

**LENGTH: 6 miles**

**CONFIGURATION: Balloon**

**DIFFICULTY: Moderate**

**SCENERY: Diabase rocks, hillside, farmland, woods**

**EXPOSURE: Mostly shade, some full sun**

**TRAIL TRAFFIC: Light**

**TRAIL SURFACE: Dirt, rocks, grass**

**HIKING TIME: 3 hours**

**DRIVING DISTANCE FROM CENTER CITY: 36.2 miles**

**ACCESS: Year-round, daily, dawn–dusk; free**

**MAPS: USGS Lambertville; maps at www.njtrails.org/printmap.php? TrailID=121**

**WHEELCHAIR TRAVERSABLE: No**

**FACILITIES: Outhouse in picnic area**

**SPECIAL COMMENTS: Inspect yourself regularly for deer ticks. For more park information, call (609) 989-6559 or see www .njtrails.org/trailguide.php? TrailID=121.**

---

## Directions ———————→

Take Interstate 95 north from Philadelphia 30 miles. Just after entering New Jersey, take Exit 1 and merge onto NJ 29 north. After 4.7 miles, turn right onto Fiddlers Creek Road, then take a left into the Green Acres parking lot. A wooden post with a blue trail blaze marks the spot. *327 Fiddler's Creek Road, Titusville, NJ 08560.*

### GPS Trailhead Coordinates

UTM Zone (WGS84) 18T

Easting 0509273

Northing 4463099

Latitude N 40° 19' 6.1"

Longitude W 74° 53' 27.2"

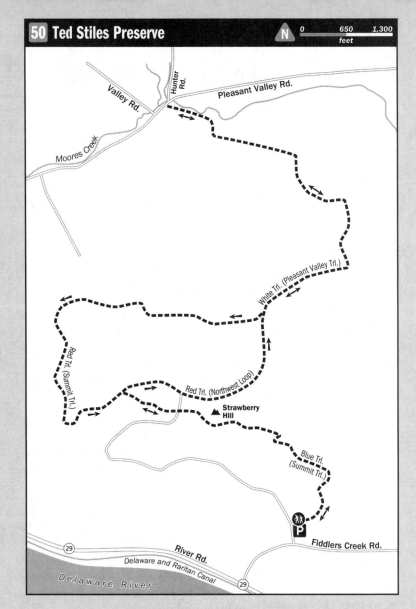

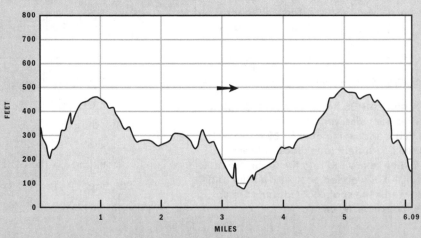

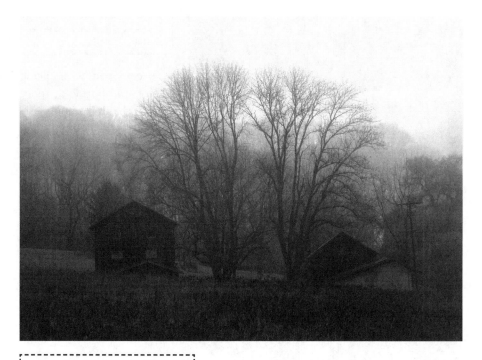

Part of the Preserve, on a misty day

you start your hike off the Green Acres parking lot, think about this great man, who loved forests and spent many days walking through the woods, watching wildlife, and gathering plant specimens in little plastic bags.

Park by the boulders and look for the kiosk across the driveway, where blue markers indicate the Summit Trail.

The trail heads uphill, northwest, through increasingly rocky terrain that twists and turns until it forms a natural rock stairway. Watch your footing; moss makes some of the rocks slippery. This section of the hike is one of the most strenuous, but you are rewarded at the top of the hill by an old farmhouse and an orchard surrounded by bushes dotted with red berries, where the birds eat their fill.

The Ted Stiles Preserve at Baldpate Mountain is part of the Sourland Mountains, a landscape of ridges and rolling farmland that's on the Atlantic Flyway for migratory birds. Migrants such as the black-throated blue warbler rely on this area for food and shelter during their annual travels.

As Stiles wandered the preserve's hills and meadows, he could identify these birds by their songs and tell you their flight patterns. He understood how birds and their environments are intertwined. In fact, birds are often the first indicators of an environmental problem, and flocks of vibrant birds can also indicate and promote a healthy environment.

So enjoy a little bird-watching as you walk along the orchard following the Blue Trail markers. They point you northwest, to a clearing lined with tall pines

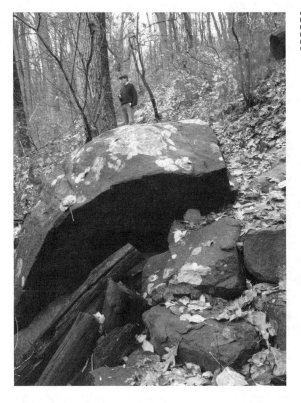

The rocky terrain ascends the side of a hill.

and equipped with picnic tables. A portable toilet here is the only public restroom on the mountain.

From the clearing, follow the white arrows to the left (north) to get on Northwest Loop, which has red markers. Ascend again until the trail turns right where it abuts the property line of a quarry. You may hear the heavy quarrying equipment in the distance as you hike up and down the hills of the Red Trail, heading northeast.

When the red markers meet the white markers, turn left and continue northeast on Pleasant Valley Trail. This out-and-back portion of the trail eventually leads to the Howell Living History Farm (see page 239). The White Trail will come to a spot where you stay right, heading east. This portion of the hike is not only rich with deer, but also dotted with 19th-century stone ruins.

The White Trail follows power lines for a short jog. More grass in this part of the trail means more deer ticks, so check yourself regularly, or let your hiking partner check you. About 25 to 50 percent of the deer ticks in this area are infected with Lyme disease, so inspect yourself during and after the hike, shower with a washcloth directly afterward if possible, and toss your clothes into a hot dryer.

As the trail turns right, heading northwest, tall grasses give way to a dirt path that parallels a winding stream amid sycamore trees. The rooster's call in the distance alerts you to the end of the trail, as it reaches a road. If you cross the road, you can hike into the Howell Living History Farm (see Nearby Activities). If you wish to save that hike for another day, turn around and head back the way you came until you see a white trail marker bearing the letter **P.** Go straight from here until you come to a **T**-intersection. Turn right, heading southwest, and continue until you come to a white trail marker bearing an **M.** From there, continue along the trail, heading northwest back to the orchard and the blue markers, which direct you down the rocky stairs and along looping paths down the mountainside toward the parking lot.

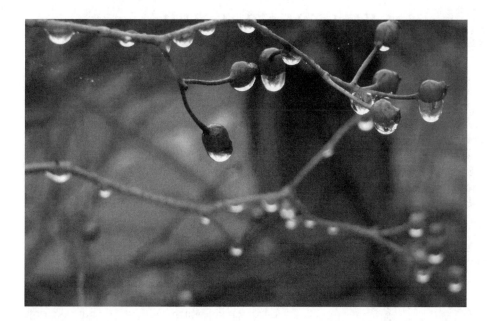

Birds just love 'em.

Before your descent, take one last look at the birds in the orchard and think about the man behind the preserve, who saw so much value in nature that he dedicated much of his life to preserving it.

## NEARBY ACTIVITIES

BULLS ISLAND RECREATION AREA
*(Park and campsite along Delaware Canal; call first as flooding can close the park.)*
Route 29, Stockton
(609) 397-2949
**www.state.nj.us/dep/parksandforests/
parks/bull.html**

HOWELL LIVING HISTORY FARM
*(See separate hike, page 239, and its nearby activities.)*
70 Wooden's Lane, Lambertville
(609) 737-3299
**www.howellfarm.org**

MERCER WILDLIFE CENTER
*(Planning a new facility, to open in fall 2009, where community members can learn more about local wildlife; call first.)*
Route 29, Titusville
(609) 883-6606
**state.nj.us/counties/mercer/
community/wildlife**

# 51 WASHINGTON CROSSING HISTORIC PARK: Continental March Plus

## KEY AT-A-GLANCE INFORMATION

**LENGTH:** 4 miles

**CONFIGURATION:** Out-and-back with a loop in the middle

**DIFFICULTY:** Moderate; can be slippery after rainfall.

**SCENERY:** Riverbank, woods, pine-lined trails

**EXPOSURE:** Full sun on the river, mostly shade on the main trails

**TRAIL TRAFFIC:** Light

**TRAIL SURFACE:** Dirt, bridge, walkway

**HIKING TIME:** 1.5 hours

**DRIVING DISTANCE FROM CENTER CITY:** 30 miles

**ACCESS:** Year-round, daily, dawn–dusk; free. See www.ushistory.org/washingtoncrossing or call (215) 862-2388 for visitor-center hours and activities.

**MAPS:** USGS Pennington

**WHEELCHAIR TRAVERSABLE:** Partially

**SPECIAL COMMENTS:** Reenactment each Christmas; dress rehearsal second weekend in December; see Web site for other special events.

## IN BRIEF

This hike, which begins in Pennsylvania, follows the path of Washington's historic crossing of the Delaware River to the woods of the New Jersey side and treks part of the Continental Army's route toward Trenton. Along this pastoral trail that hugs a glistening creek, you'll see historic homes and stone bridges, among others sights.

## DESCRIPTION

You can almost hear the marching footsteps on this hike, which follows the path taken by George Washington's Continental Army as they trod the woods on their way to attack Hessian troops, who were just waking up in nearby Trenton on that famous Christmas day that changed the course of U.S. history.

This hike starts on the Pennsylvania side of the Delaware River, where sturdy Durham boats stood waiting for General Washington's army.

Park your car by the tall flagpole and cross the street, where a statue that pays tribute to the famous general looks out toward the glistening river. Here, a sidewalk paralleling the Delaware River weaves past historic homes. This village was sparsely populated when Washington's troops made their crossing; only

## GPS Trailhead Coordinates

UTM Zone (WGS84)  18T

Easting    0510918.4

Northing   4460574.8

Latitude   N 40° 17' 44.16"

Longitude  W 74° 52' 17.52"

## Directions

From Philadelphia, go 28.8 miles on US 95 North, then take Exit 51 and turn left on Taylorsville Road toward New Hope. Drive 2.9 miles, then turn right onto PA 532 (General Washington Memorial Road). After 0.5 miles, turn left onto PA 32 (River Road). Go 0.2 miles and look for parking on the left, at the giant flagpole. *New Hope, PA 18938.*

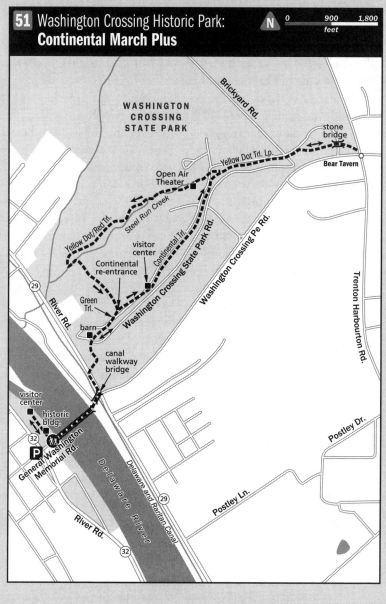

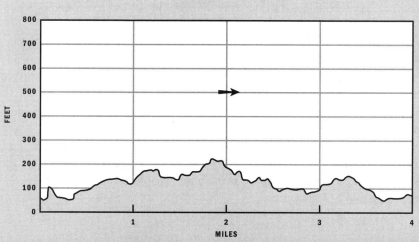

McConkey Ferry Inn stood by the river, and it is said that the general supped there before carrying out his famous attack.

Shortly after the attack, the Taylor family purchased the inn and its surrounding land and built a small village, aptly named Taylorsville. The now-preserved village includes Federal-style homes; tenant homes for a blacksmith, wheelwright, tailor, and physician; and a post office, a general store, and the Washington Crossing Inn, where a warm cup of soup and a cozy fire await winter hikers returning from their historical trek along Continental Trail.

A visitor center and store beside the village offers maps, books, shirts, and tickets for historical tours. A free 17-minute orientation film, *Of Dire Necessity*, can be viewed in the center's small theater. From here, continue your hike from the paved river walkway. Along the way, you pass historic buildings—one of them contains replicas of the long boats the troops used for the crossing and which are still used for yearly reenactments. Past these buildings, cross the street toward the bridge and turn left to cross the bridge.

Admire the mighty Delaware in all its power and glory—this river saw six floods between 1991 and 2006, leaving some locals devastated as they lost nearly everything they owned to waters racing downstream from the north.

The river stretches from the Catskill Mountains south to the Atlantic Ocean, a distance of some 400 miles. Traversing four states, this waterway has been used for centuries for fishing, transportation, and trade. Unfortunately, the river became severely polluted at the start of the Industrial Revolution, reaching its peak of putrefaction after World War II, as factories and residences dumped waste in it. The waters were further poisoned by PCB dumping and oil spills. Consequently, the river, which once provided plentiful resources for Native Americans, early settlers, and the wildlife they hunted, quickly became a giant cesspool.

Recent efforts have sought to reduce dumping and clean up the river, but unless efforts are increased to curb development and curb runoff containing pesticides and other pollutants, the river will never again flow clear. But things *have* improved, as evidenced by the yearly Shad Festival upriver in Lambertville, which features fish that have successfully been reintroduced to the river, beginning in the 1960s.

After crossing the bridge, cross the street and head to the right of Nelson House, where you take a footbridge that zigzags across NJ 546 and safely leads you to the Washington Crossing State Park, with its plethora of trails. The river and the canal, which run parallel, attract ducks, geese, gulls, and other birds. Bird-watchers can expect to see red-tailed hawks flying over nearby woodlands, an occasional Eastern screech owl, red-bellied woodpeckers, and an assortment of warblers and vireos in the warmer months. Since many bird-watchers head to nearby Princeton for the spring migration, this state park provides a secret hideaway for those wishing to peek at the birds with less interruption from the larger population of sightseers.

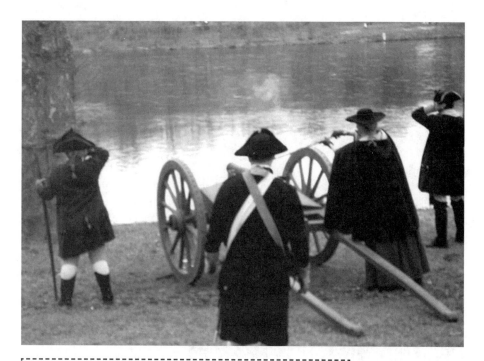

Revolutionary reenactment along the Delaware at Washington Crossing.

Continue straight after the bridge, and then head left. A stone barn welcomes you to the New Jersey trails. Here, turn right on the Continental Trail and walk due east under the towering pines. Other common trees throughout the park include maples, birches, and oaks. In fact, more than 30 species of trees can be found here, and you will not need to look far to see outstretched branches, or small groves of trees embracing one another, giving the park an almost mystical feel.

A paved trail is just right of the Continental Army's historic route—diehards stay on the dirt trail, remembering that many of the ragtag troops of Washington's brigades made this journey without shoes. Soon a marker assures you that you are on the right track, and you'll see a visitor center on the right. The trail veers right at Yellow Dot Trail and parallels the babbling Steel Run Creek, left, where white-tailed deer often stop for refreshment. At certain points, the park road can be glimpsed to your left, but, eventually, history again takes hold, as you pass under an old stone bridge near Bear Tavern.

At this point, the Continental Trail part of the hike is almost done. Beyond the bridge, the trail continues until it meets a road; park offices are nearby. Pause and imagine what this country would be like if the brave Continental soldiers hadn't waged their fight for freedom. Today, a different battle rages—the fight for open space, which has become a threatened and precious commodity, so necessary in our stressed, polluted and over-extended age.

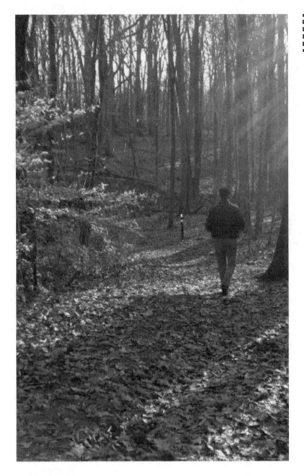

> The park has an almost mystical feel.

Retrace your route to the junction with Yellow Dot Trail. From here, bear right on the Yellow Dot Trail, signed for Green Grove. Stay on Yellow Dot Trail and enjoy the peaceful trickle of the creek as it meanders through the park. The trail eventually leads to an open-air theater on your right, where audiences enjoy main stage performances and Broadway revivals in summer, surrounded by the forest flora and fauna. A wide range of children's musical theater is offered here, too.

Continue on the trail until it hugs Steel Run Creek, and follow it to the junction of the Yellow Dot and Red trails. Here, stay beside the creek by bearing left on the Red Trail. Cross a wooden bridge and ramble through woods until you come to a majestic pine tree. This tree marks an open field that you must cross for the last stretch of the Red Trail. Return to Continental Trail by turning right to march back to the parking lot.

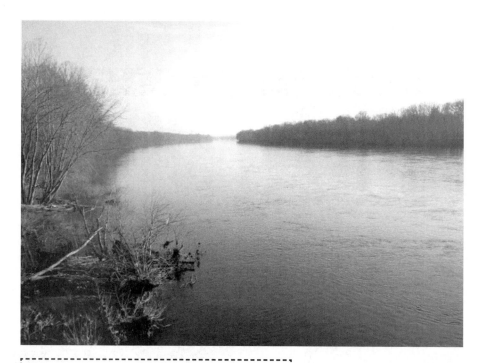

Recent efforts have sought to clean up the Delaware River.

## NEARBY ACTIVITIES

BOWMAN'S HILL WILDFLOWER PRESERVE
New Hope
(215) 862-2924
www.bhwp.org/index.php

CROSSING VINEYARDS AND WINERY, INC.
1853 Wrightstown Road,
Washington Crossing
(215) 493-6500
info@crossingvineyards.com

THE INN AT BOWMAN'S HILL
518 Lurgan Road, New Hope
(215) 862-8090
www.theinnatbowmanshill.com

WASHINGTON CROSSING INN
Routes 532 and 32,
Washington Crossing
(215) 493-3634
(215) 493-3094 (fax)
mysite.verizon.net/vzeop9gh/
washingtoncrossinginn

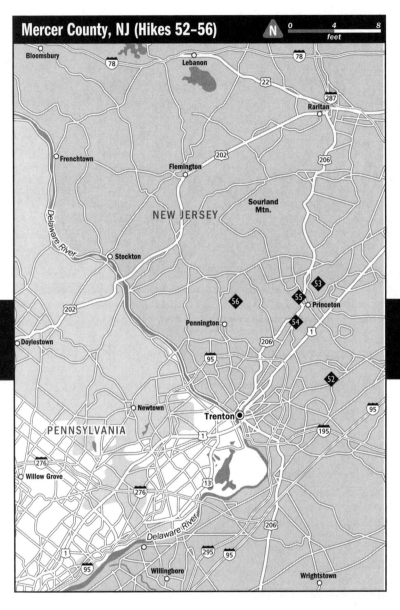

N

0    4    8
feet

Bloomsbury

78

Lebanon

78

22

287

Raritan

Frenchtown

202

206

Flemington

NEW JERSEY

Sourland
Mtn.

Delaware River

Stockton

53

202

55

56

Princeton

Doylestown

54

Pennington

1

206

95

52

Newtown

95

Trenton

PENNSYLVANIA

1

195

276

Willow Grove

276

13

Delaware River

206

1

295

95

95

Willingboro

Wrightstown

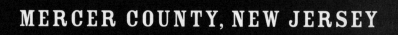

MERCER COUNTY, NEW JERSEY

# 52  HERRONTOWN WOODS

## KEY AT-A-GLANCE INFORMATION

**LENGTH:** 1.9 miles

**CONFIGURATION:** Figure-8

**DIFFICULTY:** Moderate

**SCENERY:** Woods, open meadows, old barn, stone fences, boulders

**EXPOSURE:** Mostly shade, some sun in the meadows

**TRAIL TRAFFIC:** Light

**TRAIL SURFACE:** Dirt

**HIKING TIME:** 50 minutes

**DRIVING DISTANCE FROM CENTER CITY:** 45 miles

**ACCESS:** Daily, dawn–dusk, year-round; free admission

**MAPS:** USGS Rocky Hill; www.njtrails.org/trailmap .php?TrailID=18

**WHEELCHAIR TRAVERSABLE:** No

**FACILITIES:** No restrooms

**SPECIAL COMMENTS:** Some markers on the Yellow Trail are faint and hard to see. More information: (609) 989-6559.

## GPS Trailhead Coordinates

UTM Zone (WGS84)  18T

Easting   0530473

Northing   4469357

Latitude   N 40° 22' 34.41"

Longitude   W 74° 38' 26.33"

## IN BRIEF

Combine this short hike with a day trip to Princeton. Herrontown Woods provides young, shady trees; large boulders; meadows of wildflowers; and a house that belonged to Oswald Veblen, an internationally renowned mathematician and colleague of Albert Einstein's.

## DESCRIPTION

Oswald Veblen was a complex man who taught mathematics at Princeton University from 1905 to 1932. In 1936, he accepted an appointment as the first professor at the university's Institute for Advanced Study, a center for postdoctorate research. Veblen helped select other members of the institute's mathematics faculty, including Albert Einstein, and also helped supervise work during World War II that led to development of the ENIAC—the first digital computer. In 1950, Veblen was selected as president of the International Congress of Mathematicians.

## Directions

Take Interstate 95 north from Philadelphia into New Jersey. After 23 miles, take Exit 46A to US 1 toward Morrisville. Stay on US 1 for 17 miles—the road will become Brunswick Avenue, then Brunswick Pike. Once in Princeton, you will come to a traffic circle; go three-quarters of the way around and bear northwest (right, between two gas stations) onto Washington Road, passing the Princeton University campus. After 1.6 miles, turn right onto Nassau Street. Stay on Nassau Street for 1 mile and turn left on Snowden Lane. Stay on Snowden Lane for about 1 mile; the entrance to the parking area will be on the left. *Snowden Lane, Princeton, NJ 08540.*

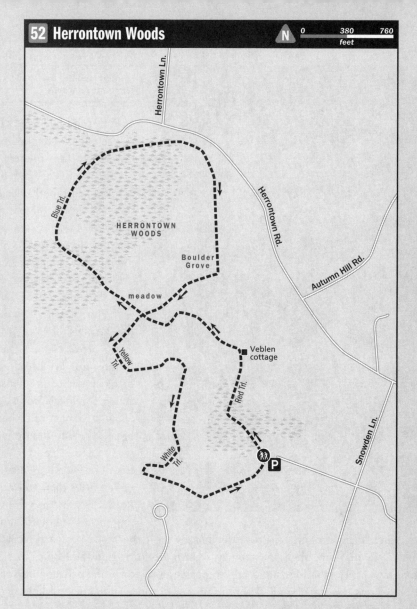

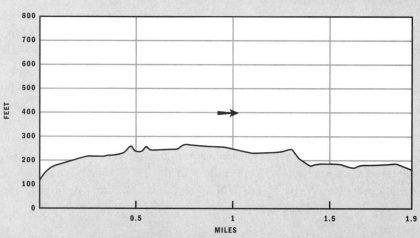

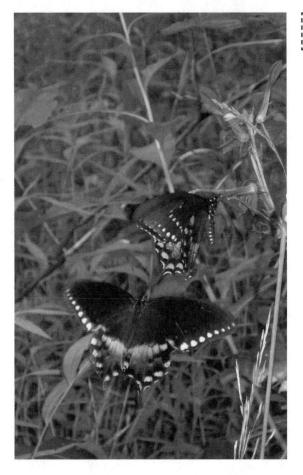

Butterflies enjoy the meadow at Herrontown Woods.

Despite Veblen's immense complexity, he loved the simple life inherent in nature. In 1957, he and his wife, Elizabeth, deeded their 81 acres of wooded land in Mercer County to the New Jersey Parks Commission, as a place where "you can get away from cars and just walk and sit."

Herrontown Woods, the Veblens' former property, provides a nearby respite for Princeton students immersed in intensive study; for local professionals who want a calm lunch break after an intense business meeting; and for tourists who need a slice of nature after their treks past Princeton's innumerable restaurants, boutiques, museums, and local attractions. Princeton buzzes with the activity of a typical Ivy League town: Young men and women wearing oxfords ride their bikes to class. Stone university buildings stand tall in the center of town like pedagogues supervising exams. Georgian and Victorian homes, set on well-manicured lawns, give the area an almost regal feel.

At Herrontown Woods, the tone of the atmosphere becomes more humble—you find an undisturbed tract of nature, marked by trees, meadows, and the small cottage where the Veblens lived. The park was enlarged in the early 1970s with a 61-acre tract of land.

The trailhead for the Red Trail is on the north side of the parking lot. The trail winds northeast to a clearing with an abandoned cottage and barn. This is what remains of the of the Veblen homestead.

After you pass the barn, head west on the Red Trail, which narrows as you walk farther into the woods. Ferns grow behind gray boulders, and young trees dot the landscape. A gypsy-moth infestation in the 1970s killed many trees in the park; unfortunately, many other New Jersey woodlands have since been

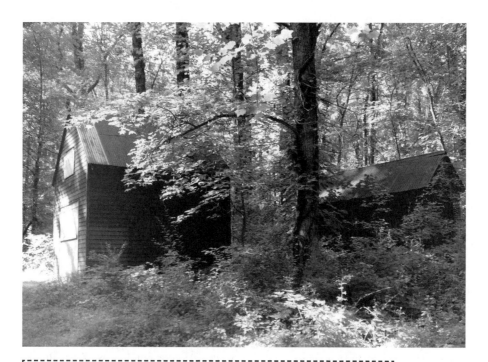

A small abondoned cottage and barn are all that remain of the Veblen homestead.

afflicted with this creeping pest. The New Jersey Department of Agriculture estimates that recent aerial treatments to control defoliation by the gypsy moth are costing the state millions of dollars.

Despite periodic infestations, the woods are making a grand comeback. Oaks, tulip poplars, beeches, sweet gums, pines, and red maples can be found in the park. In spring, dogwoods and apple trees are in flower, and woodland asters bloom in the fall. Warblers and thrushes flit from bush to tree, gathering twigs for their nests. Great-horned owls and eastern screech owls also reside here. Eastern cottontail rabbits peep from behind the underbrush, and chipmunks weave in and out between the fallen trees. Gray squirrels sink their claws in the bark of the tall trees as they search for mates in the midsummer heat, or for food come fall and early winter.

Larger boulders become more and more numerous as you proceed along this leg of the Red Trail. The boulders in this park likely resulted from a combination of sedimentary rocks from the Triassic and Jurassic periods and igneous (volcanic) rock from the Jurassic age. In this boulder-strewn, wooded area, you come to a junction with the Blue Trail. Here turn right, heading northeast.

About 300 feet from Herrontown Road, the Blue Trail turns to the right and heads southeast. You will need to look carefully to stay on the trail, since the markers are few, faint, and far between, and this section of trail is narrow and not well maintained. Continue southward until you reach a meadow.

After you cross this meadow, turn right onto the White Trail, heading southwest. The trail climbs between even larger boulders, making this the most strenuous part of the hike. Continue along the White Trail until you come to a **T**-junction, and turn right on the Yellow Trail. Now carefully hop over a narrow stream, where you can stop to look for salamanders, toads, and frogs. Once across, turn left at the white markers and head south on the White Trail, which returns you to the parking lot.

Herrontown Woods remains a simple slice of land—a place where people can set aside the complexities of daily life and, as the Veblens said, just walk and sit. Out of all the equations that Veblen solved in his life, perhaps using nature to balance life's other factors and problems proved the greatest solution of them all.

## NEARBY ACTIVITIES

PRINCETON CEMETERY
*(Graveyard dating to 1757)*
Witherspoon and Wiggins streets,
Princeton
(609) 924-1369
**www.nassauchurch.org/cemetery**

PRINCETON UNIVERSITY ART MUSEUM
*(72,000 works of art, including a
Picasso)*
Washington Road, McCormick Hall,
Princeton
(609) 258-3788
**artmuseum.princeton.edu**

PRINCETON UNIVERSITY CHAPEL
*(Third largest college chapel
in the world)*
53 University Place, Princeton
(609) 258-3047
**www.princeton.edu/~oktour/virtualtour/
english/Stop05.htm**

# INSTITUTE WOODS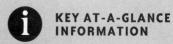

## IN BRIEF

This hike offers rich woodlands, preserved farmland, a meandering brook, and lush meadows in an area where some of the greatest minds in history rejuvenated and took solace.

## DESCRIPTION

You see them walking through the trails: some young and on fire with ideas, some sages, with wisdom and knowledge pumping through their brains with each step. Some of the greatest minds of our time have unlocked the ultimate secret to regeneration through a simple walk in the woods—in this case, the Institute Woods.

This is the Institute for Advanced Study, a center for theoretical research in Princeton, New Jersey, with close ties to Princeton University. Some of the most famous contributors to science, archaeology, history, and philosophy have called the institute their academic home. Albert Einstein, J. Robert Oppenheimer, John von Neumann, Kurt Gödel, George Kennan, and many others have roamed the woods surrounding the Institute. More than a dozen Nobel laureates have been institute faculty, and today, visiting scholars from around the world come here to pursue their academic interests amid the serenity of the Institute Woods.

### KEY AT-A-GLANCE INFORMATION

**LENGTH:** 2.68 miles

**CONFIGURATION:** Figure-8

**DIFFICULTY:** Moderate

**SCENERY:** Woodlands, cornfields, meadows, brook

**EXPOSURE:** Mostly shade

**TRAIL TRAFFIC:** Medium

**TRAIL SURFACE:** Dirt, some mud, gravel, grass

**HIKING TIME:** 1 hour

**DRIVING DISTANCE FROM CENTER CITY:** 43.1 miles

**ACCESS:** Daily, dawn–dusk, year-round; free admission

**MAPS:** USGS Princeton; www.njtrails .org/trailmap.php?TrailID=7

**WHEELCHAIR TRAVERSABLE:** No

**FACILITIES:** No public restrooms

**SPECIAL COMMENTS:** For more information, call (609) 734-8000 or visit www.ias.edu/about/ institute-grounds.

## Directions

**Access Institute Woods from Princeton Battlefield State Park: Take Interstate 95 north from Philadelphia, entering New Jersey. After 37.7 miles, take Exit 8B and merge onto Princeton Pike. After 2.3 miles, the highway becomes Mercer Street; 1.3 miles after that, the park will be on the right. Park in the lot and follow the signs for the Clarke House; the trail begins behind it. *50 Mercer Street, Princeton, NJ 08540.***

### GPS Trailhead Coordinates

UTM Zone (WGS84)  18T

Easting   0527490

Northing  4464410

Latitude  N 40° 19' 47.3"

Longitude  W 74° 40' 34.8"

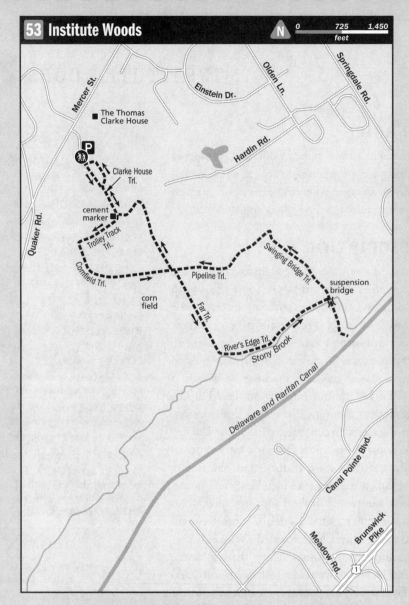

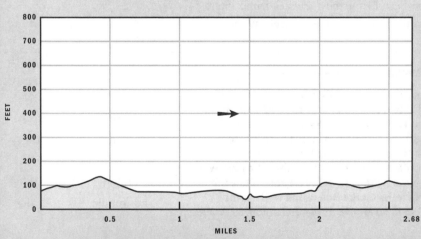

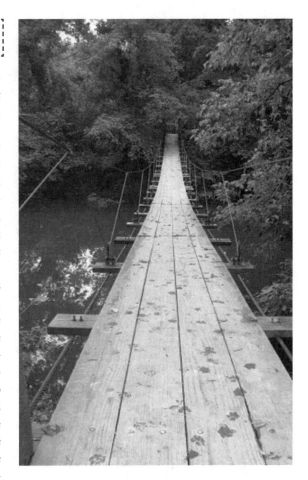

Mysterious paw prints dot the suspension bridge over Stoney Brook.

In 1997, the institute relinquished development rights to the 589-acre woods. Oak, maple, hickory, sweet gum, and other hardwoods stand alongside marshes, farm fields, and meadows. The New Jersey Green Acres program manages the property, and the trails are open to the public.

Because parking is limited at the Institute, access the woods from the Princeton Battlefield State Park parking lot, off Mercer Road. From the parking lot, follow the signs to the trails behind the 1772 Clarke House. During the Revolutionary War's Battle of Princeton in 1777, the house served as a field hospital for both British and Continental soldiers.

At the **T**-junction, turn right onto a dirt path that leads to the Trolley Track Trail, a wide gravel path. Turn right (west) at a concrete marker onto the Trolley Track Trail, and continue on it until it ends at another **T**-junction. Turn left onto the Cornfield Trail. This trail can be particularly muddy at times; markers become fewer and farther between here. After about 0.2 miles, look for a green post, which indicates that the Cornfield Trail turns left and heads east. Do not continue straight into the cornfields.

Almost a half mile after the green post, take the first right and head south on the Far Trail. Watch for turtles crossing. At the end of the Far Trail, turn left onto the River's Edge Trail and walk along the banks of Stony Brook. The brook is a popular stop for migratory birds; peak migration season occurs in mid-May, but you will find an abundance of bird-watching from March to early June. Nearly 200 species of birds have been recorded here. They include 30 different kinds of warblers, such as the American redstart, unmistakable for its rich black color and contrasting markings of bright yellow and orange.

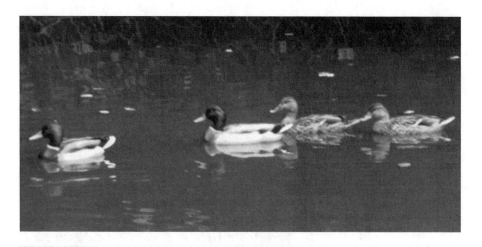

Mallards, double-dating along Stoney Brook inside Institute Woods

Mallards weave through the water. In spring, wildflowers such as pink spring beauties, purple violets, and yellow trout lilies speckle the brook side, looking like a Monet painting. When the trail ends at a **T**-junction, turn right for a short out-and-back over a suspension bridge across the creek.

When you cross back over the bridge, continue north on the Swinging Bridge Trail about 0.3 miles until you reach the Pipeline Trail. Turn left onto the Pipeline Trail and, after 0.3 miles, turn right, back onto the Far Trail. A short trek north brings you past two commemorative plaques in honor of the Revolutionary War soldiers; to the left, a concrete marker points you back to the Clarke House where you started. The Clarke House Trail brings you back to the Princeton Battlefield parking lot.

Will walking through the Institute Woods make you smarter? Will the winds of this profound collective of intelligence blow your way? Does nature nurture the mind? Maybe not—but it sure couldn't hurt.

## NEARBY ACTIVITIES

DRUMTHWACKET
*(New Jersey governor's mansion)*
Guided tours available most
Wednesdays; call first
354 Stockton Street, Princeton
(609) 683-0057
**www.drumthwacket.org**

PRINCETON BATTLEFIELD STATE PARK
500 Mercer Road, Princeton
(609) 921-0074
**state.nj.us/dep/parksandforests/parks/
princeton.html**

ROCKINGHAM HISTORIC SITE
*(Washington headquarters)*
84 Laurel Avenue, Kingston
(609) 921-8835
**www.rockingham.net**

## MERCER COUNTY PARK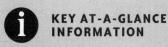

## IN BRIEF

Once you've hiked this paved trail and strolled beside the park's scenic lake, you will most certainly want to return to enjoy the other recreational and athletic activities that Mercer County Park offers.

## DESCRIPTION

Some parks claim that they have something for everyone, but Mercer County Park really does. There are 17 athletic fields for soccer, football, lacrosse, and Frisbee. A 200-foot, open-air, ice-skating rink is open year-round. The park has 24 tennis courts, 6 of them covered and lighted. There are seven basketball courts, several picnic areas, and even a dog park divided for large and small dogs. As well, there are three sand volleyball courts, two cricket pitches, ten softball fields, a nature trail, a cross-country track, and mountain-biking trails.

Lake Mercer, a 365-acre impoundment, offers fishing and boating. You can rent boats at the boathouse, and the marina provides catering services for parties of up to 150 people.

### KEY AT-A-GLANCE INFORMATION

**LENGTH:** 6.5 miles

**CONFIGURATION:** Out-and-back

**DIFFICULTY:** Easy

**SCENERY:** Woods and lake

**EXPOSURE:** Full sun–full shade

**TRAIL TRAFFIC:** Moderate

**TRAIL SURFACE:** Paved, some gravel

**HIKING TIME:** 2–3 hours

**DRIVING DISTANCE FROM CENTER CITY:** 41 miles

**ACCESS:** Year-round, daily, dawn–dusk; free admission

**MAPS:** USGS Princeton and Hightstown. Maps online at state.nj.us/counties/mercer/commissions/pdfs/mercer_county_park_map.pdf

**WHEELCHAIR TRAVERSABLE:** Yes, except on the nature trail

**FACILITIES:** Restrooms at trailhead

**SPECIAL COMMENTS:** For more information, call (609) 448-1947.

### Directions

From Philadelphia, follow Interstate 95 north 24 miles, then take Exit 46A onto US 1 northbound toward Morrisville. After 10 miles, take the Whitehead Road exit and turn right. Within a block, make a left onto Sweet Briar Avenue. This will become Sloan Avenue after 1 mile and then Flock Road after 1.5 miles. After another mile, turn left at Edinburg Road. This will continue as Old Trenton Road for 2 miles. Look for Edinburg Road again on your left. After traveling one block on Edinburg Road, look for the park entrance on your left. The trailhead is to the left of the restrooms. *334 South Post Road, West Windsor, NJ.*

GPS Trailhead
Coordinates

UTM Zone (WGS84)  18T

Easting  0532270

Northing  4456800

Latitude  N 40° 15' 39.9"

Longitude  W 74° 37' 13.6"

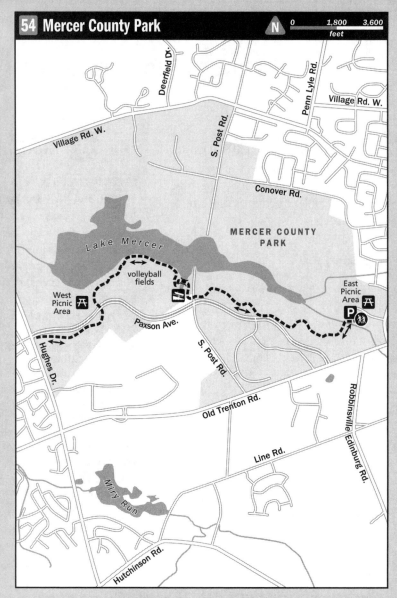

0   1,800   3,600
feet
N

Deerfield Dr.

Penn Lyle Rd.

Village Rd. W.

Village Rd. W.

S. Post Rd.

Conover Rd.

MERCER COUNTY PARK

Lake Mercer

volleyball fields

West Picnic Area

East Picnic Area

Paxson Ave.

Hughes Dr.

S. Post Rd.

Old Trenton Rd.

Robbinsville Edinburg Rd.

Line Rd.

Miry Run

Hutchinson Rd.

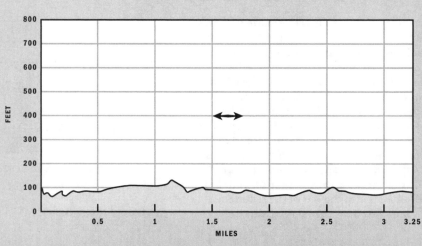

FEET

800
700
600
500
400
300
200
100
0

0.5    1    1.5    2    2.5    3    3.25

MILES

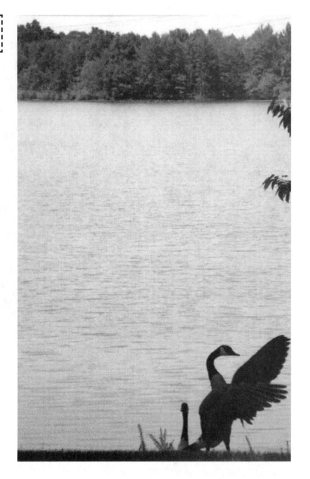

Canadian geese on Lake Mercer, doing a swan dance

The Finn Casperson Rowing Center, on the lake's north shore, is home to the Princeton National Rowing Association and provides a training venue for U.S. rowing teams.

So why hike in Mercer County Park? Not only does the park provide scenic trails with bright fields of goldenrod in spring and summer, it's also a great place to bring the whole family. The park is not far from scenic Princeton, with its quaint cafés, historic campus, and inviting ice-cream shops; and for a traditional, small-town experience, you can visit nearby Hopewell Borough, which has farm stands, antique shops, and historic homes and buildings.

This hike around Mercer County Park starts at parking lot 13, near the East Picnic Area, off Edinburg Road. Restrooms are conveniently located here; facing these, you will see the trailhead to the left of the lot. The trail starts off shaded, but after you cross a small wooden footbridge, sun dominates. Wooded wetlands are to your right, and some of the park's recreational facilities are across Paxson Road to your left.

Continue west past the ice-skating center to a wildflower meadow on your right. A trailhead for an alternate nature trail is directly across from one of the park's two cricket pitches. The nature trail is not paved and therefore not appropriate for wheelchairs. This alternate route heads northeast, then due west, turning left and heading south again to pick up the paved trail, which affords just as much pleasant scenery.

Continue west on the paved trail, which then turns north, passes the volleyball fields to your right, and heads toward Lake Mercer, where the breeze off the water may be welcome. Stop on a small footbridge to view the butterfly flowers and box turtles below, then have a snack at the West Picnic Area.

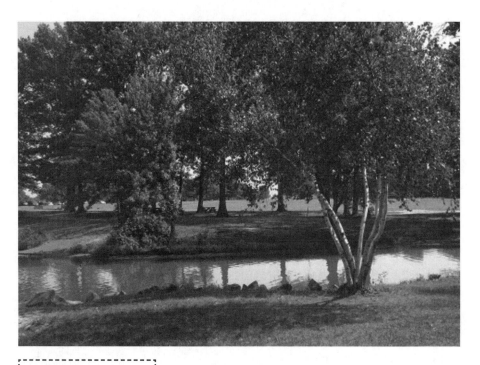

A perfect place for a picnic

This part of the park buzzes with activity: anglers cast their lines from electric-powered boats, parents teach their children to bike, and in many spots, people sit and read the newspaper by the water. Fish species in the lake include yellow perch, largemouth bass, cutthroat trout, and stocked rainbow trout.

As you head northwest for the next 0.25 miles or so, enjoy tree-lined views of the lake and the surrounding marshland. Twisty mountain-biking trails branch left and right. Young oak and ash trees arch over the trail like soldiers performing a sword ceremony. The trail heads west and then turns south, passing over Paxson Avenue via a marked walkway, which cuts through the middle of the park. Next you come to Hughes Drive and head back the way you came.

Mercer County Park was acquired during the late 1960s and 1970s. It was a win-win situation: the lake basin was excavated at no cost to the county, which sold gravel to highway contractors during the construction of I-95 and I-295. A dam was built to keep the impounded waters of Assunpink Creek from flooding the excavated lake basin. Today, the 2,500-acre park provides a plethora of recreational possibilities for hundred of thousands of park visitors each year.

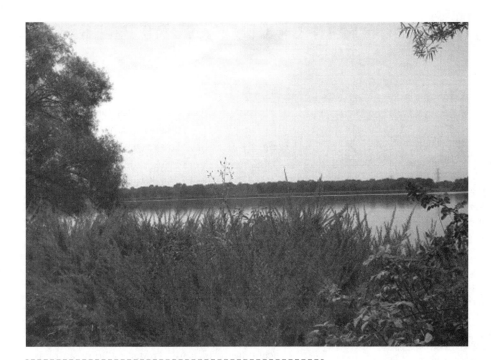

Lake Mercer has been used by the U.S. rowing team for practice.

## NEARBY ACTIVITIES

PRINCETON UNIVERSITY CHAPEL
*(Third largest college chapel
in the world)*
53 University Place, Princeton
(609) 258-3047
**www.princeton.edu/~oktour/virtualtour/
english/Stop05.htm**

SANSONE'S FARM MARKET AND
GREENHOUSES
245 Lambertville–Hopewell Road,
Hopewell
From Route 31, just 0.5 miles west on
Route 518
(609) 466-1323
**www.sansonesfarmmarket.com**

THOMAS SWEET ICE CREAM AND
CHOCOLATE
179 Nassau Street, Princeton
(609) 683-8720
**www.thomassweet.com**

# 55 MOUNTAIN LAKES NATURE PRESERVE

## KEY AT-A-GLANCE INFORMATION

**LENGTH: 3.13 miles**

**CONFIGURATION: Balloon**

**DIFFICULTY: Moderate**

**SCENERY: Woods, lake, boulder fields, meadows**

**EXPOSURE: Full sun–full shade**

**TRAIL TRAFFIC: Moderate**

**TRAIL SURFACE: Dirt, asphalt, gravel, grass**

**HIKING TIME: 1 hour**

**DRIVING DISTANCE FROM CENTER CITY: 45 miles**

**ACCESS: Year-round, daily, dawn–dusk; free admission**

**MAPS: USGS Princeton; access maps at www.njtrails.org/trailmap.php? TrailID=16**

**FACILITIES: Restrooms in parking lot, near trailhead**

**WHEELCHAIR TRAVERSABLE: No, but the pond at Community Park has a paved path around it.**

**SPECIAL COMMENTS: Call (609) 924-8720 for more information.**

## IN BRIEF

Mountain Lakes Nature Preserve, once home to an ice-harvesting company, now warms the hearts of hikers with its crystal-clear lake, mature forests, boulder fields, and open meadows—each offering a wide array of flora and fauna.

## DESCRIPTION

Rugged, brawny men worked the ice ponds of the late 19th and early 20th centuries, sawing, tugging, and hauling the huge blocks onto horse-drawn sleds, which transported the loads to the nearby icehouse. Carriages came to the icehouse to pick up chunks for home and business delivery.

Back then, the iceman cameth to your home, hauling blocks of chilly goodness to heave into your icebox, keeping your dairy cool and your meat fresh. Eventually, however, that ice melteth, and the pans under the icebox needed emptying; if you neglected to empty the pan, you might wake up to a large puddle in the middle of your kitchen floor.

Steve Margerum, who bought farm property in Princeton, New Jersey, in 1883, built dams and retaining walls to capture water from natural mountain streams on the property to

---

## GPS Trailhead Coordinates

UTM Zone (WGS84)  18T

Easting  0527954

Northing  4467542

Latitude  N 40° 21' 28.7"

Longitude  W 74° 40' 14.7"

## Directions

**Follow Interstate 95 north from Philadelphia, traveling almost 37 miles, then take Exit 7B for US 206 north toward Princeton/Lawrenceville. After less than 0.5 miles, merge onto Lawrenceville Road/US 206; continue 6 miles. Turn left at Bayard Lane/US 206. After about 0.5 miles, bear right on Mountain Avenue. The park entrance is within a block, on the left. *57 Mountain Avenue, Princeton, NJ 08540.***

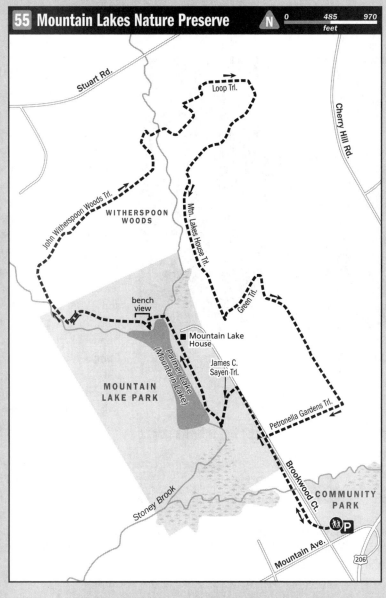

N

0    485    970
**feet**

Stuart Rd.

Loop Trl.

Cherry Hill Rd.

John Witherspoon Woods Trl.

WITHERSPOON
WOODS

Mtn. Lakes House Trl.

Green Trl.

bench
view

Mountain Lake
House

Palmer Lake
(Mountain Lake)

James C.
Sayen Trl.

MOUNTAIN
LAKE PARK

Petronella Gardens Trl.

Stoney Brook

Brookwood Ct.

COMMUNITY
PARK

P

Mountain Ave.

206

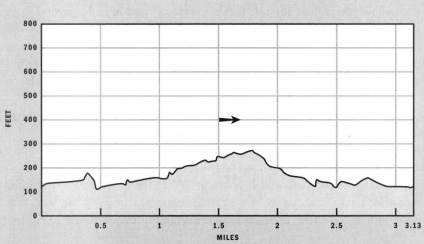

800
700
600
500
400
300
200
100
0

FEET

0.5    1    1.5    2    2.5    3  3.13

MILES

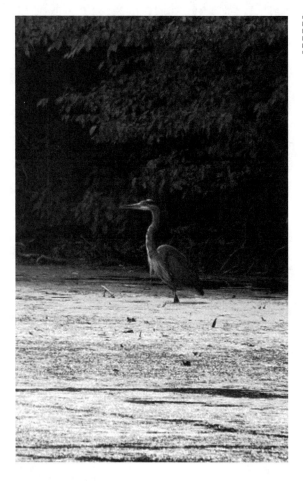

A great blue heron takes a break after searching for prey.

create a pure lake, forming the Mountain Lake Ice Company. In its heyday, the entire ice industry harvested more than 25 million tons of ice in the United States.

Margerum's son, James, inherited the farm and ice company from his father in 1901, but after a warm winter, and ice shortage in 1905 and 1906, he sold the company to businessman H. C. Bunn. In the early 1920s, Bunn's company, the Princeton Ice Company, stopped harvesting ice at Mountain Lake. Shortly thereafter, Bunn opened the lake to the public as a swimming site.

In 1987, with funding from the Friends of Princeton Open Space, New Jersey Green Acres, and private donors, Princeton Township purchased the property, saving it from development. In 2007 the Mountain Lakes Nature Preserve was entered into the New Jersey and National Registers of Historic Places.

This parcel, which was once used to harvest ice today offers a diverse natural experience, including forests, lakes, meadows, and hillsides with a large array of flora and fauna. This hike begins at the Community Park parking lot; the trailhead is on the west side of the lot, next to the water fountain and restrooms. Follow signs for Mountain Lakes House and stay on the paved trail until you reach a kiosk with information about the preserve, and a junction. Here, turn left and head southwest on James C. Sayen Trail.

About 100 yards along, turn right at the junction and head northwest, toward the upper tier of Mountain Lake. In fact, there is only one lake at the Mountain Lakes Nature Preserve, with the upper portion of the lake acting as a sediment trap, and the lower portion catching the clear water.

Continue past the dam and Mountain Lakes House, going north around the perimeter of the lake. Great blue herons, common visitors to the lake, may wade amid the cattails and marsh grass, searching for prey. The birds do not like

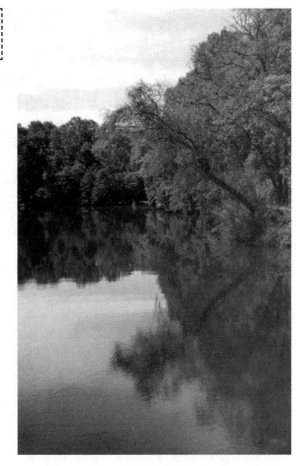

Once the site of an ice company, Mountain Lakes is now saved from development.

to be disturbed, however, and will squawk loudly and take flight if you come too close.

Round the corner, heading west, where a bench invites you to take a quiet rest and enjoy looking at the clouds in the lake's reflection before you continue. Soon, the lake gives way to wetlands, and a wooden bridge signals a left (southwest) turn. Once across the bridge, turn right and head northwest. Look for a narrow trail on your right, which will take you to John Witherspoon Woods Trail, marked with yellow hiker icons.

John Witherspoon, one of the signers of the Declaration of Independence, owned a country home nearby on Cherry Hill Road, which is today someone else's private residence. Witherspoon was the sixth president of Princeton University, which at the time was called the College of New Jersey.

Inside the Witherspoon Woods, you cross one of the park's four streams. Two enter from the northern corner of the hillside and feed the lake below. The trail soon turns east–northeast. Diabase rocks lie beside the trail, small at first and then larger as you ascend. When you come to the sign for Loop Trail, turn left and continue to follow the yellow hiker icons until you are surrounded by enormous boulders. Look for yellow markers on the rocks. Where Loop Trail veers right, go straight toward Mountain Lakes House.

Now you pass through a rich meadow and then meander through a shady pine forest. Soon, a green hiker icon indicates a left turn through another open meadow. Upon reaching a white arrow, turn right and head southeast. (If you continue southeast, you will end up in Community Park, which is on the east side of the parking lot.) Join Petronella Gardens Trail for a short way, following orange hiker icons until you come to a fork. Here, turn right (west) and continue until you reach the paved road where you picked up James C. Sayen Trail. Turn

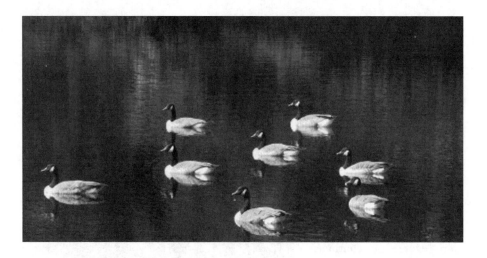

Canadian geese play follow-the-leader on Mountain Lake.

left and continue until you see the left-hand turn that leads you back to Community Park's north parking lot, where you began this hike.

Right now, in a refrigerator near you, a cold drink waits to rehydrate you after this long hike. Since the late 19th and early 20th centuries, when Mountain Lakes Nature Preserve was used for ice harvesting, the refrigeration industry has changed drastically. By the 1960s refrigerants containing chlorofluorocarbons (CFCs) had replaced the ice blocks, and a new age of refrigeration had dawned. The cost for this convenience, however, was destruction of the ozone layer by CFCs. The development of asbestos insulation led to widespread mesothelioma, a malignant cancer, and the use of lead paints and lead additives has led to neurological damage in many humans. The use of these materials has since been banned, but the effects are irreversible.

So the next time you visit Mountain Lakes, think of the household appliances and conveniences that you take for granted every day, their environmental costs, and the things you can do today to live lean, green, and clean.

For more information on energy-efficient appliances and some tips on saving energy, visit **www.greenlivingideas.com/household-appliances/household-appliances -the-new-green-standard-for-energy-efficiency.html**.

## NEARBY ACTIVITIES

Witherspoon Street, named for John Witherspoon, follows the route he took to and from Princeton University. This area is sometimes called Princeton's Greenwich Village. For more information, visit **www.princetonol.com/patron/withers**.

# STONY BROOK-MILLSTONE WATERSHED RESERVE 56

## IN BRIEF

Much of the Stony Brook–Watershed Reserve was donated by a woman who was likely the model for "Julia," the heroic and tragic title character of the 1977 film. The good news: (a) she lived to tell her story, and (b) she left 585 acres to an association that preserves and protects the watershed. The preserve boasts 14 miles of hiking trails.

## DESCRIPTION

Julia had it all—beauty, wealth, love, and intelligence. Born and raised in the United States, she moved to Vienna to study under Sigmund Freud. World War II was imminent, and the "banality of evil" and extreme economic disparity around her inspired her to fight for those less fortunate. In Austria, she became involved with a prewar anti-Fascist movement and helped Jewish citizens escape the country. Sadly, she was caught and killed by the Gestapo.

The story of Julia, which originated in Lillian Hellman's memoir *Pentimento,* is best known through the film adaptation starring Jane Fonda and Vanessa Redgrave. But many believe that the story of Julia was actually based on the life of Muriel Gardiner Buttinger,

**KEY AT-A-GLANCE INFORMATION**

**LENGTH: 3.57 miles**

**CONFIGURATION: Double out-and-back with a loop**

**DIFFICULTY: Moderate**

**SCENERY: Field, forest, pond, stream, wetlands**

**EXPOSURE: Full sun–full shade**

**TRAIL TRAFFIC: Light**

**TRAIL SURFACE: Dirt, gravel, boardwalks**

**HIKING TIME: 1.5 hours**

**DRIVING DISTANCE FROM CENTER CITY: 40 miles**

**ACCESS: Year-round, daily, dawn–dusk; free**

**MAPS: USGS Pennington. Maps at www.njtrails.org/trailmap.php? TrailID=12**

**WHEELCHAIR TRAVERSABLE: No**

**FACILITIES: Restrooms in nature center**

**SPECIAL COMMENTS: Stay on the trails. Smoking is not permitted. See www.thewatershed.org or call (609) 737-7592 for more park information.**

---

## Directions

**From Philadelphia, follow Interstate 95 north 33.7 miles, entering New Jersey. Take Exit 4 and turn left at the end of the ramp onto NJ 31. Continue through a traffic circle, driving 5.5 miles, then turn right onto Titus Mill Road. The reserve entrance is 1.2 miles ahead, on the left. Look for the trailhead at the butterfly house not far from the parking lot to the left.** *31 Titus Mill Road, Pennington, NJ 08534.*

### GPS Trailhead Coordinates

UTM Zone (WGS84)  18T
Easting  0519330
Northing  4466950
Latitude  N 40° 21' 10.6"
Longitude  W 74° 46' 20.5"

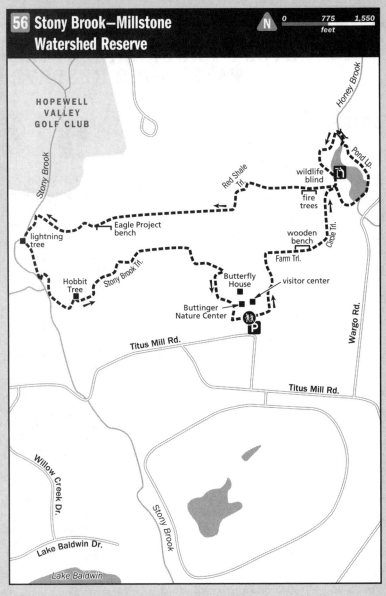

N    0    775    1,550
feet

HOPEWELL
VALLEY
GOLF CLUB

Honey Brook

Pond Lp.

wildlife
blind

fire
trees

Red Shale Trl.

Stony Brook

Circle Trl.

Eagle Project
bench

lightning
tree

wooden
bench

Farm Trl.

Stony Brook Trl.

Hobbit
Tree

Butterfly
House

visitor center

Buttinger
Nature Center

Wargo Rd.

Titus Mill Rd.

Titus Mill Rd.

Willow Creek Dr.

Stony Brook

Lake Baldwin Dr.

Lake Baldwin

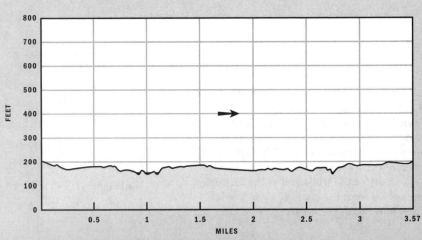

FEET

800
700
600
500
400
300
200
100
0

0.5    1    1.5    2    2.5    3    3.57

MILES

The pond along Pond Loop provides a quiet resting spot for the great blue heron.

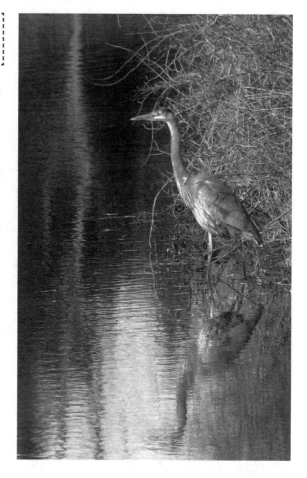

who was a friend of Lillian Hellman's lawyer—a lawyer who likely shared Buttinger's experiences with Hellman.

Fortunately, unlike the fictional "Julia," Buttinger lived and in reality settled in the United States, aiding concentration-camp refugees when she arrived in New York, later conducting research for the New Jersey Department of Health. She became a renowned psychoanalyst and an adjunct professor at Rutgers University in New Brunswick, New Jersey. She also wrote several books, including *Code Name "Mary,"* which details her brave work in the Viennese underground.

Buttinger died in 1985, but not before leaving her Pennington, New Jersey, farm and two other properties—525 acres in all—to the Stony Brook–Millstone Watershed Association, a conservation and preservation organization. The association is now headquartered at Buttinger's former Brookdale Farm. Its 860-acre reserve offers 14 miles of hiking trails surrounded by field and forest, pond and stream.

This hike begins behind Buttinger Nature Center, which is next to the association's offices and Kate Gorrie Memorial Butterfly House. Seasonally, monarchs, black swallowtails, pearl crescents, and common wood nymphs feed, breed, and fly among native wildflowers.

Find the trailhead between the butterfly house and a red shed, or access another trailhead directly behind a white farmhouse, which is now the association headquarters. Both take you onto the Farm Trail; turn right and head east. At a **T**-intersection, turn left onto Circle Trail, heading north. Sandwiched between forest and meadow, the trail turns right and enters a boardwalk. At the end of the boardwalk, turn right to stay on Circle Trail and head east.

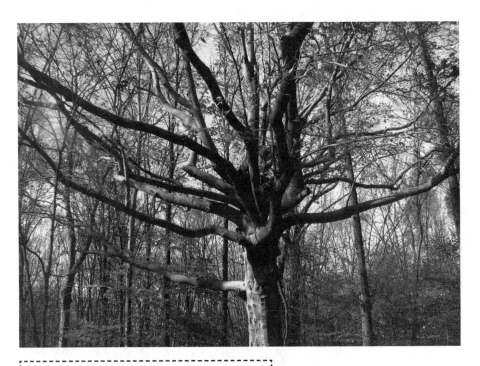

The Hobbit Tree shakes hands with its leafy neighbors.

At the **T**-intersection, take a left turn where you can glimpse Honey Brook Organic Farm across Wargo Road. This farm, part of a community-supported agricultural program, provides shareholders with fresh organic produce from May to November. Community-supported agriculture allows the land to be maintained and sustained while providing local produce for members. Less gasoline is needed for transport. Members of the community become closer as they work together toward the common goal of a healthy diet and healthy ecosystem.

The farm fades from view as the trail bends left. At a pine forest, turn left, heading northeast. Cardinals, sparrows, and robins can be seen almost any time.

A little more than 500 feet from your last turn, Circle Trail turns right. Ignore side trails to your right and continue until you see the red pond house ahead. The trail turns right and heads south, where you will see the parking lot for the Pond Loop. Walk toward the pond and head northeast on Pond Loop.

This trail circles the pond, showcasing mallards, Canadian geese, and great blue herons. A wildlife blind toward the end of the trail as you reach the back of the pond house and pier is a great place to view waterfowl.

After completing the loop in front of the pond house, head back toward Circle Trail. But instead of continuing on Circle Trail, take the first right onto Red Shale Trail, approximately 10 to 20 feet before the pond house. This narrow trail passes a variety of wetland plants. After about 500 feet, you'll reach wooden benches surrounded by tall pines, a restful place to view more birds. You have walked a little more than 1 mile to this point.

When you come to a **T**-intersection, take a right onto Stony Brook Trail and continue west. Many hawks and other birds of prey, such as eagles and osprey, fly above the trees along the beginning of this trail. The trail is muddy after rain, but the many boardwalks help keep you from slogging through marshy areas.

About 100 feet after a wooden Eagle Scout bench, the trail turns left and heads southwest to Stony Brook, which really is a stony brook. Draining from the Sourland Mountains, it flows to Carnegie Lake in Princeton, then continues to the Millstone River. The Watershed Association and its volunteers monitor the health of this brook and others throughout the watershed. The shallows provide another popular hangout for the great blue heron.

A kiosk on the trail points to where lightning struck a large American beech in 1994. The tree exploded, and its top was found about 0.25 miles downstream. After the lightning tree, the trail turns left away from the brook, leading to another interesting beech tree about 150 feet ahead, called the Hobbit Tree because its twisty shape and large crown resembles a tree one might find in a J. R. R. Tolkien story. The tree's branches spread wide, making it appear the tree is shaking hands with its leafy neighbors. Such trees are referred to as "wolf trees."

Perhaps the tree once grew in the middle of a farm field. The hike yields other hints of former use as farmland: barbed wire attached to trees, cattle paths that cut through groves, and aged apple trees.

After the Hobbit Tree, you traverse a small conifer forest. Boardwalks then lead you over a small stream; this means you are reaching the end of Stony Brook Trail. Look for the sign directing you back to the nature center, where you began this hike.

Stony Brook–Millstone Watershed Preserve reflects not the tragic story of a woman lost, but rather the gains made by a woman who understood the value of human life and its connection to this great planet.

## NEARBY ACTIVITIES

HOPEWELL VALLEY VINEYARDS
*(Winery)*
46 Yard Road, Pennington
(609) 737-4465, (866) HVV-WINE
**hopewellvalleyvineyards.com**

PENNINGTON QUILT WORKS
*(Fabric and quilts)*
7 Tree Farm Road, Suite 104,
Pennington
(609) 737-4321
**www.penningtonquilts.com**

VIVA GELATO CAFÉ
*(Gelato and coffee)*
12 South Main Street, Pennington
(609) 737-8988

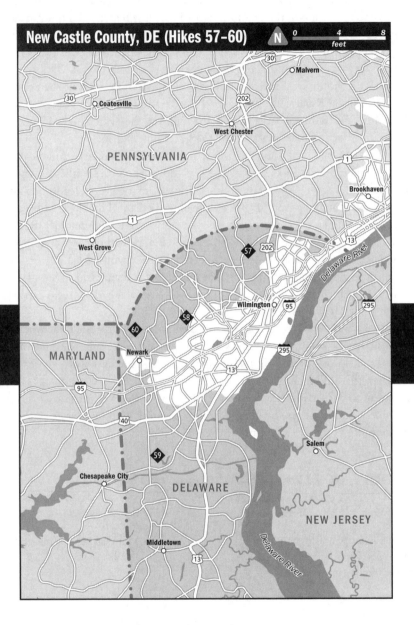

## New Castle County, DE (Hikes 57–60)

N

0  4  8
feet

Malvern

30

Coatesville

202

West Chester

PENNSYLVANIA

1

Brookhaven

1

West Grove

57  202

13

Wilmington

95

295

58

Delaware River

60

MARYLAND  Newark

295

95

13

40

Salem

59

Chesapeake City

DELAWARE

NEW JERSEY

Middletown

Delaware River

13

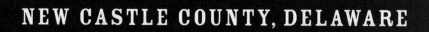

NEW CASTLE COUNTY, DELAWARE

# 57 BRANDYWINE CREEK STATE PARK

## KEY AT-A-GLANCE INFORMATION

**LENGTH:** 4 miles

**CONFIGURATION:** Loop

**DIFFICULTY:** Moderate

**SCENERY:** Tree-lined hills, stone walls, woods

**EXPOSURE:** Full sun–full shade

**TRAIL TRAFFIC:** Medium

**TRAIL SURFACE:** Dirt

**HIKING TIME:** 1.5 hours

**DRIVING DISTANCE FROM CENTER CITY:** 30.3 miles

**ACCESS:** Daily, 8 a.m.–sunset, year-round; free admission

**MAPS:** USGS Wilmington North; maps outside main office

**WHEELCHAIR TRAVERSABLE:** No

**FACILITIES:** Restrooms in nature center

**SPECIAL COMMENTS:** Bring a camera for some surprising views from 2 hilltops. More information: (302) 577-3534; www.destateparks.com/park/brandywine-creek.

## GPS Trailhead Coordinates

UTM Zone (WGS84) 18S

Easting 0450450

Northing 4406600

Latitude N 39° 48' 28.7"

Longitude W 75° 34' 43.6"

## IN BRIEF

Century-old stone walls outline a tree-lined hill and a woodlands hike with two striking high vistas.

## DESCRIPTION

Brandywine Creek, which flows through Chester County, Pennsylvania, and New Castle County, Delaware, is renowned for its rolling mountains, rural landscapes, and stone houses. The creek has also played an important role in local industry, with more than 100 mills having sat on its banks. In 1965, the state of Delaware bought the area known today as Brandywine Creek State Park.

A large white barn stands just inside the park. The park property was once a large dairy farm owned by the du Pont family. An immaculately maintained gray-stone wall runs along the right side of the park road, one of several such walls throughout the 933-acre

### Directions

Take Interstate 95 south from Philadelphia into Delaware. After 23 miles, take Exit 8B, US 202–Concord Pike. Stay in the right lane; after 0.8 miles, take the DE 261–Foulk Road exit. At the end of the ramp, turn left onto DE 261–Foulk Road. Just after crossing under US 202, turn left onto West Park Drive, then immediately turn right onto Rockland Road. After 2.2 miles, Rockland becomes Adams Dam Road. A half mile later, turn right into the park. Take the park road until it ends at the nature center and park office parking lot. The trail starts right behind the nature center. The signs will show the start of the Indian Springs and Hidden Pond trails, which share the same path for the first 1,500 feet. *41 Adams Dam Road, Wilmington, DE 19807.*

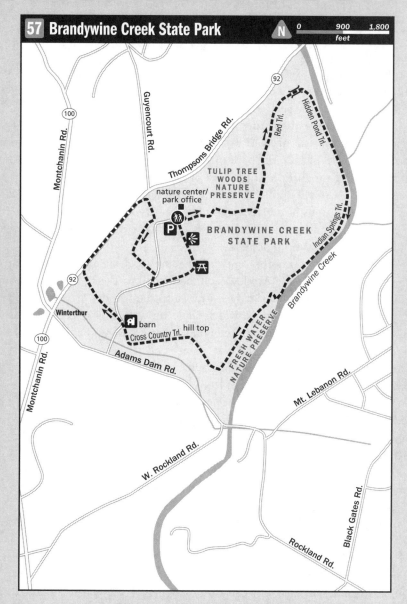

Montchanin Rd.

Guyencourt Rd.

Thompsons Bridge Rd.

Red Trl.

Hidden Pond Trl.

TULIP TREE
WOODS
NATURE
PRESERVE

nature center/
park office

P

Indian Springs Trl.

BRANDYWINE CREEK
STATE PARK

Brandywine Creek

Winterthur

barn    hill top

Cross Country Trl.

FRESH WATER
NATURE PRESERVE

Adams Dam Rd.

Montchanin Rd.

Mt. Lebanon Rd.

W. Rockland Rd.

Black Gates Rd.

Rockland Rd.

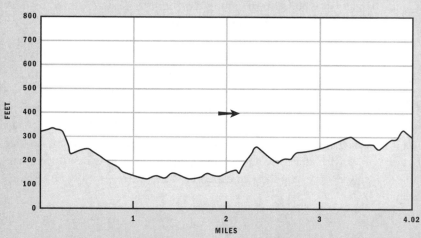

FEET

800

700

600

500

400

300

200

100

0

1          2          3      4.02

MILES

park. Built in the late 1800s by Italian workers, they are among the park's most distinctive trademarks and can be seen even within the wooded area of the hike. You will marvel at how perfectly the stones fit together.

The road ends at the nature center and park office. Inside, you can obtain a detailed trail map along with brochures for local attractions. (You can also secure a trail map outside the park office when this building is closed.) Parking is in front of the park office. At the back of the building, a large observation window overlooks a small wildlife habitat, which includes small ponds, a variety of plant life, and various bird feeders. You may see an occasional bluebird or other songbird. Behind the nature center is the Tulip Tree Woods Nature Preserve, a stand of 190-year-old tulip poplars.

The hike itself covers three distinct habitats and includes a wooded path, a creek, fields, and scenic overlooks. Immediately to the right of and behind the nature center, a sign marks the entrance to the wooded part of the Indian Springs and Hidden Pond trails, which share the same path for the first 1,500 feet. At the 1,500-foot mark, take the Hidden Pond Trail to the left (north). This trail is marked with purplish-red blazes on wooden posts. *Note:* The trail will go straight and unmarked for a short distance before the blazes resume. You will notice the occasional roar of traffic from DE 92.

After you pass a small footbridge on your left, at about the 1-mile mark, the Hidden Pond Trail turns south following Brandywine Creek. The path is well maintained and well suited for horseback riders, who are allowed on the park trails. For this reason, park officials require that all dogs be on leashes. Erosion has caused many trees to slant into the creek, some almost toppling over. In the summer, the occasional canoe drifts by and an angler may work the bank.

Stay close to the creek for the next mile. The Hidden Pond Trail turns into an unmarked path (shown in brown on the park map) that hugs the creek. At the 1.8-mile mark of the hike, a foot-high sign on your right announces that you have entered the Fresh Water Nature Preserve. At this sign, turn right. Then take the next left onto the path that follows the marsh on your left. The unmarked trail, at this juncture, becomes the Cross Country Trail, which is marked with dark-yellow blazes on wooden posts along its length; it is also marked as dark yellow on Brandywine Creek State Park maps. As you leave the marsh, the path meets a maintenance area to the left at the base of a hill. The Cross Country Trail continues up the hill on the right, which will reach more than 100 feet in elevation at the top. The hilltop, with its many large trees, is a good spot to rest and take in the beautiful view of the landscape. Beneath the trees is one of the ever-present stone walls that seem to follow the hills throughout the park. The valley lacks commercial development, and most of the wood and stone buildings look as if they have been part of the landscape for decades. You also may notice some metal poles with chains hanging from rings at the top, which form a basket. These are used for disc golf, also called Frisbee golf.

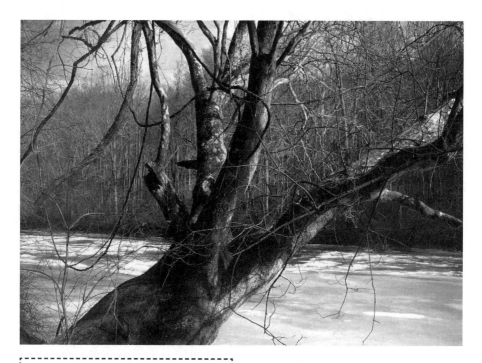

A sycamore overhangs the Brandywine Creek.

The park also hosts Civil War reenactments, for which the rolling hills and meadows certainly form a convincing backdrop. At the top of the hill, turn left (west), following the Cross Country Trail along the stone wall. After 800 feet, the trail continues to the right, and you will pass the barn you saw when you entered the park. Cross the park-entrance road and follow the trail around a large field. The path will lead back to the road. In the distance, on the left, is the nature center parking area. Cross the road and continue following the wooden markers for the Cross Country Trail. After 500 feet, the trail meets a picnic table and kiosk. Here the final part of the trail turns left (due north), and after a couple hundred feet you will reach the highest peak in the park, which offers an impressive view of the whole valley. During autumn the changing leaves make the scenery especially spectacular. Here, a stone plaque commemorates the life of Clayton M. Hoff, the first executive vice president of the Brandywine Valley Association, an early preservation group that started in Delaware. In 1987, the association established the Clayton M. Hoff Conservation Award to recognize contributions to the conservation of the valley. The hike finishes just a few hundred feet ahead, back at the nature center.

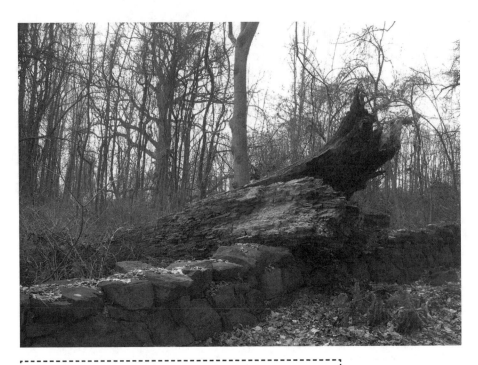

One of the many stone walls that line the Brandywine Creek State Park

## NEARBY ACTIVITIES

DELAWARE MUSEUM OF NATURAL
HISTORY
4840 Kennett Pike, Wilmington
(302) 658-9111
www.delmnh.org

GREENBANK STATION
*(Wilmington & Western Railroad
vintage train)*
2201 Newport Gap Pike, Wilmington
(302) 998-1930
www.wwrr.com

WILMINGTON STATE PARKS AND THE
BRANDYWINE ZOO
1021 West 18th Street, Wilmington
(302) 577-7020
www.destateparks.com/park/wilmington

# CAROUSEL PARK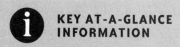

## IN BRIEF

Although not a deep-woods experience, this park offers an unusual blend of equestrian scenery and wetland greenery, plus a dog park for your favorite pooch.

## DESCRIPTION

When you drive into the equestrian center at Carousel Park, you might feel as if you've driven onto the set of a Western B-movie. The themed facade is staged and ready for a hoedown or a simulated gunfight; winter weekends give this part of the park more of a ghost-town quality. So mosey over to the white arches just off the parking lot to find the trailhead at the opening of the main outdoor horse ring, where you can watch the horses and ponies graze.

The equestrian center is only one of the features that make this 217-acre park so attractive. Riding lessons go on year-round in the indoor and outdoor arenas. The center offers pony rides, pony parties, and horse shows. Well-maintained walking trails circle the riding rings, the dog park, Enchanted Lake, and two small ponds. The lake and ponds are stocked with turtles and fish. From April through November, the park organizes hayrides and bonfires. Other attractions include

### i  KEY AT-A-GLANCE INFORMATION

**LENGTH: 3.13 miles**

**CONFIGURATION: Figure-8**

**DIFFICULTY: Moderate**

**SCENERY: Horse pastures and corral, dog park, pond, geese**

**EXPOSURE: Mostly sun, some shade**

**TRAIL TRAFFIC: Moderate**

**TRAIL SURFACE: Mostly paved, some gravel**

**HIKING TIME: 1 hour**

**DRIVING DISTANCE FROM CENTER CITY: 39 miles**

**ACCESS: Dawn–dusk; free admission, but fees apply for special programs.**

**MAPS: USGS Newark East; no maps at park**

**WHEELCHAIR TRAVERSABLE: No**

**FACILITIES: For restrooms, ask at front office**

**SPECIAL COMMENTS: Watch your small children in the dog park. More information: (302) 454-8082.**

---

## Directions

**Take Interstate 95 south from Philadelphia into Delaware. After 28.6 miles, take Exit 5B to DE 141 north, toward Newport. After 2.5 miles, take Exit 6B to DE 2. After 2.3 miles, turn right onto DE 7–Limestone Road. The park is on the left in 1.5 miles. The hike begins behind the Western-style barn.** *3700 Limestone Road, Wilmington, DE 19808.*

### GPS Trailhead Coordinates

UTM Zone (WGS84)  18S

Easting  0441841

Northing  4397903

Latitude  N 39° 43' 44.4"

Longitude  W 75° 40' 43.3"

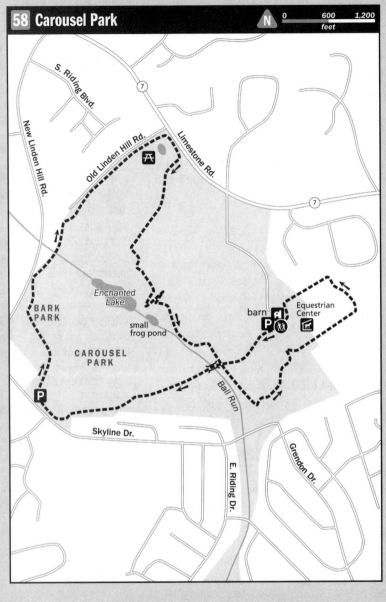

S. Riding Blvd.

New Linden Hill Rd.

Old Linden Hill Rd.

Limestone Rd.

7

7

Enchanted Lake

small frog pond

BARK PARK

CAROUSEL PARK

barn

Equestrian Center

P

Ball Run

Skyline Dr.

E. Riding Dr.

Grendon Dr.

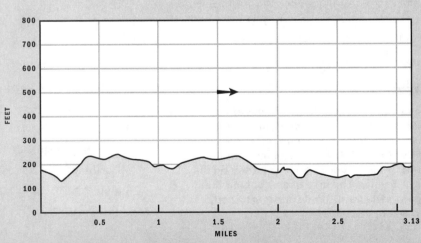

800

700

600

500

400

300

200

100

0

FEET

0.5    1    1.5    2    2.5    3.13

MILES

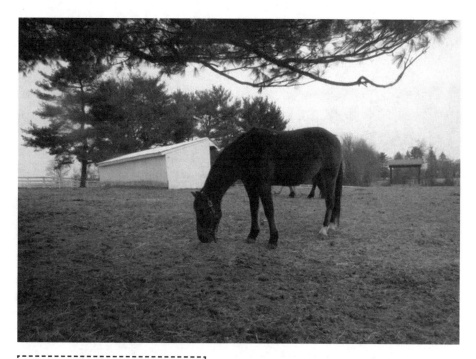

A horse grazes in the equestrian center.

fly-fishing, stargazing, and summer camps. The county also sponsors Girl Scout and Boy Scout programs.

Felix du Pont, an aviator, businessman, and philanthropist, donated the park property to New Castle County, Delaware, in the late 1960s. The county cleared brush and established the trails, and continues to maintain the park and the haying operation, which feeds the horses.

From the trailhead, turn right onto the single trail leading from the corral, and head south past the pastures and toward a small bridge that crosses a stream. After the bridge, stay southwest on a wide gravel path instead of going right or left before the bridge. This is the most strenuous part of the hike—not necessarily happy trails—so pace yourself to the top of the hill, where the path turns left and levels. Because horses sometimes share these trails, the surface can be muddy, especially in late winter and early spring.

The trail loops right and heads northwest, taking you downhill before bending right toward the entrance of the Bark Park. A major draw for local canine enthusiasts, the park provides an enormous field and a lake where dogs can run and play with wild abandon. You can see the smiles on the doggie faces as they jump, sprint, swim, and fetch.

If you wish to see the dogs at play, take a right. If you're not a dog lover, continue along the trail, staying on the outer paved path, heading northeast. Just past the entrance to the dog park, the path narrows under a grove of trees

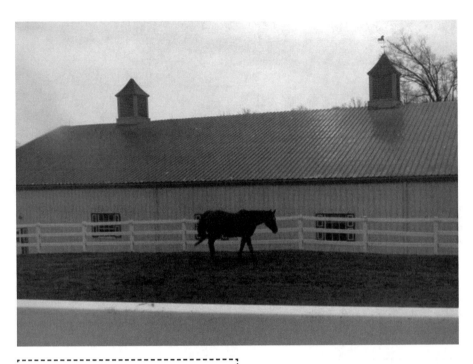

It's happy trails for the horses at Carousel Park.

where you can watch hawks fly over the meadows. As you reach DE 7, the trail passes a small pond and picnic area before turning right and heading east, then southwest. This stretch provides pastoral views of the horse pastures.

The paved trail ends, and you will cross a grassy knoll toward the seasonally stocked Enchanted Lake. The lake covers eight acres and stretches to the dog park on the other side. The geese, understandably, remain on this side of the lake so they won't end up as dog food.

Walk toward the pond to enjoy the white geese as they splash and clean their feathers, but beware of droppings. Head southeast, to your left, across the grass until you pick up a gravel trail. You will circle a small pond that has a turtle statue, then after about a quarter mile, you will reach the bridge you crossed at the beginning of this hike. Continue back toward the horse pens, but stay on the path, to the right side of the ring. In another quarter mile, turn left before you reach the road and head northeast to get close to the horses in their corral. Walk on the grass for a short time until you reach the white-fenced corral, then turn right onto a paved trail that circles the horse pen and drops you back in front of the riding ring where you began this eclectic walk.

Carousel Park may not be a deep-in-the-woods hike, but it is an interesting stop, offering a lot of community and a little slice of nature within the suburbs of Wilmington, Delaware. Besides, where else can you feel as if you have just stepped off the sets of both *Shane* and *Lassie Come Home* while remaining less than 60 miles from Philadelphia?

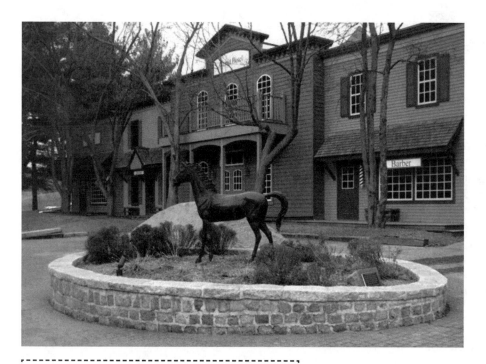

The themed facade at Carousel Park is ready for a hoedown.

## NEARBY ACTIVITIES

BRANDYWINE CREEK STATE PARK
*(See Hike 57, page 300)*
41 Adams Dam Road, Wilmington
(302) 577-3534
**www.destateparks.com/park/
brandywine-creek**

DELAWARE MUSEUM OF NATURAL
HISTORY
4840 Kennett Pike, Wilmington
(302) 658-9111
**www.delmnh.org**

WHITE CLAY CREEK STATE PARK
*(See Hike 60, page 314)*
425 Wedgewood Road, Newark
(302) 368-6900
**www.destateparks.com/park/
white-clay-creek**

# 59 LUMS POND STATE PARK

### KEY AT-A-GLANCE INFORMATION

**LENGTH:** 6.57 miles

**CONFIGURATION:** Loop

**DIFFICULTY:** Moderate

**SCENERY:** Pond and forest

**EXPOSURE:** Full sun–full shade

**TRAIL TRAFFIC:** Medium

**TRAIL SURFACE:** Dirt, concrete, planks, bridges

**HIKING TIME:** 3 hours

**DRIVING DISTANCE FROM CENTER CITY:** 47.5 miles

**ACCESS:** Daily, 8 a.m.–dusk, year-round; admission $5 May–October, otherwise free

**MAPS:** USGS Saint Georges; www.destateparks.com/downloads/maps/lums-pond/lums-pond.pdf

**WHEELCHAIR TRAVERSABLE:** No

**FACILITIES:** Restrooms at campground and boat ramp

**SPECIAL COMMENTS:** This is the largest freshwater pond in Delaware. More information: (302) 368-6989; www.destateparks.com/park/lums-pond.

## IN BRIEF

A long but relatively easy hike on a mostly flat trail with views of a large pond throughout.

## DESCRIPTION

Lums Pond State Park is north of the Chesapeake and Delaware Canal. The Swamp Forest Trail hike follows the perimeter of 200-acre Lums Pond, which offers swimming, boating, and fishing. The park also rents boats, including pedal boats, May through September.

On the trail, bridges cross small streams. The paths are well maintained and mostly devoid of roots and rocks. The flat landscape allows a brisk pace. You may encounter an occasional horseback rider or mountain biker. Campsites along the way offer picnic tables, grills, and restrooms. Three large pavilions can be rented.

Before the pond existed, Native Americans hunted here. The St. Georges River was dammed in the 1800s, and Lums Pond supplied water to the canal locks and a mill. In 1963, it became a Delaware state park.

The hike starts at the pond end of the Area 4 parking lot, just past the nature center. The pond does not seem large at first, but it branches out in many directions. In fact,

## GPS Trailhead Coordinates

UTM Zone (WGS84)  18S

Easting   0437625

Northing   4379381

Latitude   N 39° 33' 42.6"

Longitude   W 75° 43' 34.1"

## Directions

Take Interstate 95 south from Philadelphia for 37.8 miles, entering Delaware. Take Exit 1A and merge onto DE 896. After 5.9 miles, turn left onto Howell School Road. After 0.25 miles, turn right into the park onto Buck Jersey Road. After about 0.5 miles, turn right into the Area 4 parking lot. The trailhead is clearly marked at the pond end of the lot. *1068 Howell School Road, Bear, DE 19701.*

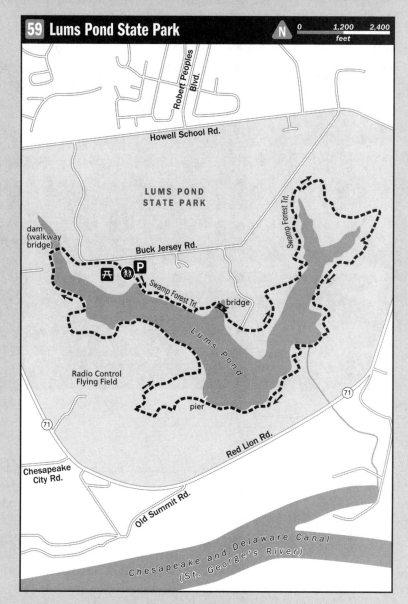

N

0      1,200      2,400
feet

LUMS POND
STATE PARK

Robert Peoples Blvd.

Howell School Rd.

dam
(walkway
bridge)

Buck Jersey Rd.

Swamp Forest Trl.

Swamp Forest Trl.

bridge

Lums Pond

Radio Control
Flying Field

pier

71

71

Red Lion Rd.

Chesapeake
City Rd.

Old Summit Rd.

Chesapeake and Delaware Canal
(St. George's River)

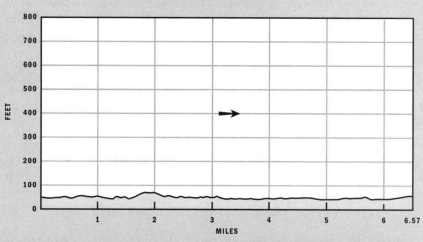

| FEET | | | | | | | |
|---|---|---|---|---|---|---|---|
| 800 | | | | | | | |
| 700 | | | | | | | |
| 600 | | | | | | | |
| 500 | | | | | | | |
| 400 | | | → | | | | |
| 300 | | | | | | | |
| 200 | | | | | | | |
| 100 | | | | | | | |
| 0 | | | | | | | |

1      2      3      4      5      6    6.57

MILES

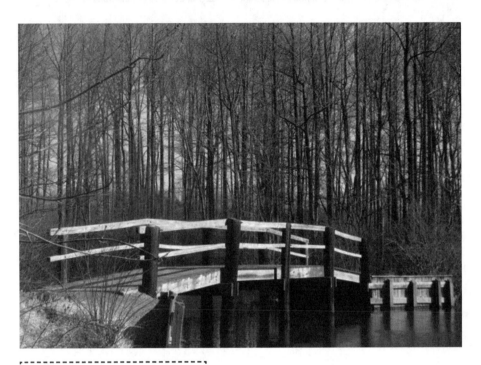

A bridge crosses an inlet of Lums Pond.

Lums Pond is the largest freshwater pond in Delaware. Many clearings along the hike allow views of the water and landscapes, including brilliant foliage displays in the fall. When the hike begins, the trail runs very close to the pond. After significant rain, flooding might be a problem. The trail continues east on a concrete walkway at the boat rental area.

Past the rental boats, turn left and follow the path as it bears right and crosses a bridge over an inlet. Within a quarter mile, the path will turn left (north).

At the 3-mile mark, there is a boat launch and an information board. Such boards are situated throughout the park and provide such useful resources as park maps and brochures. After the path turns west, there is a fishing pier. Lums Pond is renowned for its bluegill, crappie, pickerel, largemouth bass, and striped bass, and the park frequently holds fishing tournaments.

Past the pier, the path heads away from the pond, for the hike's only significant change of landscape. The path loops around tall reeds rising from wetlands, then heads back to the pond. You may hear model aircraft engines from the park's nearby Radio Control Flying Field.

The path returns to the shoreline across the pond from the boat rental site. After another quarter mile is the final bridge of the hike. The hike may be long, but the walking planks and well-maintained pathways and bridges make it easy, with minimal mud.

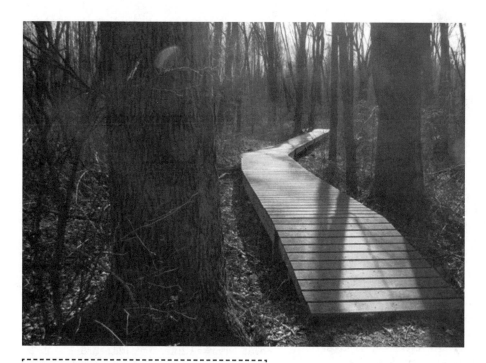

Walking planks and flat trails make for an easy hike.

During the final mile of the hike, the trail crosses the dam, bears right, and runs through the picnic area. The hike ends at the parking area where you started.

## NEARBY ACTIVITIES

C&D CANAL MUSEUM
(Original pump house with artifacts and interactive kiosks)
815 Bethel Road, Chesapeake City, Maryland
(410) 885-5621
nap.usace.army.mil/sb/c&d
.htm#attractions

LUMS POND STATE PARK
RADIO CONTROL FLYING FIELD
(For enthusiasts of radio-controlled model aircraft)
Red Lion Road, Bear
(302) 368-6989

SUMMIT NORTH MARINA
(30-foot replica of a lighthouse)
3000 Summit Harbour Place, Bear
(302) 836-1800
www.summitnorthmarina.net

# 60 WHITE CLAY CREEK STATE PARK

**KEY AT-A-GLANCE INFORMATION**

**LENGTH: 4.74 miles**

**CONFIGURATION: Loop**

**DIFFICULTY: Moderate**

**SCENERY: Creek, pond, meadows, pine groves, forests, monument**

**EXPOSURE: Full shade–full sun**

**TRAIL TRAFFIC: Light–moderate**

**TRAIL SURFACE: Grass, dirt**

**HIKING TIME: 2 hours**

**DRIVING DISTANCE FROM CENTER CITY: 41 miles**

**ACCESS: Year-round, 8 a.m.–sunset; March 1–November 30 entry is $3 for Delaware residents, $6 for nonresidents; free December 1– February 29**

**MAPS: USGS Newark West; map at www.destateparks.com/park/ white-clay-creek**

**WHEELCHAIR TRAVERSABLE: No**

**FACILITIES: For restrooms, see www.destateparks.com/downloads/ maps/white-clay-creek/white-clay-creek.pdf.**

**SPECIAL COMMENTS: For more information, (302) 368-6900 or visit www.destateparks.com/park/ white-clay-creek.**

## IN BRIEF

This park, which crosses two states, offers tall pine forests beside pastoral meadows. White Clay Creek peeks through oak and sycamore trees, and there are many hidden surprises, such as a bamboo grove, a cattail pond, and Millstone Pond, where young musicians come to enjoy the acoustics of the bordering pegmatite outcrop.

## DESCRIPTION

Mason Dixon Trail begins at Whiskey Springs, Pennsylvania, on the Appalachian Trail and continues east to Brandywine Trail at Chadds Ford, Pennsylvania, passing through three major state parks along the way: Gifford Pinchot State Park and White Clay Creek Preserve, both in Pennsylvania, and White Clay Creek State Park in Delaware. The trail is 193 miles long, but don't worry—this hike covers a mere 4.74 miles.

White Clay Creek State Park runs along White Clay Creek, offering 3,300 acres of diverse landscapes with 30 miles of nature and fitness trails. Mason Dixon Trail roughly parallels the Mason–Dixon Line, surveyed between 1763 and 1767 by Charles Mason and Jeremiah

## GPS Trailhead Coordinates

UTM Zone (WGS84)  18S

Easting   0434810

Northing  4296524

Latitude   N 39° 42' 57.9"

Longitude  W 75° 45' 37.9"

## *Directions* ⟶

From Philadelphia, follow Interstate 95 south 33 miles, entering Delaware. Take Exit 3 and turn right at the end of the ramp onto DE 273. After 5 miles, turn right at the triple fork in New London onto DE 896. Drive 2.2 miles, then turn right onto Wedgewood Road. After about 1 mile, turn left into the parking lot. Walk just beyond the blocked (gated) road to find the entrance to the Twin Valley (Mason Dixon) hike on the left. It's a short steep climb to the main trail.
*425 Wedgewood Road, Newark, DE 19711.*

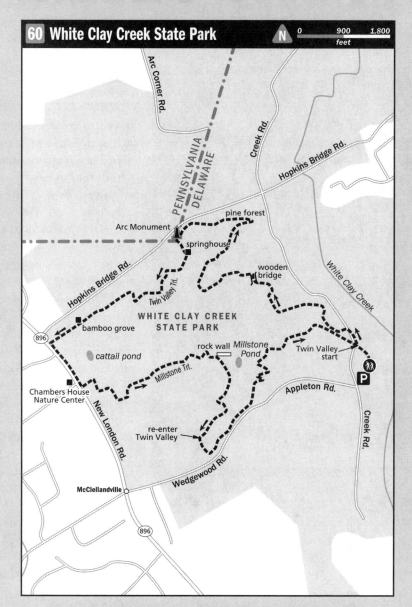

N  0    900    1,800
feet

Arc Corner Rd.

Creek Rd.

Hopkins Bridge Rd.

PENNSYLVANIA
DELAWARE

pine forest

Arc Monument

springhouse

wooden
bridge

White Clay Creek

Hopkins Bridge Rd.

Twin Valley Trl.

WHITE CLAY CREEK
STATE PARK

bamboo grove

896

cattail pond

rock wall   Millstone
Pond

Twin Valley
start

Millstone Trl.

P

Chambers House
Nature Center

New London Rd.

Appleton Rd.

re-enter
Twin Valley

Creek Rd.

Wedgewood Rd.

McClellandville

896

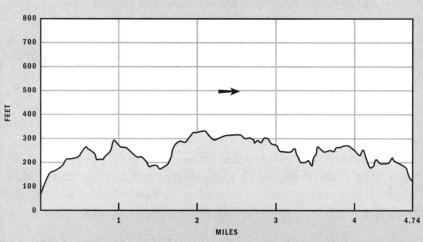

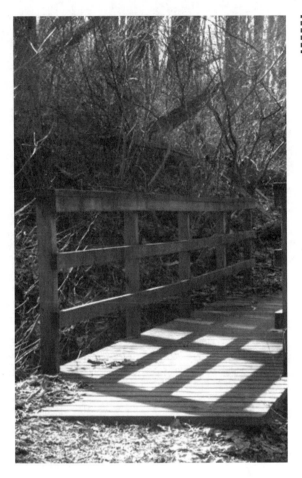

Boardwalks along the trails make for less muddy boots.

Dixon to resolve a border disagreement between colonies. The line, which forms part of the borders of Pennsylvania, West Virginia, Maryland, and Delaware, became a demarcation line between North and South in the years leading up to the Civil War.

This hike combines the park's Millstone Trail with Twin Valley Trail. Twin Valley Trail is an alternative route on Mason Dixon Trail and leads to the arc between Delaware and Pennsylvania, where a monument shows the boundary surveyed in 1892 by the U.S. Coast and Geodetic Survey. This marker, in its own small way, also symbolizes freedom: on one side of the monument, in Delaware, consumers are free from sales tax; on the other side, Pennsylvania charges a 6 percent tax.

So plan on a little shopping later, but first start the hike by picking up Twin Valley–Mason Dixon Trail just off the parking lot. At the first intersection, turn left and head northwest toward White Clay Creek until the trail turns left, away from the water, and briefly heads southwest. In winter, you can plainly see the creek. During other seasons, you will catch only glimpses. You will cross a series of wooden pedestrian bridges throughout this hike. After the second bridge stand two stone ruins, remains of 18th- and 19th-century farmsteads.

As you head up a hill, an old white farmhouse on your left adds to the pastoral scene. Continue uphill as the trail takes a sharp right and then reaches an intersection. Turn right to traverse a rich, cool pine forest with ample bird-watching opportunities.

The Carolina chickadee, the tufted titmouse, the vibrant Northern cardinal, and many other birds frequent these trails all year. For a more comprehensive list of birds, see the birder's guide to the park at **www.whiteclayfriends.org/birders_guide.php,** the Web site of the Friends of White Clay Creek State Park.

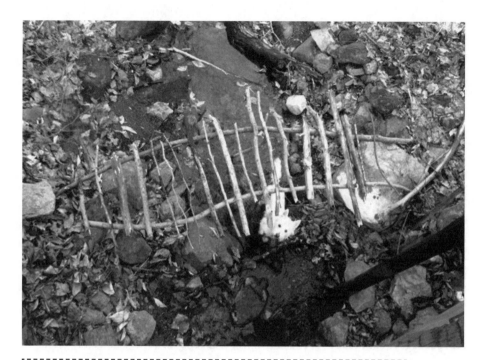

Crystal peers up at the makeshift bridge as confused as anyone to its purported use.

Watch for a sharp left turn within the pine forest. Take this left and continue north. Traffic sounds from nearby Hopkins Bridge Road indicate that you are close to the Arc Monument, where you can hop back and forth from one state to the other. Once you have enjoyed this novelty, continue south uphill.

Halfway up the hill, clear waters sparkle under a stone springhouse to the left. Turn right at the fork, almost at the top of the hill, and continue your ascent, heading southwest into another forest of tall pine trees. At the **T**-intersection, turn right onto a cross-county ski trail. You head north past a disc golf course on the left and a few residences on the right before reaching a bamboo grove that will make you feel as if you have stepped out of Delaware and into a tropical forest in Malaysia.

Bamboo is one of the strongest plants on earth. It grows faster than any other woody plant (up to a yard a day, depending on species) and has the greatest uptake of carbon dioxide. Bamboo was used in the first regreening of Hiroshima after the atomic bomb blast of 1945. It can prevent soil erosion and is used for such products as plywood, roofing, and flooring. It is also considered a viable feedstock for the production of bioethanol and biofuel.

The trail turns left to hug Hopkins Road. If you have time, cross Hopkins Bridge Road and visit the Chambers House Nature Center, about 100 feet straight ahead on Creek Road. This classic stone farmhouse, open to park visitors, contains a library on local natural resources, plus field guides, nature activity brochures, and an exhibit room.

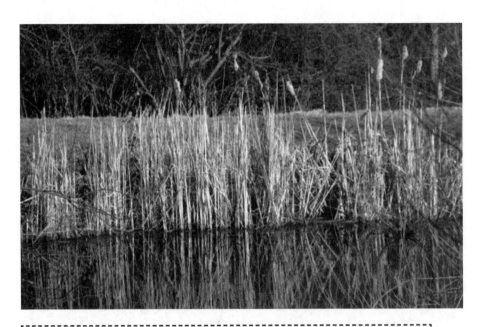

The cattail pond is just one of many natural surprises with the White Clay Creek State Park.

Recross the road to return to the trail. Follow it to a **T**-intersection, and then turn right. Follow the blue arrows and take Millstone Trail to Millstone Pond, where young local musicians sometimes go to jam and hear the sound bounce off the pegmatite outcrop on the pond's western side.

Stay on Millstone Trail, but look for a left turn that will take you back to Twin Valley–Mason Dixon Trail and toward Creek Road, where you began. Before leaving the parking area, follow the signs to a footbridge, which offers one more scenic view of the White Clay Creek.

## NEARBY ACTIVITIES

DOWNTOWN NEWARK
*(Quaint shopping and restaurants)*
Main Street, Newark
**newark.de.us/downtown/MAP.htm**

THE DAYS OF KNIGHTS
*(Fantasy and science-fiction gifts, gaming shop)*
173 East Main Street, Newark
(302) 366-0963

LETTUCE FEED YOU
*(Salads, sandwiches, wraps, soups, pasta)*
45 East Main Street, Galleria, Newark
(302) 369-3010

SWEET-SASSY CUPCAKES
*(Gourmet cupcakes and whimsical party goods)*
134 East Main Street, Newark
(302) 368-2253

# APPENDIXES AND INDEX

# APPENDIX A:
# HIKING CLUBS

**BATONA HIKING CLUB OF PHILADELPHIA**
www.batonahikingclub.org

**PHILADELPHIA HIKING & ADVENTURE MEETUP GROUP**
www.meetup.com/hiking-adventure

**SIERRA CLUB–NEW JERSEY CHAPTER, HUNTERDON COUNTY GROUP**
145 West Hanover Street
Trenton, NJ 08618
(609) 656-7612
newjersey.sierraclub.org

**SIERRA CLUB–PENNSYLVANIA CHAPTER, PHILADELPHIA OFFICE**
4100 Main Street, Suite 405
Philadelphia, PA 19127
(215) 508-3310
pennsylvania.sierraclub.org

**SIERRA CLUB–DELAWARE CHAPTER**
100 West 10th Street, Suite 1107
Wilmington, DE 19801
(302) 351-2776
delaware.sierraclub.org

**AL'S SPORTING GOODS**
210 North Market Street
Wilmington, DE 19801
(302) 655-1511

**BLACK DIAMOND MOUNTAIN SPORTS**
400 West Route 38, #1610
Moorestown, NJ 08057
(856) 778-8801
www.whatsyourmountain.com

**BLUE RIDGE MOUNTAIN SPORTS**
301 North Harrison Street, #6
Princeton, NJ 08540
(609) 921-6078
www.brmsstore.com

**BUCKS COUNTY OUTFITTERS**
64 East Swamp Road
Doylestown, PA 18901
(215) 340-0633

**DICK'S SPORTING GOODS**
www.dickssportinggoods.com
150 Commerce Boulevard
Fairless Hills, PA 19030
(215) 946-8750

20 Franklin Mills Boulevard
Philadelphia, PA 19154
(215) 637-3230

2430 Chemical Road
Plymouth Meeting, PA 19462
(610) 260-4400

2510 West Moreland Road
Willow Grove, PA 19090
(215) 657-8977

**EASTERN MOUNTAIN SPORTS**
www.ems.com
3401 Chestnut Street
Philadelphia, PA 19104
(215) 382-0930
(Plus eight other Philadelphia-area stores)

**ENDURANCE SPORTS**
1617 Big Oak Road
Yardley, PA 19067
(215) 369-0225
www.endurancesportsonline.com

**I. GOLDBERG ARMY & NAVY**
1300 Chestnut Street
Philadelphia, PA 19107
(215) 925-9393
www.igoco.com

**MODELL'S SPORTING GOODS**
www.modells.com
US 1 at Bristol Road
Bensalem, PA 19020
(215) 396-1800

283 Main Street
Exton, PA 19341
(610) 363-8432

1067 West Baltimore Pike
Media, PA 19063
(610) 565-9360

1315 New Churchmans Road
Newark, DE 19713
(302) 369-1500

# APPENDIX B:
# OUTDOOR SHOPS (CONTINUED)

### MODELL'S SPORTING GOODS
### (CONTINUED)

3400 Aramingo Avenue, #44
Philadelphia, PA 19134
(215) 634-7677

1280 Franklin Mills Circle
Philadelphia, PA 19154
(215) 824-3900

### OUT THERE OUTFITTERS
123 North Wayne Avenue
Wayne, PA 19087
(610) 688-6383
www.outthereoutfitters.com

### PHILADELPHIA SCOUT SHOP
225 North 22nd Street
(22nd Street at Winters Street)
Philadelphia, PA 19107
(215) 564-0785

### REI
200 West Ridge Pike
Conshohocken, PA 19428
(610) 940-0809
www.rei.com

### SPORTS AUTHORITY
www.sportsauthority.com
125 West DeKalb Pike
King of Prussia, PA 19406
(610) 783-1502

2375 East Lincoln Highway
Langhorne, PA 19047
(215) 946-2434

1035 Main Street
Warrington, PA 18976
(215) 918-3310

1100 Rocky Run Parkway
Wilmington, DE 19803
(302) 479-7560

### SPORTSMAN'S OUTPOST
2517 Fries Mill Road
Williamstown, NJ 08094
(856) 881-3244
www.sportsmansoutpost.com

### SPORTSMEN'S CENTER
69 Route 130
Bordentown, NJ 08505
(609) 298-5300
www.sportsmenscenter.com

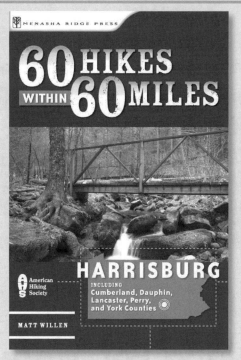
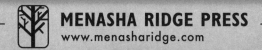

# Best In Tent Camping: Pennsylvania

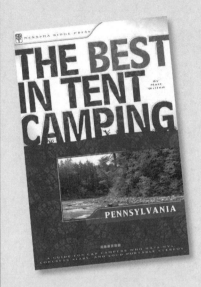

by Matt Willen
$14.95, 1st Edition
ISBN: 978-0-89732-613-1
6x9, paperback
208 pages, maps, photographs, index

This guide provides outdoor enthusiasts with all of the information needed to choose a perfect site in any section of Pennsylvania. With local camping experts as authors the very best camping sites in the state are only a read away. We provide a detailed profile and useful at-a-glance information, our maps show campground layout, individual sites, and key facilities. Driving directions and GPS-based coordinates make sure you don't get lost.

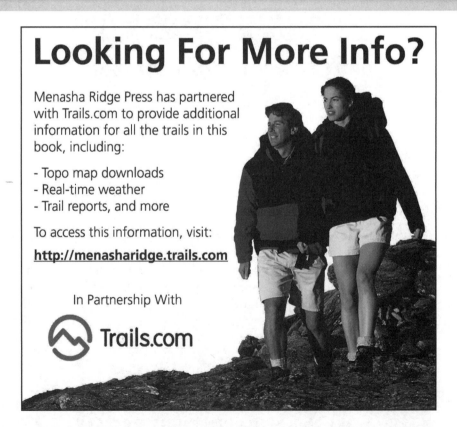

# Looking For More Info?

Menasha Ridge Press has partnered with Trails.com to provide additional information for all the trails in this book, including:

- Topo map downloads
- Real-time weather
- Trail reports, and more

To access this information, visit:

**http://menasharidge.trails.com**

In Partnership With

**Trails.com**

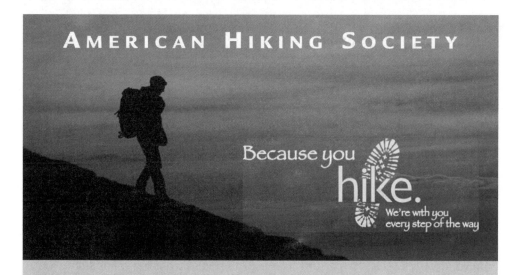
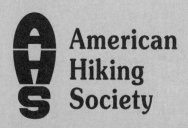

**DEAR CUSTOMERS AND FRIENDS,**

**SUPPORTING YOUR INTEREST IN OUTDOOR ADVENTURE**, travel, and an active lifestyle is central to our operations, from the authors we choose to the locations we detail to the way we design our books. Menasha Ridge Press was incorporated in 1982 by a group of veteran outdoorsmen and professional outfitters. For 25 years now, we've specialized in creating books that benefit the outdoors enthusiast.

Almost immediately, Menasha Ridge Press earned a reputation for revolutionizing outdoors- and travel-guidebook publishing. For such activities as canoeing, kayaking, hiking, backpacking, and mountain biking, we established new standards of quality that transformed the whole genre, resulting in outdoor-recreation guides of great sophistication and solid content. Menasha Ridge continues to be outdoor publishing's greatest innovator.

The folks at Menasha Ridge Press are as at home on a white-water river or mountain trail as they are editing a manuscript. The books we build for you are the best they can be, because we're responding to your needs. Plus, we use and depend on them ourselves.

We look forward to seeing you on the river or the trail. If you'd like to contact us directly, join in at www.trekalong.com or visit us at www.menasharidge.com. We thank you for your interest in our books and the natural world around us all.

**SAFE TRAVELS,**

*Bob Sehlinger*

**BOB SEHLINGER**
**PUBLISHER**